TREATING ADULT SURVIVORS
OF CHILDHOOD EMOTIONAL ABUSE AND NEGLECT

Treating Adult Survivors of Childhood Emotional Abuse and Neglect

Component-Based Psychotherapy

Elizabeth K. Hopper
Frances K. Grossman
Joseph Spinazzola
Marla Zucker

Foreword by Bessel A. van der Kolk

Introduction by Christine A. Courtois

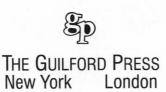

THE GUILFORD PRESS
New York   London

Library of Congress Cataloging-in-Publication Data

Names: Hopper, Elizabeth K. (Elizabeth Kay), 1973– author.
Title: Treating adult survivors of childhood emotional abuse and neglect :
  component-based psychotherapy / Elizabeth K. Hopper [and three others].
Description: New York : The Guilford Press, [2019] | Includes bibliographical
  references and index.
Identifiers: LCCN 2018015007 | ISBN 9781462537297 (hardback)
Subjects: LCSH: Adult child abuse victims—Treatment. | Psychotherapy. |
  Psychotherapist and patient. | BISAC: PSYCHOLOGY / Psychopathology /
  Post-Traumatic Stress Disorder (PTSD). | MEDICAL / Psychiatry / General. |
  SOCIAL SCIENCE / Social Work. | PSYCHOLOGY / Psychotherapy / Counseling.
Classification: LCC RC569.5.C55 H67 2018 | DDC 616.85/822390651—dc23
LC record available at https://lccn.loc.gov/2018015007

About the Authors

Elizabeth K. Hopper, PhD, is a clinician, supervisor, and member of the training faculty at the Trauma Center at Justice Resource Institute (JRI) in Brookline, Massachusetts. She is Senior Administrator and Director of Supervisory Services at the Trauma Center and served as Associate Director of Training for a decade. As the Chief Program Officer for the Trauma Center's anti-trafficking programs, Dr. Hopper oversees several regional and national counter-trafficking programs and networks, including programs that provide direct services to survivors and that improve service delivery through outreach, training, and consultation. She has collaborated with cross-discipline agencies and organizations in developing trauma-informed care systems. Dr. Hopper is coauthor of a book on yoga as a body-based intervention for trauma and has written numerous articles and chapters on complex trauma, trauma-informed care, homelessness, and human trafficking. She has a strong interest in integration across treatment models and in interventions that can be individually adapted.

Frances K. Grossman, PhD, ABPP, is a senior supervisor and member of the training faculty at the Trauma Center at JRI, with which she has been affiliated since 2001. She is Professor Emeritus in the Clinical Psychology program at Boston University, having taught there for over 30 years, and was an adjunct faculty member in the Lesley University Master's in Counseling Psychology program for a decade. Dr. Grossman has published and presented on topics including resiliency in women and men with histories of childhood sexual abuse. With a particular interest in dissociation, she teaches a dissociation seminar at the Trauma Center and has developed an imagery technique for engagement with dissociated parts of self. She is highly engaged in the national dialogue about implicit and explicit racism and has participated in the development of a Trauma Center working group on issues related to diversity.

Joseph Spinazzola, PhD, a clinical psychologist in private practice, was a clinician, researcher, clinical supervisor, and national trainer for the Trauma Center at JRI for over 18 years, including 12 years as Executive Director of the Trauma Center. He is Adjunct Professor at Richmont Graduate University, a member of The Forensic Panel consulting practice, and Executive Director of the Foundation Trust. Dr. Spinazzola founded the Complex Trauma Treatment Network of the National Child Traumatic Stress Network, coauthored the International Society for Traumatic Stress Studies' expert guidelines for the treatment of complex posttraumatic stress disorder, served as Co-Principal Investigator of the developmental trauma disorder national field trials, and has published over 60 peer-reviewed journal articles and book chapters. He is also the lead developer of the Trauma Drama intervention for youth and young adults.

Marla Zucker, PhD, CMPC, is a clinical psychologist and certified sport psychologist in private practice in Brookline, Massachusetts. She is a supervisor and lecturer in the Sport Psychology specialization at Boston University within the Counseling Psychology program. Dr. Zucker worked with the Trauma Center at JRI for 15 years, including 11 years as Director of Clinical Services and then Program Director, and 8 years as Program Director at JRI's Metrowest Behavioral Health Center in Acton, Massachusetts. At the Trauma Center, she was also on the training faculty and worked clinically with traumatized children, adolescents, and adults. Dr. Zucker has published and presented widely in the areas of trauma and trauma treatment and developmental learning and attention disorders.

Foreword

Bessel A. van der Kolk

Helping people recover from trauma, abuse, and neglect has always struck me as being vastly more complicated than the most intricate brain surgery that I witnessed as a medical student and as a surgical intern, but without the technical tools or the financial support that are provided to neurosurgeons to accomplish their arduous tasks. In this book, my colleagues at the Trauma Center have taken on the formidable challenge of presenting one aspect of the complexity of this undertaking: the personal and technical skills it takes for a psychotherapist to accomplish the task of returning people who have been exposed to unspeakable betrayal, abandonment, and assaults to feeling fully alive in the present.

When psychiatry and psychology first started to grapple with the fact that much of human suffering is the result of living with the legacy of trauma, we thought that trauma simply consisted of intrusive memories of bad experiences. Hence, our initial approach was based on the naive assumption that we could simply help people return to normalcy by "dealing with" or "processing" particular traumatic events. Gradually, we came to realize that trauma, particularly trauma that occurs early in life in the context of caregiving relationships, changes how mind and brain mature, affecting one's perceptions, physical sensations, physiological reactivity, and, perhaps most profoundly,

Bessel A. van der Kolk, MD, is Medical Director of the Trauma Center at Justice Resource Institute in Brookline, Massachusetts; President of the Trauma Research Foundation; and Professor of Psychiatry at Boston University School of Medicine.

one's relationship to oneself. As a result, we came to realize that recovery from prolonged trauma requires a profound reorganization in multiple domains of functioning.

People rarely come for therapy to deal with childhood trauma. They take the brave step of talking with a complete stranger about their shameful and terrifying inadequacies because they are desperate. Nothing seems to work: they can't sleep, their appetite is off, they have extreme emotions in response to the slightest challenges—the basic housekeeping functions of their bodies have broken down. They also tend to hate themselves; they often enrage the people around them, they have trouble feeling relaxed and intimate with others, they feel generally out of synch, or they feel dead to the world.

Few people who enter therapy make a conscious connection between their current distress and past trauma. All they know is that they feel heartbroken and that their guts are tied in a knot. In recent years, we have gained a great deal of understanding about the physiological basis of those sensations, that alienation and that lack of self-control. We have learned that "the body keeps the score" and that trauma is not a story about an event that happened a long time ago, but that the traces of long-ago experiences continue to be experienced right now in body, mind, and brain. The entire "organism" has become stuck in the past and has trouble getting adjusted to living in the present. Pioneering French psychologist Pierre Janet (1859–1947), who wrote the first extensive treatise about trauma back in 1889, entitled his work l'Automatisme Psychologique—psychological automatism. He observed that traumatized individuals automatically keep reenacting and reexperiencing sensations, emotions, and behaviors that are rooted in the past. In fact, he called "le traumatisme" a "maladie de présentification"—an illness of not being able to feel fully alive in the present.

Janet also was the first to notice that the overwhelming nature of traumatic experiences interferes with one being able to mentally "process the event," that is, put it behind oneself as belonging to the past, and that overwhelming experiences leave people speechless and unable to tell the story of what happened. Not only that: trauma then causes further changes that make it difficult to learn from subsequent experiences and to absorb new information. All of this further amplifies the power of the past over the present. (I have discussed our attempts to deal with these issues in much greater detail elsewhere; see van der Kolk, 2014). We at the Trauma Center were fortunate enough to be part of the team that did the first neuroimaging studies of posttraumatic stress disorder. These showed what happens in the brains of traumatized individuals while they relive their traumatic past in a brain scanner, and we found exactly what Janet had described, namely, that during their reliving of the experience the speech center of the brain, Broca's area, shuts down.

Of course, trauma has been with us ever since humankind first walked on the face of this earth: we are a troubled and violent species, and throughout history our great poets and playwrights, like Homer and Shakespeare, have described the effects of human tragedies, including how people keep engaging in wars and family calamities, and how they keep responding in the same way that we do today. This includes the age-old awareness that trauma renders people dumbfounded; they are plunged into a state of speechless terror. Our brain scans and our clinical experience made us realize that resolving trauma may sometimes have to bypass the use of language and that at times it may be necessary to deal with trauma's legacy indirectly, bypassing telling a story that may be too overwhelming to be told. Eye movement desensitization and reprocessing and yoga proved to be highly efficacious methods to accomplish that.

In the course of developing a discipline of traumatic stress studies, many of us quickly became aware that the vast majority of traumatized people we see in clinical practice have been severely hurt in the context of their own families. The bulk of our clientele was made up of people who had been abused, neglected, or abandoned as children by their own caregivers. That was not an easy admission for our clients to make because it seems to be a universal human trait to want to be proud of one's family, and most people instinctively blame any unpleasant childhood experiences on defects in their own character rather than on having had terrifying, intrusive, or frozen parents. After first meeting John Bowlby and Mary Main, we started to pay attention to the field of attachment research, as exemplified by the work of our contemporaries Dante Cicchetti, Alan Sroufe, Karlen Lyons-Ruth, Beatrice Beebe, and Ed Tronick, who were studying attachment patterns between infants and their caregivers. Gradually, it became clear that the greatest damage in our patients was the direct result not of specific traumatic incidents, but of chronic patterns of impaired caregiving, in which adults who were responsible for the child's growth and development simultaneously were their greatest sources of threat. The therapeutic challenge was not so much the resolution of specific horrendous events, but healing chronic relational patterns of abuse and neglect.

This realization brought our therapeutic endeavors more closely in line with traditional psychotherapeutic methods and schools of thought, but with an entirely new angle—namely, we now were able to expand our skills by incorporating what we and our colleagues had learned in our research about the effects of disorganized attachment and chronic interpersonal danger on mental, somatosensory, and physical development. We came to fully appreciate that, as human beings, our nature is rooted in our nurture. Or, as my friend and attachment researcher Ed Tronick taught me: the brain is a cultural organ.

This research clarified that the primary function of our minds and brains is to be productive and cooperative members of our families, tribes, and larger social groups; that we are social creatures through and through, whose purpose is to live in synch with our surroundings. This angle on child development demonstrated that terrifying early caregiving experiences interfere with one's ability to be in tune with one's surroundings, regulating emotional responses, paying attention and concentrating on nonthreatening stimuli, and engaging in mutually satisfying relationships. Without a trauma or attachment perspective, kids who suffer from these problems tend be given diagnoses such as "oppositional defiant disorder" (meaning "You're a pain in the ass"); "conduct disorder" (which simply means "I can't stand you"); or "bipolar disorder" (which means you're emotionally all over the place). Those vernacular descriptions have about as much scientific validity as these so-called diagnoses.

Obviously, taking good care of your kids has evolutionary advantages: if you shower them with consistent and predictable care, they are much more likely to grow up to become playful, joyful, and productive members of your family. We gradually learned that early abuse, neglect, and abandonment literally reorganize core neurobiological, perceptual, and integrative patterns in the brain that later are expressed in difficulties in relationships between oneself and others, as well as in a person's sensory perceptions, self-regulatory capacities, and awareness of oneself and others. These are capacities that we literally learn at our mothers' knees.

In the past 30 years neuroimaging studies, including some that came from the Trauma Center itself and from students who graduated from our program, have shown that terrifying attachment experiences as a child are likely to result in impaired functioning of brain areas devoted to self-reflection (the medial prefrontal cortex). These experiences can lead to an inability to distinguish dangerous from safe or pleasurable stimuli (the amygdala), to be aware of the consequences of one's actions over time, and to understand that feelings and experiences have a beginning, middle, and end (the dorsolateral prefrontal cortex). Also affected can be the capacity to filter out relevant from irrelevant stimuli (the anterior cingulate) and to develop an integrated relationship to the demands, warnings, and comfort of one's bodily sensations (the insula). Most recently, neuroscience research is beginning to show how prolonged early childhood trauma is associated with damage in brain areas devoted to learning, sensory integration, long-term planning, and even the capacity to feel safe while looking at other people's faces. The therapeutic challenge is to normalize these functions, all of which are necessary to have a self that is in harmonious relation to others and that can be in charge of a self's actions and emotions.

One of the things you learn at your mother's knee is to identify and express your feelings in words and not in actions. Seeing yourself reflected in the facial expressions and vocal responses of your caregivers seems to be a necessary ingredient for developing those skills. Self-knowledge depends on being able to find words for your sensations and reactions, and on being affirmed in your observations, movements, and intentions by seeing yourself reflected in the movements, facial mirroring, and language of the people around you. Clearly, abuse, neglect, and abandonment make it impossible to feel you are reflected in those around you: you are likely to be met with an angry or frozen face, and you often are ignored, shamed, silenced, or sworn to secrecy. The great attachment researcher John Bowlby once said, "What cannot be told to the [m]other cannot be told to the self."

That is where psychotherapy comes in: belatedly, you need to experience what happens when you feel reflected in the hearts, minds, and physical reactions of others; in this way, you can learn that feeling upsetting emotions does not mean you will fall apart, go crazy, or be unable to function. By being met with curiosity and compassion, one can gradually find words to describe one's internal experiences. Words are essential not only for self-knowledge, but also for determining what is going on with you and what you want to do about it.

Now that we know how early abuse, neglect, and abandonment all interfere with knowing what you're feeling, being able to communicate what is going on with you, and identifying the origin of your emotional reactions (or even knowing where your body is—its location and position in the world), we can recognize the vast therapeutic challenges that face us to repair the damage of the greatest public health issue in the United States: the long-term effects of abandoning, neglecting, and brutalizing children. As the Adverse Childhood Experiences (ACE) study has shown, this public health issue is more expensive than the cumulative costs of cancer or heart disease.

Psychotherapy is only one part of reversing the damage. In the Trauma Center, we have studied numerous other modalities as well, including yoga, neurofeedback, sensory integration, and theater. We also don't underestimate the potential therapeutic effects of learning martial arts, becoming a tango dancer, or being able to put experience to music, but those interventions cannot currently be studied within the context of medical and psychological research. We also are aware of the transformative power of experiences such as basic training in the military, religious conversions, psychedelic experiences, or competence in a particular skill.

In order to fully own ourselves, however, we need to learn to accept, tolerate, and even understand what is going on inside of us—our sensations, emotions, and reactions. Mindfulness is central to being able to observe, tolerate, and understand what is going on inside. Attentive parents and thoughtful kindergarten teachers help children acquire the ability to enjoy one's own company and not drown out awareness of oneself with blaring televisions or constant visits to social media or computer games. But mindfulness is not enough: the research of the German neuroscientist Tanya Singer has shown that mindfulness becomes transformative only if it is accompanied by self-compassion. Therein lies the rub. Children create an inner map of who they are in relationship to their surroundings based on their experiences. Abuse and abandonment become hardwired in the brain. A child who is abused, unwanted, neglected, or abandoned cannot help but attribute the misery of his or her existence to who he or she fundamentally is. To me, one of the most profound findings of the ACE study relates to the prevalence of behaviors that indicate a fundamental lack of self-care and self-respect: smoking, drug taking, indiscriminate involvement with sexual partners, and a general inability to arrange for a playful life marked by self-protection and self-care. Childhood abandonment and brutalization makes people prone to self-loathing, self-blame, and chronic shame: "I don't deserve any better—it's all I am good for."

If you are not known, seen, and appropriately responded to as a child, you will find it difficult not only to know *who* you are—what you feel like and what your purpose is—but also to feel safe in intimate relationships, understand how you affect other people, and safely negotiate the effects other people have on you. You apply what you have learned: maybe compliance worked, or perhaps you were always on guard, or were the toughest kid on the block, or managed your feelings by burning yourself with cigarettes or by cutting yourself with razor blades. These behaviors then become the stuff that needs to be "fixed." However, reason and understanding don't fix these behaviors—they originate in the most primitive self-preserving part of our nervous system, and in order to resolve them, we need to revisit and restructure the drama of the unwanted child. You need to come to a point that you can lovingly and compassionately observe what you had to endure as a child and give the part of yourself the care that was lacking back then. Getting there always is an arduous process. One keeps hoping that other people will love that wounded kid that you yourself can't stand. Most therapists I know sooner or later come to love their patients, or at least feel a deep affection for them, but as long as *you* can't stand who you are, other people's affection tends to fall on fallow ground.

Working with traumatized children and adults confronts us with "the life force": the incredible drive of people to carve out the best possible life for themselves. As one of my patients once told me, "I pay, I pay, and I pay. I paid with my childhood, I paid with my innocence, I paid with my adolescence, and I paid for all sorts of different forms of therapy, often by inadequate therapists. I have trained dozens of therapists how to treat people like me, but it was I who had to pay the bills." But my patient never gave up trying.

My spiritual ancestor Pierre Janet said, almost 150 years ago, that "every life is an act of creation, cobbled together with whatever means people have at their disposal." That is true for all of us, including our traumatized clients. They do what they can. Sometimes they do it in ways that have a transformative effect on the world, like Maya Angelou or Nelson Mandela; sometimes they do it by hiding and shutting down. But if anything has become clear in my 40 years of doing this work, it is the fundamental truth of my friend Richard Schwartz (the inventor of internal family systems therapy): "All parts are welcome." All of their behaviors can be understood as ways in which they originally protected themselves, and all of them can be assumed to have contributed to their survival. The now ill-fated behaviors of traumatized individuals do not respond well to the power of positive thinking or simplistic solutions to "fix" the problem: sooner or later you must go to the source and discover that wounded person inside, the child you once were, whom, upon closer examination, you may find you despise because of how compliant, weak, seductive, terrified or frozen he or she was. The perpetrator once lived outside, but for most people with childhood trauma the persecutor now resides inside. As Pogo famously said, "We have met the enemy and it is us."

Becoming a trauma therapist means signing up to go on a roller-coaster ride of intense reactions, violent response, frozen disappearances, often speechless fear and anger, and powerful feelings of love, passion, and dependency. As this book so carefully describes, these reactions will be played out in the space between the therapist and the patient. In order to manage this space successfully, the therapist needs to be intimately familiar with the same issues that her client now faces: delving deep into him- or herself and dealing with his or her own issues involving fear, rage, abandonment, passion, and intimacy. No therapist should do this work alone: that would only replicate the tragedy of the traumatized and isolated child who cannot safely talk about his or her feelings, observations, reactions, and emotions. At the Trauma Center we spend almost as much time examining our clinical work with our colleagues and supervisors as we do in direct care. We also have a tradition that requires most clinicians to simultaneously function as researchers. The tradition calls for psychotherapists to become deeply identified with a particular school of thought that is then often uncritically followed, much like the faithful adhere to a particular sect or religion. But make no mistake: therapy is not a religion; we simply are getting paid to help our patients live life to its fullest in whatever way is useful to them.

When you come from a place where you were not allowed to know what you know or feel what you feel, it can be extraordinarily difficult to find a language for yourself and your inner experience. The presence of a compassionate, safe, and reflective therapist is essential to help you discover who you are and what is going on inside. This is never an easy process, and the main task of the therapist is to create physiological stability and the necessary safety to activate the "watchtower of the mind" (van der Kolk, 2014), where we can compassionately observe ourselves and examine our warring fears, longings, and impulses.

At the Trauma Center we have resisted the impulse to follow only one model by trying to adhere to the dictate of my principal teacher during my training as a psychiatrist, namely: "There is only one textbook, and that is your patient." By researching what we do, we keep discovering that one size never fits all: some clients may be ready to engage in an intense course of self-exploration in an insight-oriented therapy; others need to be helped to get in touch with their bodies first and to acquire a yoga practice. Yet other people first need to have a relationship with a dog before they can engage with a member of that much more treacherous species: people. Others may be so flustered and terrified by human contact that a course of neurofeedback is indicated to prepare them to be able to tolerate the journey inside and negotiate the intimacy that is at the heart of every good therapeutic relationship.

In this book, my colleagues have developed a model for psychotherapists in an "attempt to describe what *actually happens* in the room with our complex trauma clients, guided by our own and our colleagues' extensive collective practice at the Trauma Center over the past four decades, and informed by the empirical literature on treatment outcome and evolving best practices guidelines for intervention with adults affected by complex posttraumatic stress" (p. 17).

Their model incorporates four core, intertwined components *within both* the client and therapist: *relationship* (working within a relational frame); *regulation* (increasing self-regulatory capacity); *parts* (working with dissociative parts); and *narrative* (identity development, integration, and meaning-making of traumatic and other life experiences through narrative work). Effective treatment of the relational traumas of emotional abuse and neglect involves a collaborative process between the client and therapist. Inevitably, psychotherapy with relationally traumatized adults sooner or later involves relational dysregulation. That is where the roller-coaster ride begins and the potential for a reparative experience starts: through the presence of emotional attunement where there was abandonment before, hopefully leading to establishing a new experience of the self as being valued, seen, and known. Sigmund Freud beautifully summarized the goal of therapy: "Where it was I shall come to be"; where that stuff of terror, abandonment, and invisibility once dominated, somebody appears and runs his or her life.

Introduction

Christine A. Courtois

The inclusion of posttraumatic stress disorder (PTSD) in 1980 as a new diagnosis in the third edition of the *Diagnostic and Statistical Manual of Mental Disorders* (DSM-III; American Psychiatric Association, 1980) included three primary symptom categories: (1) reexperiencing, (2) numbing, and (3) physiological hyperarousal, derived primarily from the study of war trauma. Perhaps if the symptoms of posttraumatic stress had been identified in a context other than combat, the effects of trauma resulting from child abuse and interpersonal violence would have been more readily accepted as having additional and different categories of expression. The inclusion of the PTSD diagnosis was nonetheless historic in many ways and welcomed by those who were involved in the nascent contemporary study of trauma at the time. However, it was not long before researchers and clinicians who were investigating the immediate and long-term effects of child abuse and other forms of prolonged interpersonal violence noticed that the PTSD criteria were not an ideal fit for these more *complex* and *developmental* forms of trauma. These were

Christine A. Courtois, PhD, ABPP, is a consultant and trainer in the psychology and treatment of trauma; cofounder and past Clinical and Training Director of The CENTER: Posttraumatic Disorders Program, in Washington, DC; chair of the American Psychological Association's (APA) Guideline Development Panel for Posttraumatic Stress Disorder; past president of APA Division 56 (Trauma Psychology); and past founding Associate Editor of the Division's journal, *Psychological Trauma: Theory, Research, Practice, and Policy*. She has published a number of books on the topic of trauma.

the types that occurred early in life and over the course of childhood; were often pervasive, repeated, and progressive; and were characterized by gross interpersonal betrayal by family members and others in significant relationships with the child victim. They markedly interfered with the child's ability to develop a secure attachment bond with caregivers and had enormous potential to negatively impact his or her psychosocial development over the entire life course.

In 1992, one of these clinical researchers, Dr. Judith Herman, published *Trauma and Recovery* along with a companion article (Herman, 1992a, 1992b) delineating differences in the circumstances and effects of combat and domestic/developmental trauma exposures (what she labeled men's and women's trauma, or nondomestic and domestic warfare, respectively). Based on the research findings on the effects of child abuse and domestic violence, Herman articulated a stressor criterion of a history of subjection to totalitarian control over a prolonged period (months to years) and seven additional symptoms categories: (1) alterations in affect regulation; (2) alterations in consciousness; (3) alterations in self-perception; (4) alterations in perception of the perpetrator; (5) alterations in relations with others; (6) alterations in somatic responses, including medical illness; and (7) alterations in systems of meaning. She suggested a new diagnosis, complex PTSD (CPTSD), for inclusion in DSM-IV to account for these additional criteria, a diagnosis that was voted in by the relevant committee but then mysteriously was never included in the finished product.

This noninclusion likely occurred in part because of the controversy surrounding the terms "complex trauma" and "complex PTSD" (perhaps they were interpreted as implying that "classic" PTSD constitutes a "simple" form, certainly not the intention of the developers of the CPTSD nomenclature) and because they were not supported by adequate research, among a number of other reasons (Resick et al., 2012). Partly to correct for this noninclusion, researchers (including those associated with the National Child Traumatic Stress Network, whose organizational mission was to systematically study traumatized children and to develop effective treatment approaches) used the term "developmental trauma" (also "attachment" and "relational" trauma) to distinguish it from adult-onset trauma. As there was no diagnosis of childhood PTSD in any of the DSM editions (other than the text suggestion that children responded much as adults did, yet according to their age and stage of maturation), based on their research with traumatized children, they suggested criteria for what they termed "developmental trauma disorder" (DTD) (D'Andrea et al., 2012; van der Kolk, 2005). This diagnosis has come to be seen as the childhood precursor to the CPTSD diagnosis in adults, since many of the same diagnostic criteria articulated by Herman were found in children exposed to prolonged trauma, and these symptoms often lasted into adulthood (Cloitre et al., 2009). Despite this, DTD was also rejected for inclusion in DSM due to a lack of research support.

Fast forward to the present: CPTSD has been included as an *associated feature of PTSD*—rather than as a freestanding diagnosis—in DSM-IV, DSM-IV-R, and DSM-5 (American Psychiatric Association, 1980, 1994, 2013). Notably, in DSM-5, PTSD has been broadened from three to four sets of criteria and include some of the symptoms most associated with CPTSD, such as emotional dysregulation, negative self-concept, additional emotional responses such as shame and anger, changes in beliefs and cognitions, and dissociative responses (Friedman, 2013). Two PTSD subtypes, dissociative and early childhood (6 years or younger), were also included. Finally, although the stressor criterion for the diagnosis has been modified between editions, it continues to emphasize physical and shock forms of trauma (usually of adult-onset and time-limited events) rather than their less evident and more hidden counterparts, such as emotional abuse and neglect, the types highlighted in this text.

The exclusion of the DTD and CPTSD diagnoses from the DSM and the lack of recognition of the often debilitating effects of attachment/relational and emotional forms of abuse trauma as legitimate trauma have effectively left victims in a state of nonrecognition and "diagnostic homelessness." Such a state has many negative consequences and implications. Consider, as the authors of this book have, that many victim/survivors continue to be unable to identify what is wrong in their lives or to understand the origin of the symptoms they experience. Instead, they most often blame themselves and believe themselves to be flawed and deserving of bad things. Moreover, these feelings and beliefs get reinforced by misunderstanding and stigmatization on the part of helping professionals who frequently blame the clients for their complicated and intransigent symptoms (which may be chronic or may emerge spontaneously when triggered in some way, including by life crises and transitions—labeled as onset of "delayed expression" PTSD in DSM-5). Because their true origins are often obscured by the passage of time and therefore are disconnected from their posttraumatic aftereffects and symptoms, and because the majority of helping professionals receive little or no training in psychological trauma, these individuals and their symptoms regularly go unrecognized and unassessed. The unfortunate result is that these clients are commonly misdiagnosed as schizophrenic, bipolar, or borderline or antisocial personality disorder, and are considered untreatable or unable to heal. Not uncommonly, this misdiagnosis results in overmedication and mismedication, accompanied by a host of negative side effects.

As the diagnostic debate has continued in the DSM, a most important development has occurred on another front. The World Health Organization has determined that enough evidence exists to differentiate "classic or standard" PTSD from "complex" forms and includes CPTSD as a distinct diagnosis in the latest edition of the *International Classification of Diseases* (ICD-11), which was just published (June 2018). The organizing principle of the ICD is clinical utility; that is, it must facilitate communication among clinicians, patients, and administrators; have good implementation characteristics; and be useful in the selection of interventions and in clinical management and decision making (Reed, 2010). In contrast to the DSM system, diagnoses in the ICD have a limited number of symptoms (three to five) and no subtypes. Based on research findings, the CPTSD diagnosis was condensed to four main symptom clusters that occur after exposure to prolonged and pervasive forms of trauma: (1) PTSD core symptoms; (2) affect dysregulation, ranging from heightened reactivity to alexithymia and anhedonia; (3) "defeated/diminished," disturbed, or deformed sense of self; and (4) disturbed relationships involving the inability to get close to others, social alienation and distancing, and failure to maintain relationships.

In my view and that of many of my like-minded colleagues who treat adults with a history of developmental trauma, this is a diagnosis whose time has come, in both its child and adult forms. CPTSD encompasses the symptoms of PTSD but also extends beyond them. Its primary utility is in helping clients and their therapists understand the confusing array of aftereffects of developmental trauma from a "whole that is greater than the sum of its parts" perspective (Herman, 2009). Recent findings from the neurosciences and developmental/attachment studies strongly support these findings and document how abuse and neglect by a parent or other caregiver impacts not only a child's psychosocial development but his or her neurobiological and physiological development (Schore, 2003a; Siegel, 1999; Teicher & Sampson, 2016). These findings also reinforce the utility of dissociation as a coping mechanism most available to children, one that can occur fairly automatically in the context of repeated and chronic traumatization and that may continue into adulthood, even when it is not needed. What began as coping mechanisms and adaptations to traumatic circumstances that were life- and sanity-saving at the time they were first deployed later became symptoms that interfered with identity and quality of life. Their impact on the developing child (and later the adult) included interfering with his or her ability to (1) experience and regulate emotions, behaviors, and cognitions/attributions; (2) develop a positive identity and self-worth; and (3) engage in satisfying, mutual, and close relationships with others.

So, the bottom line is that the aftereffects of developmental trauma are complex and that their treatment is similarly complex and must involve a variety of treatment approaches customized to the needs of the individual client (Cloitre, 2015; Courtois & Ford, 2009, 2013). These approaches incorporate evidence-based practices for the treatment of the symptoms of classic PTSD, but they extend beyond them to include the additional symptom classes that have been identified in CPTSD. Starting with Herman's reformulation of Pierre Janet's original three-stage model of treatment (Herman, 1992b; Janet, 1889/1973), complex trauma treatments have developed over time. As the authors of this book document, they can be catalogued into several "generations" according to the focus and types of treatment that were utilized and according to their recommendations for the sequencing of treatment and a general hierarchy of treatment goals, starting with stabilization and emotional regulation. In 2012, two sets of professional practice/treatment guidelines for CPTSD were published, both of which recommended sequenced and multimodal approaches (Adults Surviving Child Abuse, 2012; Cloitre et al., 2011).

These recommendations have not been above controversy, however. Developers of trauma-focused cognitive-behavioral treatments—those studied predominantly with adult-onset trauma that involves hyperarousal, which focus primarily on the extinction of fear responses (i.e., those with the strongest evidence base at present)—have recently challenged the need for sequencing and the ethics of not immediately offering traumatized clients the most efficacious treatments that are available (De Jongh et al., 2016). The jury is still out on these issues, with complex trauma advocates continuing to press the need for sequencing of treatment and stabilization before approaching traumatic memories, and classic trauma advocates arguing for the immediate treatment of the trauma using evidence-based trauma treatment, such as prolonged exposure or cognitive processing therapy. Many of those studying and treating complex trauma have developed some short-term (15–20 session) "hybrid models" that incorporate the best of both worlds, namely, a first phase devoted to stabilization, relational development, and skill building in emotional regulation, followed by a second, narrative exposure-based stage. These include the emotion-focused therapy (EFT) model developed by Paivio and Pascual-Leone (2010) and Paivio and Angus (2017); the skills training in affective and interpersonal regulation (STAIR) model developed by Cloitre, Cohen, and Koenen (2006); and the trauma affect regulation: guide for education and therapy (TARGET) model presented by Ford (2015), all of which have research supporting their efficacy.

The model in this book, components-based psychotherapy (CBP), has been under development for more than 40 years at the renowned Trauma Center in Boston. It is the latest of the longer-term treatment models and is notable for its sophistication and its flexible approach to the complexities of treating CPTSD. Developed specifically to address the effects of emotional abuse, this model shows how this less evident and more hidden form of abuse ("the unseen wounds") is highly damaging in its own right and potentiates the effects of other forms of childhood abuse and trauma. CBP is not a sequenced model per se, but it deliberately attends to the following four components in roughly the following order: (1) relational, focused on client and therapist attachment styles and relational patterns with the intent of building a secure attachment as the context of the remaining work; (2) self-regulation, not only of emotions but of cognitions and behavior; (3) dissociative parts of self and their identification and elicitation; and (4) narrative construction of a coherent self. CBP does so in a way that is client-centered, flexible, and fluid, yet it is also systematic and has a structure.

In this model, the process is the content and the content is the process. Incorporating somatic, neurophysiologically based, and creative narrative techniques that expand on other treatment models, clients are actively encouraged in self-exploration through experiential awareness and in interaction and enactments with the therapist. Using a variety of techniques from a number of affective and somatosensory treatment models, the therapist seeks to actively attune to and reflect the client in order to provide reparative relational experiences that include high degrees of sensitivity and acceptance—a major counter to the neglect and shaming of the past. Clients learn to self-regulate across a number of domains (emotional, physical, behavioral, and cognitive) with the therapist's active support and education. Quite specific to the model is the emphasis placed on the therapist and, per the authors, "putting the therapist back in the therapy." The therapy is seen as a joint venture, a codevelopment between therapist and client that transforms them both. The therapist's use of self is emphasized and encouraged, as is ongoing supervision to assist the therapist in his or her own personal and professional development and in understanding and therapeutically working with the intricacies of the treatment and the expected impasses that develop. Supervision and consultation also give needed support and perspective to the therapist, helping him or her stay grounded in what is often a fluid and ever changing atmosphere—what Loewenstein (1993) defined as the posttraumatic and dissociative relational context of the treatment that can confuse the therapist and obfuscate the treatment process and goals.

Two additional components of CBP are noteworthy: the attention to dissociative process and "parts" of the client (wherever the client is on the dissociative diagnostic spectrum) and the emphasis placed on developing a narrative that is coherent and by which the client tells his or her own story. Clients are encouraged to learn about their "part-selves" along with their unique functions and to communicate and empathize with them over time. These efforts are in the interest of integrating the experiences and emotions held by each and creating collaboration through association (vs. separation through dissociation). As communication increases and dissociation breaks down, hidden or missing parts of the individual's narrative begin to fill in, creating consistency and coherence rather than disparate fragments and threads. The brain actually begins to regenerate and to make new neuronal connections as a result of the relationship and the integrative work. This is what Schore (2003b) and Siegel (1999) have termed "interpersonal neurobiology."

The authors of this text creatively use the metaphor of the abyss (or black hole of trauma, per van der Kolk & McFarlane, 1996) in describing clients' experiences and the treatment process. Clients are first engaged in the work by relational approaches that begin to take them out of the abyss of aloneness and nothingness and into relational space. With the support of the therapist using experiential and somatically based focusing and self-exploration along with attunement and reflection, they begin to learn to define and "take themselves back." This is supported by the development of skills in self-regulation across various domains of self (emotions, cognitions, behaviors). Working with dissociated information and parts of self brings the therapist into the depths of the abyss with clients. Gradually, the missing pieces of the storyline get filled in and the story gets told in a much more coherent form. This is not enough, however. For change to occur, the story must be understood differently, optimally from a position of self-compassion rather than shame and self-hatred. The more complete narration allows for transformation of story and self, changes that affect both the client and the therapist-in-relationship. As the client develops and differentiates, he or she begins to transcend and transform the past by getting out of the abyss and creating a coherent rather than disjunctive narrative, in the process opening many more options for the future.

With its sophisticated understanding of the needs of the emotionally abused client with CPTSD, its emphasis on the ever developing relationship between the therapist and client as the crucible of the learning process and the backbone of the treatment, its identification of other core components of treatment, and its integration and fluid application of a wide variety of treatment approaches, CBP provides an update on and expansion of previous models. It is a most welcome addition to the treatment literature for complex trauma, specifically as it addresses what has previously been an often underidentified component: the insidious and damaging effects of emotional abuse in childhood. These adults are homeless no more.

Acknowledgments

In writing this book, we've been reminded of the old adage "It takes a village. . . ." Though conceived by the four lead authors of this book, the intervention model presented herein, component-based psychotherapy (CBP), is the conceptual outgrowth of four decades of psychotherapy with adult survivors of complex childhood abuse and neglect at our Center. Accordingly, we have a long list of people to acknowledge, without whom this book would not have been possible.

Foremost among these is Bessel van der Kolk. Along with Judith Herman, Bessel is indisputably one of the two most important figures in shaping our field's understanding of the complexity of adaptation to psychological trauma and essential elements of effective treatment. In founding the Trauma Center in 1982, Bessel cemented his vision by establishing a vibrant community to undertake this challenging and important work.

The pages that follow constitute the third attempt to produce a coauthored book capturing the essential facets of our Center's collective approach to adult complex trauma intervention. Dating back to the early 1990s, two earlier writing groups traversed similarly challenging terrain to that undertaken here. While neither ultimately generated a published manuscript, the present book shares common ancestry and mission and owes a debt of gratitude to our colleagues and predecessors involved in these efforts, including Jodie Wigren, Dawn Balcazar, Bessel van der Kolk, Steve Krugman, Sarah Stewart, Denise Elliott, Charles Ducey, Patti Levin, Janina Fisher, Diane Englund, Deborah

Korn, and Frank Guastella-Anderson, with apologies for omitting any names that may have eluded us in the annals of time. The work of the first of these groups yielded an important paper on narrative completion in trauma treatment written by Jodie Wigren (Wigren, 1994). Fittingly, Jodie returns here to contribute an important chapter (Chapter 9) on the narrative component of CBP.

Formal articulation of the CBP model began in 2009 following intensive focus groups with current and alumni supervisors and clinicians from our Center in which they shared their wealth of applied knowledge on adult complex trauma treatment. Our own thinking and writing process was immeasurably enriched by this launching-off point. Ultimately, this book was guided by the entire clinical team of the Trauma Center as we developed this model over the past 8 years, through these initial focus groups, ongoing editorial feedback, and, above all, through engagement with us in this work, as our colleagues, supervisors, and supervisees. To the extent that we have successfully captured the essence of their voices and perspectives in the pages that follow, we have done our job. We wish to acknowledge and extend our gratitude to two of our Trauma Center contemporaries for their written contributions to individual chapters of this book: Hilary Hodgdon (Chapter 1) and Margaret Blaustein (Chapter 3). We are indebted to several additional colleagues who offered conceptual support and writing for an early draft of an edited volume on this topic: Richard Jacobs, Frank Guastella-Anderson, Kari Gleiser, Janina Fisher, Pat Ogden, Erika Lally, Michelle Harris, Wendy D'Andrea, Dawn Balcazar, Ritu Sharma, and Jana Pressley. Their wisdom and expertise informed our thinking considerably. We give special thanks to Kari Gleiser for suggesting what became the working title of this book, *Reaching across the Abyss*.

Elizabeth is indebted to the Trauma Center and the many gifted and impassioned people at its core for their role in the evolution of this book, as well as their immense influence on her professional and personal development. She extends her appreciation to her supervisors and mentors over the years, including Bessel van der Kolk, Frances Grossman, Richard Jacobs, Deborah Korn, Frank Guastella-Anderson, Sarah Stewart, Patti Levin, Kevin Becker, Roslin Moore, Leslie Lebowitz, Terri Weaver, and Honore Hughes. She expresses deep thanks to Joseph Spinazzola for his mentorship and leadership at our Center and to Margaret Blaustein for her ongoing guidance and support, as well as for her innovations in the treatment of complex trauma in children and adolescents. Elizabeth's understanding of culture and context has been heavily influenced by her antitrafficking work with Paola Contreras, Jose Hidalgo, Sujata Swaroop, Cynthia Kennedy, Margaret Dunn, Elizabeth Gruenfeld, Naomi Azar, and Sriya Bhattacharyya. She extends her thanks to Bessel van der Kolk, David Emerson, Pat Ogden, Janina Fisher, Elizabeth Warner, Alex Cook, and Anne Westcott for their influence on her understanding of trauma and the body; to Fran Grossman for her understanding of dissociation; and to Deborah Korn, who greatly impacted her thinking about integration across treatment models. She thanks her friends and colleagues for bringing some light into this work and expresses sincere appreciation to her coauthors for their collaborative commitment and dedication to this text over the course of many years. Finally, she expresses her deepest love and gratitude to her family, who make everything worthwhile.

Fran acknowledges the important lessons she learned from Roy Schafer, MD, who supervised her work at the Student Health Center at Yale University and supported her in her early days as a psychotherapist. She learned about trauma therapy from Faye Snider, LICSW, and her early trauma clients. Fran is deeply appreciative of all she has learned from Jodie Wigren about many things, including being an open, generous, and collegial therapist. Fran wants to acknowledge her early learning about resiliency in traumatized individuals from the participants in the men's and women's studies and from her coauthors, Alex Cook, Selin Kepkep, and Karestan Koenen, of *With the Phoenix Rising*. She has learned more than she could ever have imagined from the staff and trainees at the Trauma Center in discussions of clinical work as well as from participants in her dissociation seminar over many years. She wants to express her appreciation to her three coauthors for what we have developed together, usually laboriously but also at times with great satisfaction. With great appreciation, Fran thanks her husband, Hank, her daughter, Jenny, her son-in-law, Aaron, and her grandson, Ethan—who has taught her to play "snow balls" in her office when it is not otherwise in use—and her son, Ben, her daughter-in-law, Jackie, her grandson, Elijah—who also participates in the above-mentioned game in her office—and her granddaughter, Julia, for their love and support and often patience with the long process of writing a book.

Joseph is indebted to the many clinical supervisors and mentors who supported his professional development and personal growth over the past three decades. Foremost among these he acknowledges Susan Roth, Leslie Lebowitz, Frances Grossman, Jodie Wigren, Roslin Moore, Sarah Stewart, Ron Batson, Philip Costanzo, Karla Fischer, and the many supervisors who guided him during his formative clinical internship year at Bellevue Hospital. He would like to express his deep respect for his three coauthors, as well as his great appreciation for their tolerance of the pace he set throughout the journey they shared in writing this book. Joseph acknowledges the invaluable camaraderie and guidance he received from members of the Complex Trauma Workgroup of the National Child Traumatic Stress Network and the Complex Trauma Taskforce of the International Society for Traumatic Stress Studies. Special mention needs to be made of the following colleagues for their friendship and influence on his thinking and work: Bessel van der Kolk, Margaret Blaustein, Julian Ford, Alexandra Cook, Lisa Amaya Jackson, Christine Courtois, Kristine Kinniburgh, Elizabeth Warner, Mandy Habib, Joshua Arvidson, Bradley Stolbach, Cassandra Kisiel, Chandra Ghosh Ippen, Jana Pressley, Victor Labruna, Tori Reynolds, Shirley Collado, Steven Gross, Kevin Smith, Dicki Johnson-Macy, Glenn Saxe, Cheryl Lanktree, John

Briere, Rosalie Suescun, Sean Rose, John Gatto, Douglas Brooks, Lisa Gold-
blatt Grace, Jenifer Maze, Ernestine Briggs-King, Melissa Brymer, Robert
Pynoos, Christopher Blodgett, Marylene Cloitre, Beth Niernberg, Jim Hopper, Deborah Korn, Christopher Layne, Mimi Sullivan, Amy Fingland, Steve
Sawyer, Prasanna Kariyawansa, Robert Macy, Michael Welner, and Susan
Miller. Joseph expresses love and appreciation for his parents, siblings, and
large extended family, not only for their loyalty, support, and belief in him,
but also for their manifold natures. They afforded him an early understanding
of human complexity and propelled him to discover the taproots to perseverance,
ingenuity, and playfulness. Above all, Joseph dedicates this book to the
great loves of his life: his sons, Balian and James, and his wife, Deanne. No
thanks he can offer will ever approach what they have given him.

Marla thanks her parents, Barbara and Leonard Zucker, first and foremost, for supporting her in all ways possible. She would not be on this road
without them. The Trauma Center has had an immeasurable influence on
Marla's development, and she is deeply grateful to her coauthors and Trauma
Center Management Team for the many complex and important ways they
have contributed to her growth and learning. She would also like to thank her
mentors, teachers, and supervisors from across her professional development
for their care, teaching, and passion: Joseph Spinazzola, Bessel van der Kolk,
Margaret Blaustein, Alexandra Cook, Mary Morris, Gregory Jurkovic, Richard
Jacobs, Kristine Kinniburgh, Roslin Moore, Frances Grossman, Toni Luxen-
berg, Deborah Korn, Elizabeth Warner, Patti Levin, Nadine Kaslow, Ernestine
Briggs-King, and Amy Baltzell. Marla acknowledges the commitment of Justice Resource Institute (JRI) and support of Andrew Pond, Mark Schueppert,
Catherine McDermott, Richard LieBerman, Jenn Miguel, and Kari Beserra.
Marla thanks her colleagues at the Trauma Center and Metrowest Behavioral
Health Center with whom she has had the pleasure of working since 2003 for
their dedication, compassion, and hard work on behalf of our clients, as well as
for the much needed support, guidance, and laughter they have brought to her
life. In particular, she would like to acknowledge Elizabeth Hopper, Heather
Finn, Dawna Gabowitz, Rona Sandberg, Janice Stubblefield-Tave, Lee Fallon-
towne, Sinead McLaughlin, Elizabeth Warner, Jamie Chiarelli, Susan Lerner,
Julie Thayer, Amie Alley-Pollack, Hilary Hodgdon, and Jana Pressley. Marla
thanks her friends, especially Allison Williams, for making life meaningful
and fun, even when the road is hard, and, finally and with continued amaze-
ment, Jane Knell for teaching her about love, trust, and the way out of the
abyss.

.We are grateful to Senior Editor Jim Nageotte at The Guilford Press for
his insight and extensive editorial contributions to this book and to Senior
Assistant Editor Jane Keislar for her organizational support and patience with
us throughout this long and not infrequently arduous process. We thank two
future bright stars in the field of psychology, Anne Sposato and Maggi Price,
for providing instrumental assistance with literature review and summary for

select chapters. Our colleague and friend Beau Stubblefield-Tave offered valued feedback on cultural sensitivity. Our nonprofit organization, JRI, has provided a safe and stable haven for this work and has enabled us to realize and expand the full extent of our mission. We extend our gratitude and respect in particular to Andrew Pond and Susan Wayne, current and former presidents of JRI, for their compassion, acumen, and stewardship.

Finally, we thank the many clients at the Trauma Center and beyond who, across our decades of clinical practice, most directly informed this book and to whom this book is dedicated. Your courage and perseverance as you have fought your way through and out of the darkest places has cast a guiding light on this book and has been our chief inspiration throughout.

Contents

Parts

Chapter 7   Fragmentation of Self and Dissociative Parts   145

Chapter 8   Working with Dissociative Parts   160
               in the Depths of the Abyss

Narrative

Chapter 9   Constructing a Narrative, Constructing a Self   179
               with Jodie Wigren

Chapter 10   Transcending the Abyss: Life Narrative   199
               and Identity Development

PART III. THE COMPONENT-BASED PSYCHOTHERAPY
MODEL INTEGRATION: OUT OF THE ABYSS

Chapter 11   Tailoring Treatment with CBP: 229
               Individualized Adaptations and Effective Pacing

Chapter 12   Applications of CBP: Revisiting David and Nicole   248

Appendix   Component-Based Psychotherapy: 267
               Clinician Self-Assessment
               with Jana Pressley

               References   275

               Index   287

PART I

OVERVIEW
AND BACKGROUND

CHAPTER 1

Component-Based Psychotherapy with Adult Survivors of Emotional Abuse and Neglect

with Hilary B. Hodgdon

At least three million children are victims of abuse or neglect each year in the United States. The vast majority of this maltreatment is perpetrated by the same adults these children rely upon for nurturance, protection, and, quite often, their very survival: parents and other primary adult caregivers or their romantic partners (Sedlak et al., 2010). Among maltreated children, more than half endure *psychological maltreatment*, characterized by repeated or ongoing exposure to severe *emotional abuse* or *emotional neglect* (Spinazzola et al., 2014). The American Professional Society on the Abuse of Children (APSAC) defines psychological maltreatment as "a repeated pattern of

Hilary B. Hodgdon, PhD, is a clinical psychologist and researcher specializing in the study and treatment of traumatic stress. She is Director of Research Operations at the Trauma Center at Justice Resource Institute and Research Assistant Professor of Clinical Practice in the Department of Psychology at Suffolk University. Dr. Hodgdon is also Co-Director of the Complex Trauma Treatment Network, a National Child Traumatic Stress Network training and technical assistance center. Her research focuses on the sequelae of childhood trauma, elucidating mechanisms that convey risk for psychopathology among vulnerable populations, and evaluation of trauma-informed treatment approaches.

caregiver behavior or a serious incident that transmits to the child that s/he is worthless, flawed, unloved, unwanted, endangered, or only of value in meeting another's needs" (Myers et al., 2002, p. 81). It may also involve the terrorizing, rejecting, spurning, or exploiting of children (Kairys, Johnson, & Committee on Child Abuse, 2002), as well as the "persistent or extreme thwarting of the child's basic emotional needs" (Barnett, Manly, & Cicchetti, 1993, p. 67).

While the term "psychological maltreatment" is sometimes referred to interchangeably as psychological abuse, in this book and elsewhere, the former term is primarily used because it more intuitively subsumes emotional neglect in addition to verbal or emotional abuse as an integral component of this form of maltreatment.

Relational in nature, psychological maltreatment represents a fundamental disruption in the attachment bond through both a lack of attunement or responsiveness and overt acts of verbal and emotional abuse. These "attachment injuries" harm children by (1) undermining their development of an internal sense of psychological safety and security and (2) impeding their cultivation of capacities essential to successful life functioning, including emotion regulation, self-esteem, interpersonal skills, and self-sufficiency (Wolfe & McIsaac, 2011). In Table 1.1, we inventory various forms of emotional abuse and emotional neglect, along with some of the contextual factors that influence variability in the expression and effects of psychological maltreatment.

UNSEEN WOUNDS

Overlooked, underreported, and unsubstantiated in comparison to more overt or tangible forms of childhood maltreatment such as sexual or physical abuse, psychological maltreatment has historically constituted a "blind spot" for families, providers, researchers, and government agencies (Rosenberg, 1987). For example, one study examining child protective service case records revealed that while 50% of maltreated children had experienced psychological maltreatment, this abuse was officially noted in only 9% of cases (Trickett, Mennen, Kim, & Sang, 2009). In contrast to state and federal reports on the prevalence of psychological maltreatment, research studies on the prevalence of emotional abuse and emotional neglect in clinical and community samples most always reveal much higher rates of exposure, with community estimates ranging as high as 80% of children surveyed (Chamberland et al., 2005). An important study of over 11,000 trauma-exposed children and adolescents receiving treatment services across the United States through the National Child Traumatic Stress Network (NCTSN) found that impaired caregiving (impacting 40% of all youth assessed), psychological maltreatment (38%), and gross neglect (31%) were the third, fourth, and fifth most prevalent of 20 types of trauma assessed (Briggs et al., 2012).

TABLE 1.1. Variability of Emotional Abuse and Emotional Neglect Based on Type, Context, and Individual Factors

Variability in emotional abuse and emotional neglect
• Inflicted by part or all of caregiving system
• With or without co-occurring abuse or other trauma
• With associated affection (unintentional, inconsistent, or reactive psychological abuse or neglect) or negativity (intentional or malicious abuse or neglect)
• Caregiver's capacity, resources, presence, and impairments

Types of emotional neglect (absence of warmth, support, nurturance)	Types of emotional abuse
• Caregiver is not physically present ▫ Forced to be physically absent due to work, military service, hospitalization, or incarceration ▫ Choosing to be absent due to substance or alcohol abuse or prioritizing another family • Caregiver is emotionally absent due to dissociation, severe depression, chronic mental illness, or developmental delays • Extreme family stress due to poverty, lack of social supports, or dangerous neighborhood interferes with caregiver's emotional availability • Caregiver ignores child's bids for attention or shuns child • Caregiver abandons the child for periods of time with no indication of when he or she will return or imposes extended periods of isolation from others	• Caregiver calls the child derogatory names or ridicules or belittles the child • Caregiver blames the child for family problems or abuse of the child • Caregiver displays an ongoing pattern of negativity or hostility toward the child • Caregiver makes excessive and/or inappropriate demands of the child • Child is exposed to extreme or unpredictable caregiver behaviors due to the caregiver's mental illness, substance or alcohol abuse, and/or violent/aggressive behavior • Caregiver uses fear, intimidation, humiliation, threats, or bullying to discipline the child or pressures the child to keep secrets • Caregiver demonstrates a pattern of boundary violations, excessive monitoring, or overcontrol that is inappropriate considering the child's age • Child is expected to assume an inappropriate level of responsibility or is placed in a role reversal, such as frequently taking care of younger siblings or attending to the emotional needs of the caregiver • Caregiver undermines child's significant relationships • Caregiver does not allow the child to engage in age-appropriate socialization • Child is exposed to relationship conflict between caregivers

Historically, emotional abuse and neglect have been understudied compared to other forms of trauma and interpersonal victimization. And yet, whenever empirical research has shined light on these unseen wounds, "sepsis" has been uncovered. For example, one of the first studies comparing the longitudinal effects of physical abuse, neglect, and psychological maltreatment found maternal verbal abuse and emotional unresponsiveness to be equally or more detrimental than physical abuse to attachment, learning, and mental health (Erickson, Egeland, & Pianta, 1989). Another early study found verbal, not physical, aggression by parents to be most predictive of adolescent physical aggression, delinquency, and interpersonal problems (Vissing, Strauss, Gelles, & Harrop, 1991).

Despite the proliferation of nearly 100 evidence-based or promising treatment models tailored to survivors of other forms of trauma designed to target particular posttraumatic symptoms or disorders, until now none have been specifically developed to treat adult or even child survivors of psychological maltreatment. In fact, many well-established, evidence-based, and widely disseminated treatments of adult traumatic stress omit assessment of exposure to childhood emotional abuse or emotional neglect entirely when conducting otherwise comprehensive trauma histories to identify clinical targets for intervention. Presumably, this is because these forms of trauma continue to be left out of the *Diagnostic and Statistical Manual of Mental Disorders* (DSM-5; American Psychiatric Association, 2013) as adverse life experiences that "qualify" as causal (or "Criterion A") stressors for posttraumatic stress disorder (PTSD), the prevailing psychological trauma-related diagnosis in the United States since the establishment of this guide in 1980.

The lesser attention paid to psychological maltreatment is likely due to a confluence of societal and cultural factors. Notwithstanding compelling research from our Center revealing that psychological maltreatment typically serves as a "driver" of subsequent familial physical abuse and assault (Hodgdon, Suvak, et al., in press), in and of itself psychological maltreatment is less likely to result in harm to the child that leaves overt physical "evidence." In contemporary Western societies, child sexual abuse and, increasingly, physical abuse have finally attained the status of consensus social taboo, motivating adults to intercede. Conversely, psychological maltreatment perpetrated by parents or other adult caregivers still largely remains in a gray area of (mis)perception regarding familial and cultural differences in parenting practices, or at worse as the unintentional consequence of ineffective or "stressed" parenting. Thus, it often fails to generate the larger systemic response from schools, pediatricians, child welfare, or law enforcement that is often necessary to result in intervention. Interestingly, as a society, we have a much easier time recognizing psychological abuse for what it is—and refusing to tolerate it—when it occurs outside the home, be it in our children's schools or communities perpetrated by peers (where we have renamed it "bullying") or when perpetrated against adults in the workplace (where we are quickest to condemn it as "harassment"). In contrast, valid assertions of the psychological maltreatment of children are often met with resistance, minimization, and even outright dismissal.

This societal "astigmatism" against recognizing psychological maltreatment clearly for what it is enables emotional abuse, and especially emotional neglect, to remain unseen or at least avoided by therapists, case workers, and other adults within a child's broader caregiving system. Perhaps more than for any other form of childhood maltreatment, providers can become complicit in "looking the other way" rather than defining emotionally aversive parenting behavior as psychologically abusive or neglectful and risk immersing themselves in a contentious and potentially ambiguous situation. Tragically, these patterns of familial and societal denial of the reality and consequences of psychological maltreatment heighten risk trajectories and exacerbate mental health disparities for this highly vulnerable subpopulation of trauma survivors. They contribute to the perpetuation of emotional abuse and neglect, with reduced likelihood of prevention, detection, and protective response, accurate understanding, or adequate intervention prior to adulthood.

A TURNING OF THE TIDE

Psychological maltreatment is finally beginning to receive greater recognition as a widespread and dangerous form of trauma in its own right and an important target of health disparities research and policy. Neuroscientific research has convincingly demonstrated specific and deleterious effects of emotional abuse and neglect perpetrated in childhood on brain development (for a seminal review, see Teicher & Sampson, 2016). The foremost leader in this research, Teicher has found parental verbal abuse to be an especially potent form of maltreatment, associated with large negative effects comparable to or greater than those observed in other forms of familial abuse on a range of outcomes including dissociation, depression, limbic irritability, anger, and hostility (Teicher, Sampson, Polcari, & McGreenery, 2006). Notably, when coupled with witnessing domestic violence, parental verbal abuse was found in that study to be associated with more severe dissociative symptoms than those observed in any other form of familial trauma or their combination, including sexual abuse. In 2012, the American Academy of Pediatrics released a special report identifying psychological maltreatment as the most challenging and prevalent form of child abuse and neglect (Hibbard, Barlow, MacMillan, & Committee on Child Abuse, 2012). Statements such as these echo emerging research findings from our Center documenting equivalent or greater immediate and long-term negative effects of childhood psychological maltreatment as compared to other forms of child victimization.

In our research using the Core Dataset (CDS) of the NCTSN, a large national sample of trauma-exposed children and adolescents, we found that psychological maltreatment was not only the most prevalent and earliest onset form of maltreatment, but also the most chronic form of trauma exposure out of 20 types of trauma assessed in the CDS (Spinazzola et al., 2014). Compared to physical and sexual abuse, psychological abuse, despite rarely being the focus of treatment, was the strongest predictor of symptomatic internalizing behaviors, attachment problems, anxiety, depression, and substance abuse and was equally predictive of externalizing behaviors and PTSD. In addition, psychological abuse was associated with equal or greater frequency than both physical and sexual abuse on over 80% of risk indicators assessed, and it was never associated with the lowest degree of risk across these three forms of maltreatment. Strikingly, experiences of emotional abuse or emotional neglect were found to carry greater "weight" or "toxicity" than other egregious forms of childhood abuse. Specifically, children and adolescents with histories of only psychological maltreatment typically exhibited equal or worse clinical outcome profiles than youth with combined physical and sexual abuse. In contrast, the co-occurrence of psychological abuse significantly potentiated the outcomes associated with either of those forms of maltreatment.

ADULT TRAUMA TREATMENT: CAN ONE SIZE REALLY FIT ALL?

The developmental disruptions that result from psychological maltreatment place children on a trajectory of continued difficulty over time. Interruption of one developmental step undermines mastery of subsequent developmental tasks, leading to an unfolding of impact that manifests over the course of the lifespan. In our clinical work, we have long regarded this form of childhood maltreatment as also having some of the most pervasive, complicated, and enduring effects on individuals across all aspects of identity and functioning. Accordingly, our approach to psychotherapy with adult clients contending with the aftermath of profound childhood psychological maltreatment differs in many important ways from traditional treatments for PTSD.

A large number of intervention models have been recognized as evidence-based treatments for PTSD based on carefully controlled clinical efficacy research (Foa, Keane, Friedman, & Cohen, 2010). However, much of the data on which these designations are based have been demonstrated to be constrained by conclusions derived from highly exclusionary study designs with adult survivors of acute traumatic events or those presenting with less complex clinical profiles and fewer risk indicators than is typically observed in clinical practice settings (Spinazzola, Blaustein, & van der Kolk, 2005). This raises fundamental questions about the generalizability of this body of research and the actual effectiveness of those treatments with real-life people who are seeking treatment for trauma, especially those suffering from more complex or treatment-resistant adaptations to trauma. This concern has led prominent trauma theorists and clinical researchers alike to challenge the adequacy of one-size-fits-all approaches to trauma treatment (e.g., Cloitre, 2015; Stein, Wilmot, & Solomon, 2016; Sykes, 2004).

In our experience working across the range of treatment settings with adult survivors of childhood emotional abuse and neglect—from community mental health centers and general outpatient clinics to trauma-specialty treatment centers and private practices, to inpatient, residential, and day-treatment settings—PTSD is the tip of the iceberg, if present at all. Through the accumulation of a substantial body of clinical wisdom, research, and scholarship over the past four decades, we have come to understand the legacy of chronic and severe childhood interpersonal violence, exploitation, attachment disruption, and neglect as a problem of *complex trauma.*

COMPLEX TRAUMA: THE MANY-NAMED FIEND

The quintessential unifying feature observed in our adult therapy clients with histories of chronic childhood trauma is this: their current difficulties are not merely linked to early life adversities; rather, the essence of these struggles, along with the core of their current identities and life narratives, cannot be meaningfully understood outside of the context of these formative experiences. For many of our clients, past experiences and present existence can appear to be hopelessly, inextricably entangled. Courtois (2004) articulated the first formal definition of *complex trauma* as a *recurrent* and *escalating* form of trauma occurring primarily within familial or intimate relationships. More recently, she elaborated on this definition in her excellent treatment book with Julian Ford:

> traumatic attachment that is life- or self-threatening, sexually violating, or otherwise emotionally overwhelming, abandoning, or personally castigating or negative, and involves events and experiences that alter the development of self by requiring survival to take precedence over normal psychobiological development. (Courtois & Ford, 2013, p. 25)

The Complex Trauma Workgroup of the NCTSN (Cook et al., 2007; Spinazzola, Ford, et al., 2005; Spinazzola et al., 2013) has a similarly developmentally anchored definition of complex trauma as—a *dualistic,* pernicious, and *progressive relationship between exposure and adaptation,* concepts that have guided our thinking about the treatment of adult complex trauma.

Nearly as many other names and clinical conceptualizations have been offered in an effort to describe and define the problem of complex trauma as there are clinical experts, researchers, and scholars in the realms of traumatic stress, victimology, and public health. First among these was Terr's (1991) highly influential differentiation of *Type I* (exposure to *single, shocking, intense* traumatic events associated with more focal intrusive symptoms and cognitive misperceptions) and *Type II* (exposure to *multiple, long-standing, or repeated extreme* traumatic events associated with broader psychological consequences and coping deficits, including numbing, dissociation, aggression, self-hatred, and personality/character impairment) trauma. While Terr did not use the term *complex trauma* per se, her conceptualization of Type II trauma has subsequently been attributed by some to be the origin of the complex trauma construct (e.g., Ford & Courtois, 2009). Even a largely overlooked conceptualization of complex trauma as constituting *Type III trauma* has been offered in the criminology literature (Solomon & Heide, 1999).

Foremost among conceptualizations of complex trauma is Herman's (1992a, 1992b) articulation of a diagnostic construct of the complexity of adaptation to trauma: *complex posttraumatic stress disorder* (*CPTSD*). For some time, this diagnostic construct was also described as *disorders of extreme stress not otherwise specified* (*DESNOS*; Pelcovitz et al., 1997; van der Kolk, Roth, Pelcovitz, Sunday, & Spinazzola, 2005) in an effort to differentiate it from PTSD during and for some time following the DSM-IV field trials. An impressive body of empirical research on CPTSD has been amassed over the past two decades to bolster the widespread clinical support for and international recognition of this diagnostic construct (Cloitre et al., 2009, 2011; Cloitre, Garvert, Brewin, Bryant, & Maercker, 2013; de Jong, Komproe, Spinazzola, van der Kolk, & van Ommeren, 2005; Ford & Kidd, 1998; Ford & Smith, 2008; Ford, Stockton, Kaltman, & Green, 2006; Karatzias et al., 2017; Zucker, Spinazzola, Blaustein, & van der Kolk, 2006), despite lingering debate that the symptoms captured by CPTSD may more accurately be conceptualized as clinical correlates of a more severe form of PTSD (Wolf et al., 2015). More recently, a parallel stream of research and advocacy has been directed toward delineating and pursuing official nosological classification of *developmental trauma disorder* (*DTD*; D'Andrea, Ford, Stolbach, Spinazzola, & van der Kolk, 2012; van der Kolk, 2005), a diagnosis designed to capture the negative consequences of childhood complex trauma exposure on core regulatory capacities, domains of functioning, and risk trajectories (Ford et al., 2013).

Other complex trauma experts, most notably John Briere, have resisted establishment of a unitary diagnostic construct for complex trauma, emphasizing instead the variable expression of impairment across clusters of symptoms and domains of functioning influenced by the nature, number, and timing of trauma exposure in conjunction with individual differences in physiology, personality, temperament, and social context (Briere & Scott, 2015). Such researchers have focused instead on the effects of complex trauma exposure on phenomenological constructs such as *symptom complexity* (e.g., Briere, Kaltman, & Green, 2008; Hodges et al., 2013) and *complex posttraumatic states* (e.g., Briere & Spinazzola, 2005). Still other trauma and victimology researchers have created clinical constructs emphasizing the number of different types of trauma exposures in general (e.g., *cumulative trauma*; Agorastos et al., 2014; Karam et al., 2013) or else the number of different types of particular victimization experiences (*polyvictimization*; e.g., Finkelhor, Ormrod, & Turner, 2007) on the breadth and severity of clinical outcomes and risk trajectories. In turn, Ford and Courtois (2009) provide a useful differentiation of *complex psychological trauma, complex posttraumatic sequelae,* and *complex traumatic stress disorders.*

Finally, preventive medicine and public health researchers have independently generated constructs that overlap with facets of complex trauma exposure and adaptation. Paradigms such as *early life stress (ELS), toxic stress,* and *adverse childhood experiences* (ACEs) emphasize medical outcomes related to compounded experiences of maltreatment, neglect, or absence of a protective adult figure during childhood. Research on ELS (e.g., Garner et al., 2012) and toxic stress (e.g., Pechtel & Pizzagalli, 2011) has primarily focused on the effects of living with chronically activated bodily stress response systems on brain architecture, organ systems, and cognition. In a similar vein, the ACE framework has produced groundbreaking studies documenting the explicit link between an exponentially predictive risk of exposure to 10 different forms of familial trauma during childhood and a startlingly wide range of serious health conditions, diseases, and premature mortality in adulthood (e.g., Felitti et al., 1998).

ON THE SHOULDERS OF GIANTS

This book is intended primarily for clinicians as an applied guide to practice. Attempting an exhaustive review of the now rather extensive literature on adult complex trauma intervention would detract from this aim (for this purpose, we recommend Courtois & Ford, 2009). Nevertheless, this book would not exist without the foundation of four decades of complex trauma treatment theory, model development, and empirical validation that preceded it, and without the numerous luminaries in the field whose formative insights and essential groundwork guided our thinking and set the stage for the model introduced here. Prominent among these influences are Putnam's (1989) seminal book on the diagnosis and treatment of dissociation and the groundbreaking early writings on treatment of complex trauma by Herman (1992b) and van der Kolk, McFarlane, and Weisaeth (1996b). Chu (2011) offered an early practical guide for the treatment of CPTSD and dissociative disorders. Brown (Brown & Fromm, 1986) paved the way for modern understanding of the intersection between childhood trauma and altered states of consciousness in adulthood and provided innumerable strategies for working with dissociative self-states. Courtois (2010) and Roth (Roth & Batson, 1997) greatly expanded understanding of treatment of adult survivors of childhood incest. Pearlman and Saakvitne (1995a) and Perlman (1998) produced lasting works exploring the effects of trauma treatment on the practicing therapist. In addition to being developers of major complex trauma treatment models in their own right (Cloitre et al., 2006; Ford, 2015), Cloitre and Ford have spearheaded vital clinical research advancing the empirical basis for complex trauma intervention paradigms and diagnostic constructs (e.g., Cloitre et al., 2010; Ford et al., 2013). Most recently, Courtois and Ford (2013) have published the most sophisticated book to date on the nuance and sequencing of relational treatment of complex trauma.

Childhood emotional abuse and neglect leave behind a powerful residue. These experiences can shape survivors' attributions of self and perceptions of others, undermine their establishment of healthy attachment relationships, and obstruct their capacity to tolerate the receipt and expression of emotional intimacy. These effects can lead some survivors of psychological maltreatment to internalize an innate sense of failure or shame to a more global extent than that observed in response to nearly any other form of trauma. We find that adult survivors of severe and prolonged childhood emotional abuse and neglect present with clinical profiles and therapeutic needs that overlap with (but that are in important and nuanced ways distinct from) those observed in adults with other complex childhood traumatic experiences. As a result, it is our experience that adult survivors of childhood emotional abuse and neglect typically require therapeutic approaches that not only diverge from those offered by traditional PTSD-focused intervention models, but that also vary in focus and degree from those offered by existing complex trauma intervention paradigms. Accordingly, whereas the new framework we describe in this book has been designed for use in treatment with adult survivors of all forms of complex trauma, we pay particular attention to adults with pronounced histories of childhood emotional abuse and neglect.

MODELS AND MYTHS

Essentially, all models are wrong, but some are useful.
—GEORGE P. BOX

The question of how to facilitate psychic healing in adults suffering from the legacy of familial maltreatment has drifted in and (often been driven) out of the forefront of psychotherapeutic theory and practice, since the advent of psychology as a science in the late 19th century. In that time, many specific treatment models have been developed or adapted to address posttraumatic sequelae. Most of these interventions fall to a greater or lesser extent within one of what we loosely conceptualize as three predominant paradigms that emerged over more than a century of traumatic stress inquiry and research, acknowledgment and denial, remembering and forgetting. Each of these paradigms has made pivotal—and to our mind, essential—contributions to the evolution of our field.

The first and most enduring of these paradigms has concentrated on the intentional activation and processing of traumatic memories as the primary mechanism of intervention. This paradigm spanned and survived the major political and ideological regime shift from psychoanalysis to behaviorism boo! that took place in psychology in the middle of the 20th century. From Janet and Freud to Foa, disclosure and catharsis became repackaged and abridged as exposure and desensitization with surprisingly little actual change in the focus, targets, and desired end result of the work (e.g., see Foa, Chrestman, & Gilboa-Schectman, 2009; Freud, 1896; van der Hart, Brown, & van der Kolk, 1989). In fact, the first formal treatment outcome study for PTSD in adults compared the relative efficacy of three very distinct approaches to engaging traumatic memories and sequelae—psychodynamic group psychotherapy, hypnotherapy, and flooding—and found all three approaches to achieve equivalent outcomes (Brom, Kleber, & Defares, 1989).

In its position then and now as the dominant paradigm of trauma treatment, traumatic memory processing is often maligned as an approach by competing paradigms: its merits are questioned, its limitations emphasized, its contraindications inventoried, and its demise is repeatedly portended (Wylie, 2004). Nevertheless, the great contribution of this paradigm to the lives of those impacted by traumatic experiences cannot be questioned. Exposure-based interventions and their proponents, beyond providing viable means of relief from suffering for many survivors of some forms of trauma, will ultimately be most remembered for their importance to victim advocacy, policy, and public awareness. In response to a century characterized by cyclical periods of societal minimization and denial of the prevalent reality of maltreatment and its devastating effects, this paradigm's champions—and none more authoritatively than Foa—have played a critical role in amassing an extensive body of empirical research that proves once and for all that violence and abuse constitute undeniable, tangible, and serious sources of human affliction that directly cause psychiatric distress and impairment of life functioning.

The birth announcement of the second paradigm arrived swaddled within the covers of Judith Herman's seminal book, *Trauma and Recovery* (1992b). This book was the first to emerge from the members of the Boston Trauma Study Group. This fecund think tank of clinicians and researchers had come together to examine and stretch the parameters of the nascent traumatic stress field. They were driven by their collective challenges to safely and successfully utilize the various emerging trauma exposure and memory processing treatment models for adults with more chronic and severe histories of childhood abuse or neglect. The three-phase model succinctly and eloquently proffered by Herman resonated deeply with clinicians for over a generation. It provided an organizing, guiding framework for what was otherwise routinely experienced by clinicians as a challenging, confusing, and chaotic treatment process. Her model restored the primacy of the therapeutic relationship to trauma treatment and illuminated the importance of establishing an internal sense of safety before engaging clients in processing traumatic memories. Shortly thereafter, van der Kolk and colleagues (van der Kolk, McFarlane, & van der Hart, 1996a) elaborated a five-phase version of treatment for complex

PTSD that emphasized the importance of fostering affective and somatic regulation capacity as a critical precursor to deconditioning traumatic memories and restructuring meaning-making.

Although complex trauma treatment in routine practice often does not smoothly progress through such clear, linear stages, these phase-oriented paradigms provided something that is sorely needed: more hopeful, better tolerated, and more affirming approaches to trauma treatment for this large subgroup of trauma survivors—the growing numbers of adult women and men bravely coming forward with disclosure—and acknowledgment of chronic childhood victimization and intrafamilial trauma. Moreover, these models recognized that the clinical needs of complex traumas change and evolve over the course of treatment, and thus so must the focus of therapeutic intervention. Initially relegated by the academic community to a status subordinate to that ascribed to the exposure-based paradigm, two decades later, the phase-oriented trauma intervention paradigm has finally attained sufficient empirical validation to receive formal endorsement as the best-practice approach to treatment of CPTSD in adults (Cloitre et al., 2011, 2012).

More recently, contemporary vanguards in the field have heralded what we regard collectively as an innovative and exciting third paradigm for recovery from traumatic stress. This emerging third paradigm is physiologically and neurobiologically driven, focusing on the critical importance of mind–body approaches to trauma recovery. Recognizing the limits of traditional forms of psychotherapy, proponents of this mind–body paradigm have pursued nonconventional approaches that target the somatosensory imprint of trauma, particularly with the sizable subset of psychotherapy-resistant adults living with chronic, complex traumatic stress and related conditions and disorders (Levine, 1997; Ogden, Minton, & Pain, 2006; van der Kolk, 2014). Intervention models falling within this paradigm revive, retool, and blend ancient, largely eastern, physical arts such as yoga, meditation, and acupuncture with advanced new technologies, including clinical biofeedback and neurofeedback, in an effort to build regulatory capacity and "retrain" brains "wired" by chronic early trauma exposure to exist in fixed or oscillating states of hyper- and hypoarousal.

While the model we introduce in this book, component-based psychotherapy (CBP), has been informed by and draws heavily from all three of these paradigms, it ultimately does not fit neatly within nor subscribe fully to any of them. In our view, successful complex trauma intervention in real-life practice—particularly when conducted with adult survivors of the kind of pervasive and profound deprivation and debasement that comes from living through chronic and severe emotional abuse and neglect in childhood—can almost never be accomplished through adoption of a singular clinical target, follow a consistently linear process, or result from adherence to one specific clinical technique. In contrast, it is tangled, precarious work, work that is predictable in its unpredictability, that inevitably requires the therapists'

extensive use of themselves in the treatment process, and that simultaneously demands attention to the body and all that usually goes unspoken in trauma and in psychotherapy. Out of necessity, then, CBP has been designed as a multi-tiered, multitargeted, component-based approach to complex trauma treatment (Grossman, Spinazzola, Zucker, & Hopper, 2017).

To be clear, with the introduction of CBP, we do not profess to be forging a new paradigm for traumatic stress intervention. Our work has most accurately evolved from a long-standing, potent, but often overlooked paradigm or "undercurrent" in mental health treatment that is hardly new at all, but rather is in line with a long-standing recognition of *common factors* or *core components in psychotherapy* dating back to the 1930s (Rosenzweig, 1936) and bolstered by decades of empirical research (e.g., Barth et al., 2012; Duncan, Miller, Wampold, & Hubble, 2010). In this vein, with the publication of their book *Psychological Trauma and the Adult Survivor*, McCann and Pearlman (1990a) quietly introduced the first theory of change and a model for treatment of relational trauma in the contemporary era: constructivist self-development theory. While their book was well respected, their delineation in it of a complex, relationally driven, component-based model of change received limited overt attention. Perhaps their important contribution to the traumatic stress field was inadvertently eclipsed by the ascendance shortly thereafter of Herman's book, with the irrefutable definitiveness of its title and the brilliant clarity of its intuitively resonant three-phase course of recovery.

Nevertheless, many of the advances made in the traumatic stress field toward understanding the intervention process have been influenced, directly or indirectly, by McCann and Pearlman's articulation of their approach to treatment with adults impacted by interpersonal trauma. Over the past decade, a resurgence of interest in applying core components-based principles of psychotherapy has been witnessed in the child traumatic stress field, spearheaded by the NCTSN (Layne et al., 2011). Inspired by this movement, colleagues at our Center developed the ARC (attachment, regulation, competency) model, a components-based approach to complex trauma treatment in children for which this book serves as a complementary companion (Blaustein & Kinniburgh, 2010; Kinniburgh, Blaustein, Spinazzola, & van der Kolk, 2005).

We wish to claim several additional companions, whose important work we seek to build on by using what we casually refer to as a "fourth paradigm" of "messy, relational" complex trauma treatment. CBP has been significantly influenced by Davies and Frawley's (1994) and Pearlman and Saakvitne's (1995a) efforts to integrate psychoanalytic models with traumatology and their strong emphasis on the therapeutic relationship in trauma therapies. Moreover, the relational psychoanalytic school, best represented by Bromberg (2001), has enriched our understanding of the complex relationships and enactments that occur in the treatment of traumatized adults, especially those with histories of complex childhood emotional abuse and neglect.

CBP intentionally delves deeply into certain problem areas and intervention components, particularly in the realm of dissociation; these components were barely understood at the time of publication of some of the formative trauma treatment models mentioned earlier. In contrast, CBP offers less extensive consideration of certain intervention components than other previous trauma treatment models, particularly in the realm of cognitive processing. Nevertheless, in its emphasis on the pivotal role of the therapeutic relationship in complex trauma treatment, its concurrent implementation of a multi-tiered set of core components, and its unwillingness to downplay the inherent idiosyncrasies and lack of "neatness" of this work, we hope that the intervention model introduced in this book helps to inspire the next generation of trauma treatment innovation.

COMPONENT-BASED PSYCHOTHERAPY: NEW MODEL, NEW MYTH?

Psychological trauma is seemingly ubiquitous to the human condition, and the prototypical adult who presents for psychotherapeutic services comes with a history of exposure to trauma. For a minority of clients, trauma occurred in the form of a single, impersonal incident: a terrible accident, an unexpected injury, or a natural disaster. For most, trauma was chronic or recurrent, began in childhood, and involved episodic or chronic exposure to often-interconnected experiences of maltreatment, exploitation, or neglect. The impact of these experiences on neurobiology, emotional development, and identity is profound and requires complex adaptations that routinely result in enduring psychological disturbance and associated social and functional impairment. Moreover, when childhood emotional abuse and/or emotional neglect constitutes the primary form or "organizing thread" of an adult survivors' trauma history, the consequences tend to be most global, the infiltration into self-appraisal and meaning systems most insidious, and the response to traditional psychotherapy most recalcitrant.

CBP is an evidence-informed framework designed to guide clinical intervention with adult survivors of complex interpersonal trauma, especially adult survivors whose trauma histories include prominent exposure to childhood emotional abuse or neglect. Conceived by senior faculty of the long-standing Trauma Center in Brookline, Massachusetts, founded by Bessel van der Kolk, CBP represents the outgrowth of four decades of extensive clinical practice, supervision, training, and research. Development of CBP was predicated on integration of perspectives and strategies from virtually all of the Center's current and alumni senior clinicians and supervisory staff members through intensive focus groups, editorial review, and multiauthored contributions to this book.

CBP is a relational intervention that offers what we regard as the next juncture in sequential approaches to complex trauma intervention. A core-components treatment model, it provides intervention targets, strategies, and techniques designed to address what we consider to be the four primary components of this work: relationship, regulation, dissociative parts, and narrative. CBP bridges trauma-focused, psychoanalytic, feminist-relational, humanistic, and mind–body theories of therapeutic action to a greater extent than any other trauma treatment model. Notable among contemporary approaches to psychotherapy—and certainly unique among evidence-based, trauma-focused interventions—is the extent of CBP's emphasis on the therapists' internal experience, relational challenges, and movement and growth within and across the four primary components of the model as work unfolds and evolves between client and therapist. Accordingly, much emphasis is placed on the role of supervision in CBP, as well as on constructively working with and through the frequent enactments that inevitably emerge in the context of this work.

CBP reflects an attempt to describe what *actually happens* in the room with our complex trauma clients, guided by our own and our colleagues' extensive collective practice at the Trauma Center over the past four decades and informed by the empirical literature on treatment outcome and evolving best-practice guidelines for intervention with adults affected by complex posttraumatic stress (Cloitre et al., 2012). We endeavored to develop CBP in accordance with contemporary perspectives on the evidence-based practice of psychotherapy (Kendall & Beidas, 2007). Nevertheless, as readers will frequently encounter throughout this book, we find this therapy to entail a complex, fluid, evolving, and at times convoluted process—one that can be hard to capture and sometimes not even within our conscious awareness. CBP is a framework designed to provide a sufficiently containing structure to support and tolerate this inevitably challenging undertaking.

As noted earlier, the CBP model incorporates four core, intertwined components within both the client and therapist: relationship (working within a relational frame), regulation (increasing self-regulatory capacity), parts (working with dissociative parts), and narrative (identity development, integration, and meaning-making of traumatic and other life experiences through narrative work as both therapist and client come to construct a shared understanding of the client's story). As we underscore repeatedly throughout the chapters that follow, clinicians' own competencies and struggles in regard to their personal relationships, emotion regulation, integration of self-states and narrative, and identity development invariably affect this work. These therapist-specific factors can advance or impede therapeutic progress through their influence on therapeutic attunement and rupture, healthy connection, detachment, and enmeshment. Moreover, CBP considers how each of these components is embedded within the unique and shared cultures and contexts of client and therapist. Above all, CBP attends to the interactive nature of each of these elements within and between the therapist and client (see Figure 1.1).

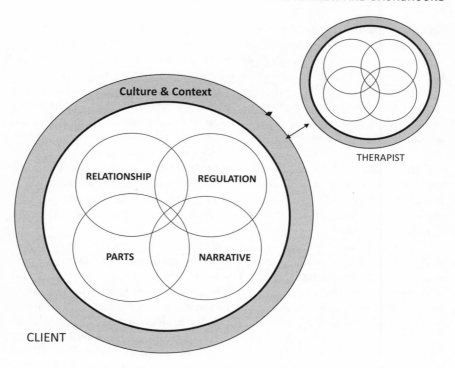

FIGURE 1.1. CBP components and context within both client and therapist.

Relationship

As we have said, the therapeutic relationship is the cornerstone of this work, and that fact is reflected throughout this book. Relational trauma requires, and seeks, relational healing; thus, complex trauma treatment should happen within a relational frame. The healing of relationally inflicted wounds occurs within the context of a holding environment, with another person to witness the client's suffering and to provide support and validation. Adults who have experienced chronic emotional abuse, neglect, and other forms of trauma have generally been deprived of this type of holding relationship. Therapy provides a partial surrogate—a parallel frame or container within which to develop self-knowledge and self-regulatory capacity.

We believe effective treatment of the relational traumas of emotional abuse and neglect involves a collaborative process between the client and therapist. The therapist guides the client in being able to go to and sit in dark places. To do so, the therapist needs to have the ability to create internal quiet and to sit in his or her own dark places. CBP is interactive and collaborative, as the therapist's and client's inner processes drive them to connect, move apart, and come back together, codeveloping the therapeutic process over time. In our view, much of what happens in this relationship is nonverbal, and much of it occurs outside the conscious awareness of the client and therapist.

Because early neglect and abuse often disrupt people's capacity for attachment, the therapeutic relationship provides a context in which the client can build relational capacity. The repair of disruptions in attunement and attachment are as important as the development of a trusting therapeutic relationship. In addition to Pearlman and Bromberg's guiding contributions noted earlier, CBP has been heavily influenced by Fosha's (2000; Fosha & Slowiaczek, 1997) delineation of specific dyadic attunement techniques and strategies for therapeutic use of self to build the relational and regulatory capacities of adult trauma clients.

Regulation

If the research of our Center and that of our colleagues over the past two decades has established anything, it is that a complexly traumatized client is a dysregulated client. Be it disturbance in regulation of affect, impulses, cognition, physiology, self- and relational attributions, or, most often, the cascading confluence of dysregulation across many or all of these domains, disrupted capacity of self-regulation has come to be heralded as the sine qua non of complex trauma. Practitioners tend to recognize dysregulation most readily when it is "loudest": in clients with pronounced bursts of hyperarousal—such as explosive and often fragmented states of rage, terror, or panic—activated by perceived threat and traumatic reminders, and perhaps followed by states of extreme hypoarousal such as social withdrawal and isolation, emotional numbness, or amnesia.

While these are undoubtedly hallmark manifestations of dysregulation, to some extent they belie the ubiquity of dysregulation in its more "quiet" expressions: the chronic unease, the hair-trigger irritability and surges of shame and loathing of self and others, and, above all, the baseline inability to self-soothe or restore equilibrium in response to internally or externally generated shifts in arousal. Particularly for adults whose adaptation to trauma has been shaped by the neurobiological sequelae of impaired caregiving, emotional abuse, and neglect in infancy and early childhood, it is often these less dramatic, more perfidious forms of dysregulation that underlie their lasting difficulties and demand primary focus in treatment (Schore, 1996).

Therapy with relationally traumatized adults almost invariably begins in a place of relational dysregulation. Given repeated past experiences of relational betrayal, abandonment, violence, or rejection, these clients are primed to distrust their trauma-specialty therapists and to discount or feel threatened by engagement in whatever new trauma-focused strategies or techniques these well-meaning practitioners introduce to help their clients learn to identify, tolerate, and modulate their distressing emotions, reactive behaviors, and troubling states of arousal. Moreover, the process of developing self-regulatory capacity with such clients takes place within this challenging relational context and is unavoidably influenced by the therapist's ability to monitor and effectively modulate his or her own regulatory systems in general, and particularly in response to his or her interactions with the client.

Important influences on CBP within this component of treatment include Linehan's (1993) and Cloitre's (Cloitre et al., 2006) approaches to emotion regulation, distress tolerance, and interpersonal skill building; Ford's (2015) integration of mindfulness and present-focused approaches to regulation; Ogden's (Ogden et al., 2006) strategies for promotion of somatic regulation; and Korn and Leeds's (2002) use of guided imagery–based techniques to cultivate internal resources for self-regulation and facilitate client readiness to access fragmented parts of self and undertake trauma processing and narrative construction.

Parts

Therapy with survivors of early childhood neglect and abuse involves bringing to awareness that which has been discounted and bringing together that which has been fragmented. Therapy with adults exposed to early deprivation and abuse is not just interrelational but also intrarelational. Dissociation and fragmentation of aspects of experience and aspects of self are common coping mechanisms for children facing violence and interpersonal deprivation. In recent years, increasing numbers of trauma therapists and theorists (e.g., Chefetz & Bromberg, 2004; van der Hart, Nijenhuis, & Steele, 2006) have come to understand that full healing of individuals suffering physical and sexual abuse requires working with dissociative "parts"—aspects of self that are to some degree disconnected from conscious awareness. We have found that working with parts is at least as essential in working with clients with histories of chronic neglect and emotional abuse as with victims of physical and sexual abuse, whether or not their histories include sexual and/or physical abuse as well.

We view parts work to be an almost universal component of intervention with adults struggling with the aftereffects of these complex forms of childhood trauma. This is a unique feature of our model and a clear departure from traditional treatment approaches for psychological trauma, which either entirely omit consideration of the presence of and response to dissociative experience or else regard this as a distinct, "comorbid condition" present in only a subset of trauma clients and needing to be addressed separately from other forms of treatment. In contrast, in our work, we have come to understand the fragmentation of traumatic experiences and posttraumatic accommodations as integral to the prototypical adult survivor of chronic and severe childhood emotional abuse and neglect. By necessity, then, CBP considers parts work to be an essential ingredient in routine clinical intervention with this complex subset of trauma survivors. Consistent with CBP's relational approach, the therapeutic process often involves interactions between parts of the therapist and parts of the client. Successful navigation of this complex process requires that the therapist be willing to explore aspects of self routinely held outside of conscious awareness. It also requires that the therapist examine his or her own overt and implicit identities and self-narratives, as both a person and a therapist, and their influence on the treatment process.

Narrative

Treatment models for adult complex trauma vary considerably in their position on when, whether, and how to integrate a memory processing or narrative component of intervention. These questions have become the nexus of a lively and long-standing debate in the traumatic stress field. A small but important body of empirical literature has documented (1) poor tolerance of exposure to traumatic memory processing interventions in emotionally dysregulated, highly avoidant, or dissociative adults; (2) better tolerance and modest gains associated with stabilization-focused treatment; and (3) enhanced outcomes associated with adherence to a phasic approach to treatment comprising the sequential combination of emotion regulation–based intervention followed by traumatic memory processing (Cloitre et al., 2010; Cloitre, Koenen, Cohen, & Han, 2002; McDonagh et al., 2005).

We view narrative work as an integral component of treatment for the majority of adult complex trauma survivors. It is our viewpoint, however, that narrative work with complex trauma clients in general, and adult survivors of childhood emotional abuse and neglect in particular, involves much more than the processing of or desensitization to discrete traumatic memories. Much of our narrative work in CBP is directed toward helping clients come to understand how their chronic difficulties stem from survival-based adaptations that they developed in response to early life adversity, and to then organize these experiences into a cohesive, meaningful, and forward-looking life narrative that transcends trauma and instills a sense of purpose and hope.

As such, the focus and end goal of narrative work in CBP goes beyond the telling of one's trauma story (or, more commonly, stories) toward constructing a comprehensive life narrative that integrates, nurtures, and helps to mature previously fragmented, underdeveloped, or compartmentalized aspects of self and identity. Another facet of CBP that is relatively unique among adult complex trauma interventions is its recognition of the implicit omnipresence of the narrative process throughout all stages of treatment, as well as its prioritization of pursuing some explicit form of trauma experience integration and life narrative work with even the most complexly traumatized adult survivors of emotional abuse and neglect. In this vein, CBP departs from a tendency of some complex trauma practitioners who display in their approach to practice a strong tendency to restrict intervention, sometimes indefinitely, to the stabilization phase of treatment

Similarly, therapists possess their own personal and professional identities and life narratives. Often implicit, these narratives and identities inevitably enter the treatment room, for better or worse, interacting with and becoming influenced by the therapeutic relationship. As with those of their clients, clinician narratives and identities change and evolve over time, affecting what they attend to and overlook in the work, how they respond to their clients, and what biases, motivations, and needs of their own seep into and complicate the treatment process. CBP places great importance on ongoing examination of these therapist-specific factors as the critical focus of the supervisory process; emphasizes recognition of the influence of the clinicians' personal experience on the treatment process; and grapples with strategies for constructive use of these experiences in working through therapeutic reenactments.

CULTURE AND CONTEXT

CBP teaches therapists to listen for gaps and omissions in the stories they are told, to attend carefully to the cultural and social contexts within which trauma and life narratives are constructed by clients, and to increase their awareness of the shared and disparate contexts from which they hear and interpret this information. There has been an increasing call to action regarding therapists' responsibility to be culturally sensitive and to cultivate awareness of institutional barriers that may prevent people from receiving and benefiting from mental health care (La Roche, Davis, & D'Angelo, 2015; Pedersen, Crethar, & Carlson, 2008). In an effort to capture in an inclusive manner the range and complexity of cultural influences and identities of potential salience in psychotherapy, Hays (2001) delineated the ADDRESSING framework: Age and generational influences, Developmental or acquired Disabilities, Religion and spiritual orientation, Ethnicity, Socioeconomic status, Sexual orientation, Indigenous heritage, National origin, Gender. CBP elaborates on and expands Hays's framework to include consideration of additional contexts that are important to the treatment of complex trauma: gender identity (Singh & Dickey, 2016) and trauma exposure group membership. Recent scholarship on cultural influences on the psychotherapy process counterbalances early efforts in the mental health field regarding culture-specific knowledge accumulation (e.g., see Sue, 1998), with emphasis on the importance of respect for subcultural diversity and of the therapist's recognition that personal identity and group membership is highly individualized even for clients sharing cultural contexts (Nezu, 2010).

CBP prioritizes adoption of an *intersectional* understanding of cultural context, namely, that these categorizations are heavily interconnected social constructs put in place by systems of power and enforced, explicitly and implicitly, to impart and maintain privilege and advantage to members of dominant cultural groups while serving to enforce and justify discrimination and oppression of others (Crenshaw, 1989). Of central importance to all mental health practice, intersectionality is critically relevant in the treatment of victims of interpersonal trauma and maltreatment. Racism, discrimination, and poverty are fundamentally experienced in and of themselves as forms of trauma (e.g., see Smith, 2009). Likewise, the history of exposure to interpersonal trauma itself functions as a societally engendered layer of oppression, serving to further subordinate, isolate, or condemn impacted individuals existing within often already marginalized cultural contexts. We believe that the historical minimization, denial, and, at times, outright mockery of childhood emotional abuse and neglect and reframing of associated difficulties as innate defects in character are part of the deepest and most treacherous layers of social ostracism.

In this book, we devote considerable attention to the ways in which perceived and actual commonalities and differences in cultural context between CBP therapists and their clients can have a significant impact on the therapeutic relationship and the course of treatment, often serving as drivers of misattunement, enactments, and therapeutic ruptures. Critiquing the status of academic multicultural training in psychology and social work and its failure to demonstrate empirical benefit for the psychotherapy outcome, Holmes (2012) identifies therapist self-awareness of implicit cultural biases as the true goal of cultural competence in therapy. CBP seeks to illuminate the early-installed, often deeply buried, prejudices and emotional misconceptions of therapists and clients alike. These underlying biases may be particularly hard for therapists to recognize because of our tendency to consciously value egalitarianism and our typical need to regard ourselves as empathic, compassionate, and generally unselfish. To avoid making inaccurate assumptions about our clients and to gain some understanding of their cultural identities and the contexts informing their exposure and adaptation to traumatic life experiences, we need to begin by striving to identify our own explicit and especially implicit prejudices, biases, and assumptions about culture (Hays, 2001). As we highlight throughout this book, this type of self-examination can engender considerable avoidance, fear, discomfort, and ultimately growth on the part of the therapist. Finding ways to manage and endure the anxiety that can ensue from engaging issues of bias and prejudice is an essential part of successful treatment in CBP, especially as effective intervention typically involves bringing conversations about issues of racism, discrimination, and other forms of oppression and marginalization to the surface with our clients. The capacity to engage these challenging topics in an authentic way with clients has been found to be beneficial not only to the therapeutic alliance but also to treatment retention and outcome (Cardemil & Battle, 2003).

Likewise, in CBP we endeavor to attend to the ways in which trauma survivors' experiences have been shaped by and viewed from the vantage point of the immediate and larger ecological contexts within which they occur (Bron-fenbrenner, 1989). These contexts are layered and change over time. For adult survivors of childhood maltreatment and neglect, this entails consideration of pivotal childhood, adolescent, and current adult ecological contexts. Most often, these contexts prominently include the client's past and present immediate environments or *microsystems* (e.g., family of origin; current adult family living situation); expanded personal environments or *mesosystems* (e.g., school and peer relationships; adult work relationships); external factors relevant to their broader communities or *exosystems* (e.g., youth drug culture; geographically linked adult political climate); and larger factors at play at the time of the trauma and currently in the society at large or the *macrosystem* (e.g., prevailing social beliefs about child development; current mental health policies and health care practices). Accordingly, CBP is predicated on a belief that effective intervention requires awareness of and ongoing exploration of the intersection of these ecological contexts and the challenges faced by clients. Building on the work of Harney (2007), CBP places particular emphasis on "the first context": the enduring gravitational pull of formative attachment relationships in the lives of adult survivors of complex childhood trauma.

INTO THE ABYSS

In his seminal book on complex trauma, our colleague Bessel van der Kolk introduced the metaphor of the *black hole of trauma* (van der Kolk et al., 1996b). For van der Kolk, the black hole represented survivors' consuming fixation on traumatic memories and their associated physiological and affect sequelae. Unable to sustain meaningful engagement in present-focused and future-oriented experience because of the continual triggering of trauma-related memory networks, survivors were recognized by van der Kolk to be caught in time, lost in the gulfs and crevasses of their past.

Since that time, we have come to recognize in our complex trauma clients, especially in adult survivors of chronic childhood emotional abuse and neglect, other poignant intrapsychic and interpersonal dimensions of this phenomenon. Through the metaphor of *the abyss,* CBP revisits the black hole of trauma as the predominant state of being experienced by adult survivors of childhood emotional abuse and neglect and thus, too, as the primary nexus of treatment. This book explores the shifting meaning and mutable protean expressions of the abyss in each component of CBP. From the simultaneous longing for and dread of closeness in *relationships* to the roller coaster of annihilating eruptions of intense affect states and utter eradication of emotional experience in *regulation*, the abyss is the central motif of this book. In *parts*, CBP invokes the abyss metaphor in the form of zones of the ocean to reframe and refine clinical understanding of awareness and integration of fragmented aspects of self. In *narrative*, CBP's rendering of the abyss motif echoes Courtois and Ford's (2013) "void of self" as the embodiment of the most desolate state of identity development: the complete absence of self. Strategies for recognizing manifestations of the abyss and for effectively engaging treatment on its precipice and in its chasm are the primary concern of CBP.

WHAT WE SEE, WHAT WE DO: CONCEPTUALIZATION AND INTERVENTION

The CBP framework is not a one-size-fits-all approach, and we try to attune to the nuanced differences among individuals as we approach case conceptualization and intervention. We view each component as being comprised of numerous dimensions, with each individual falling at a different place along these dimensions at different points in time. The first chapter on each component (Chapters 3, 5, 7, and 9) includes a table that identifies several dimensions for that component; we provide examples of how different clients might be conceptualized using these dimensions, establishing the groundwork for treatment planning. Therapeutic change can be assessed by reconsidering where a client falls along these dimensions of each component over time. Similarly, we are well aware that there are many paths to a common goal. Because CBP has emerged from a rich history of various intervention modalities, many of the intervention strategies or tools might be familiar to clinicians. To help place these strategies within the context of CBP, the second chapter on each component (Chapters 4, 6, 8, and 10) includes a table that provides examples of intervention techniques that target that component or interactions between that component and others. Chapter 11 includes a final integrative table that describes intervention strategies addressing all of the components in CBP. These tables can be used to assist clinicians in considering *why* they are doing *what* they are doing in the room, supporting meta-awareness of the therapeutic process over time.

THE STORIES WE TELL: A NOVEL APPROACH TO TEACHING COMPLEX TRAUMA TREATMENT

Introduction to the CBP approach to complex trauma treatment revolves around the stories of two adult trauma clients: David and Nicole. These cases, together with our collective struggles in understanding and treating them, are the heart of this book and serve as its organizing thread. Both vignettes are case composites reflecting core themes, histories, and challenges encountered in the many complexly traumatized adult survivors of childhood emotional abuse and neglect whose treatment we have conducted or supervised. Also featured throughout are Nicole and David's therapists; these therapists represent facets of ourselves at various stages of our professional development, as well as aspects of the many novice and experienced clinicians we have supervised. The crafting and function of these vignettes intentionally deviate from those of traditional case illustrations. They are not composed of typical categories of information of relevance to conceptualization and treatment planning, and they are delivered in a more or less sequential, orderly fashion. No attempt is made to provide comprehensive information, exhaustive history, or "objective" rendering of the clients' experiences. Instead, clients are revealed in vivo, in glimpses and fragments representing discrete moments at various stages of treatment, from vantage points that alternate between client and therapist. Written in literary form, the chapter introducing these characters tells stories: about this approach to treatment, about the clients immersed in it, and about the therapists struggling to provide it. In this book, we have set out not only to elucidate the fundamental elements of the CBP model but also to absorb the reader in an in-depth exploration of the complexities of this work.

Like ourselves and our colleagues, the therapists depicted in these vignettes at times demonstrate deep compassion or attain moments of great insight or attunement; in other instances, they miss the mark entirely. Like all of us, they are as intrinsically flawed in their capacity to understand themselves and others as they are filled with profound potential for growth and connection. CBP is equally concerned with the clinician's internal processes of relationship, regulation, parts, and narrative. At times these are strikingly parallel to those of their clients and at other times markedly divergent. Invariably, the therapists' internal systems and schemas become activated and challenged by engagement in this complex relational work. Accordingly, these vignettes are as much about the clinicians as about the clients they are struggling to treat.

The vignettes are taken up in each ensuing chapter, intermingled with brief consideration of other cases, to illustrate key aspects of CBP. Each chapter offers observations of false starts, missed opportunities, pivotal interactions, and alternate approaches in response to particular exchanges between therapist and client and highlights and builds on interactions and interpretations perceived to bear promise. In the final chapter, we revisit David and Nicole and offer an integrative consideration of their treatment using the CBP framework. Our aim is for the reader to arrive, in a manner as close as possible to actual supervised treatment itself, at successively deeper understandings of the CBP approach to complex trauma intervention. If this book's somewhat unorthodox narrative device sufficiently intrigues you to sustain the openness and curiosity necessary to remain "experience-near" to this rich but often opaque subject matter, then we will have succeeded in our intent.

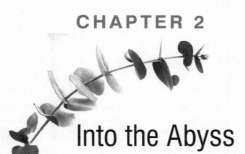

CHAPTER 2

Into the Abyss

A Series of Moments in the Clinical Process for Client and Therapist

DAVID

Prologue

The little boy sits hunched over the curb, elbows on his knees, forehead slumped in his hands. He wants to throw a really big stone into a car window or something worse. Trouble is, the street is so clean he can't find a pebble to kick, never mind the giant potholes he liked to jump over where he used to live. The boy wants to yell really loudly, but he's afraid that if he makes a commotion in a place like this—which is cleaner and quieter than anywhere he's ever been except for church—he'll get in big trouble for sure. He turns and looks up at the big hill of grass behind him. It belongs to the gigantic white house he was brought to by the man and woman who picked him up from the terrible place and told him they were his new parents. He wants to roll down it but knows he'd get stains on the stiff pants and itchy white shirt they make him wear and is afraid that he'd be punished by the lady with the big scary smile who keeps telling him to call her "mother."

The little boy doesn't want to call her that. He used to have his own mama. He tries hard not to think about her; it hurts too much when he does. He doesn't understand why he couldn't have just stayed with his real family, with his auntie and cousins? He misses them so much but worries in his heart that it's his fault. If he hadn't been such a bad, useless boy, maybe his auntie wouldn't have gotten sick and stopped loving him and sent him away.

He wishes he could just disappear. Maybe if he tries really hard, if he's really good and does everything they ask him to do, maybe these new parents won't send him back to that awful place where all the little boys with no mommies and daddies to love them have to stay. It's really hard to behave though when these people keep taking away all his things from before and saying bad things about them: his old clothes, his favorite toy (a little broken but still good!), even his thick, curly hair that his mama always loved. They told him they had to shave it off so he could make friends with the other boys in the neighborhood. That made no sense to the little boy at all. They even told him that the plain old words he's always used are no good and that he has to learn new words now that he lives with decent people.

The only thing the boy still has of his own is his name. *David*. He remembers the morning they sent him away, how his auntie gave him a long, hard hug and whispered a secret to him about his name. She told him it came right out of the special book she always keeps by her bedside. That it is the name of the bravest boy of all: the boy who slayed the giant. She told David he was her brave little boy but then started crying and hurried off into her bedroom and closed the door. That was the last time he saw his auntie.

David does not feel brave, only sad, and scared, and terribly angry.

1. The First Session

David Stapleton sits in the waiting room of Dr. Susan Thalman's private practice, located in an affluent, tree-lined neighborhood of a metropolitan city in the northeastern United States. Classical music streams into the room from small speakers tastefully concealed from view. The chair is surprisingly comfortable, and several magazines that match his interests rest on the coffee table in front of him. David is not at all sure he wants to be here. He and his wife are talking more heatedly now about getting a divorce. His daughter is out of control. Worst of all, David's work, which has always been his anchor and his refuge, has somehow started falling apart. All of this is his doing, or at least this is what has been hammered into his brain by his wife, Joyce.

Vexed, David ruminates about how all this came to be. He is pretty certain that for years he had been appreciated by his wife and daughter as a hardworking and devoted husband and father. Morning after morning David would awake, unchanged, the exact same man. Somewhere along the way, though, his family apparently grew frustrated with his reserved nature. David can't pinpoint when, or for that matter understand why, being quiet and deferential to how his wife runs the household and disciplines their daughter suddenly became a source of resentment and evidence of his being emotionally vacant and neglectful. Lately he's even managed to stumble blindly into a hornet's nest of entitlement and retribution with the new generation of up-and-coming engineers at his firm. Since when does nearly two decades of being task-oriented, highly productive, and minding your own business lead people to question whether you "continue to be aligned with the values of the team"? Is all this headache because I raised my voice one time at that totally incompetent, snotty new Ivy League recruit they ended up letting go just a few months later?! And where the hell does Joyce get off telling me that I'm the one that needs therapy? Maybe she should take a closer look in the mirror!

David has the urge to get up and walk out and leans forward in his chair. He notices that his chest has tightened and his heart is racing. He takes a slow, deep breath and wills his head to clear.

The door opens. A gray-haired woman with bright, inquisitive eyes gently smiles at him and invites him to enter. Dr. Thalman strikes David as shorter, frailer, and older than she looked to him from her website photo. Dr. Thalman offers him coffee. He declines. David chooses the chair furthest from the one she clearly uses.

After some niceties and introductions, Susan Thalman asks David what has brought him in. He inhales deeply and then launches into a story that strikes Susan as simultaneously rehearsed and exhausting. David portrays his 20-year marriage as one constant argument with his wife, typified by her chronic objections and righteous complaints and his sullen resignation and inward retreat. He describes always feeling criticized by his wife no matter what he does—never feeling accepted by her, nor ever being able to stand up for himself. And now that their once demure, obedient daughter Grace is exhibiting what he imagines is typical teenage rebellion and exploration, his wife is a nervous wreck and attributing Grace's "acting out" to his failure to be emotionally available as a father. David tells Susan, "My wife insisted that I either get into therapy to work out my issues, or else maybe it's time we just throw in the towel. Well, those weren't precisely Joyce's words," David corrects. "No, it was some equally annoying cliché about her being 'ready to wave the white flag.' Now that I think of it, I'm sure she slipped that comment in as a subtle jab." Susan responds with a look of puzzlement. "Because I'm only half-white, obviously." David clarifies, widening his eyes to emphasize the obviousness of this point.

As David pauses and shifts in his seat, Susan attempts to synthesize three emerging observations. First, despite how articulately this man conveyed his predicament and the poignancy of the details surrounding his marital conflict, his opening story was rendered with such affective flatness that she finds herself feeling emotionally detached and wonders whether she might be getting an initial glimpse into one aspect of David's dynamic with his wife. The second has to do with his physical presentation. A lean but fit-looking man of above-average height in his early 40s, David nonetheless carries himself with an almost droopy meekness, accentuated by his conservative and somewhat bland, white-collar office attire.

Susan finds herself most curious about her third observation—the realization that despite his relatively light complexion, this man is visually recognizable to be of mixed African American descent. However, it was not until he brought this matter of race up that she noticed David was anything other than one more of the many emotionally constricted Caucasian men she had treated over the past two decades. David speaks and carries himself in the manner of other clients she feels she knows so well. And yet the act of his bringing up this aspect of his identity in the context of a perceived devaluation, coupled with the fact of her initially overlooking it, signals to Susan that David's relationship to his ethnicity will hold some kind of relevance to whatever work is to ensue between them and could ultimately pose a challenge to the comfort zone in which she has grown accustomed to practicing. Did she not already detect in David a hint of annoyance with her for missing the boat on this? Susan notices a rustle of energy in her limbs and a brief clenching of her stomach and feels momentarily unnerved. Attempting to sit more deeply in her chair, Susan is uncertain this challenge will be one she welcomes wholeheartedly.

Susan replies by asking David how he feels about his wife pushing him to come to therapy. He responds that he is willing to give it a try for the sake of his family. When she asks him if he has ever been in therapy before, David tells her he saw someone last year for a few sessions but didn't feel connected to the therapist. He then curtly informs Susan that he expects to be in treatment for 2 to 3 months tops and wants a road map for how she is going to help him. Susan says that they will need to meet several times before she will be able to provide much in the way of specific treatment recommendations, so he can get a sense of how she works, and so that she can start to understand what is and is not working for him. David lets out a defeated-sounding sigh and replies, "Alright I guess, but I wish I knew where we're going with all this," his voice trailing off to almost a mumble and his head turning downward and away from Susan.

2. Clinical Consultation

Susan tells her supervisor about her first session with David, describing his request for a road map and the highly ambitious time limit he has set. They share a brief laugh over this, but then Susan admits that she is worried that he will quit once he realizes that she cannot give him what he has asked of her. Susan shares what she describes as a "bumbling oversight" regarding David's ethnicity and her apprehension about whether she is truly qualified to take on this particular client. Furthermore, because of his marital conflicts, Susan wonders whether she should recommend couples therapy or at least give David a "consumer warning" that individual therapy can be hard on a marriage when the presenting problem centers on partner conflict. "Wow! If you're feeling such pressure right now, imagine what he's feeling!" Her supervisor then provides her with a solid round of encouragement, reframing, and recommendations for initial approach and pacing at this very early stage of treatment. Although the advice is more or less what Susan expected to hear, the recommendations are the same ones she would give were the roles reversed, and the feedback is of the kind she usually welcomes, Susan notices that in this instance none of this provides much relief.

Driving home following the clinical consultation, Susan finds herself perturbed, anticipating that she will continue to struggle to get a foothold with this client. Even though only one session has transpired, every time she tried to test the limits by encouraging David to consider his feelings, he launched into another angry but flat diatribe. As Susan pulls into her driveway, she lets out a short whistle and muses to herself, "Let's hope I'm not getting in over my head with this one."

3. David's Story

When David returns for the next session, Susan asks him to tell her about his history. David tells her that as a young child he had to fend for himself a lot until he was adopted at age 6. Before his adoption, he grew up in a poor neighborhood in Georgia, born to a white mother and an African American father. The neighborhood was primarily black, most of his friends were black, and he grew up speaking the southern black vernacular. David's dad was in and out of the house, and his mother, who had gotten pregnant with him when she was 17, was struggling. He remembers his mother sleeping on the couch a lot during the day. She would go out frequently with friends or sometimes with a man, and when she came home, she would slur her words. He recalls being scared when she went out because often he was left home alone. Susan stops David mid-story to ask about this fear. His memories are vague, and he cannot really say anything else.

David brushes this question off and continues with his story. He acknowledges that it bothers him that he can no longer picture what his mother's face looked like. He remembers once his mother asking him to comb her pretty, straw-colored hair while she lay on the couch, but that is all. David concludes this story by informing Susan of the abrupt death of his mother when he was around 5 years old. He acknowledged a hazy recollection of the details surrounding his mother's death and limited memory fragments. "Looking back as an adult, I assume it had something to do with drugs or alcohol and the troubled men she spent time with, although I think this may have been complicated by her having some kind of chronic illness. Anyway, I came home from school, and there were lots of people and cars outside my house. My dad wasn't there. I never saw him again either. A neighbor lady took me to stay with an aunt, my dad's older sister. Not long after that I was sent to a kind of orphanage for boys. I guess I must have been too much trouble for my aunt to manage on top of her own kids. I don't remember too much about that orphanage either, other than hating it, and wanting to leave, and these big rough hands and a stern voice that would shake me awake each morning and loudly remind me to make by bed and stay on my best behavior and tuck in my shirt and keep my face clean and stuff like that or else I would have to stay there until I was all grown up. There was no way I was going to let that happen, and to this day I am obsessively organized, tidy, and punctual. Next thing I remember I was picked up by this very white family who drove me away from that place in what I thought at the time was a broken-down, ugly gray-colored station wagon—turns out it was an expensive Volvo, which sounded noisy to me because of its diesel engine. I drive one myself now. That's about it," David finishes with a shrug.

When David finishes speaking, he notices that Dr. Thalman is regarding him silently and that a tear has formed in one of her eyes. He supposes she is responding empathically to his story, which he recognizes is objectively sad, although certainly not nearly the worse of what he imagines she's heard. He feels frustrated and defective, almost alien, that he can't join her in these feelings. David regards Susan with a look that perplexes her, leading her to pause and consider the most effective way to respond in this fragile early juncture to the heartbreaking but powerfully dissociated story of loss and resilience she has just heard.

4. Everything and Nothing

Weeks more have gone by in therapy. Susan is pleased that David has been willing and able to explore his feelings more, but something else has begun to nag at her. She likes him but continues to feel little, and at times no, emotional connection to him. Usually she feels strongly engaged with her clients. Susan tells her supervisor, "I feel like I'm everything and nothing to David all at the same time. Like he's absolutely desperate for my help, answers all my questions, comes to every session . . . but I could disappear from his life tomorrow, and it would barely register. I just feel so far away from him."

5. Nowhere Man

A couple of months have passed since David began treatment with Susan. David always comes in with an agenda, written down in bullet points. He tells Susan that his wife Joyce has been complaining that he isn't "working" in therapy and that he hasn't gotten to his "core issues." David quickly runs through a life of topics his wife put together for him to address in therapy: (1) your adoption, (2) your parents, (3) your anger, and (4) your inability to be intimate.

Susan is a little taken aback and cannot decide whether to be grateful to David's wife for encouraging him to explore these difficult topics or annoyed at her for trying to direct the therapy. Wondering if David's wife is addressing her own issues in her own therapy, Susan considers how little she knows about her. In their second or third session, David had only briefly described his wife Joyce, an attorney, as a woman he met during college who also came from a biracial family background. Today Susan decides it's time to express some curiosity about wanting to get a better picture of Joyce as a person.

David replies by labeling Joyce as the "opposite of me in almost every sense." He describes her as extroverted, funny, and messy. Eventually, he reveals that they differ most in regard to their upbringing and background. David informs Susan that Joyce comes from an intact stable family headed by a Lebanese American mother and a Peruvian father. Her parents shared similar enough Christian backgrounds, their families accepted each other, and they went on to raise Joyce and her siblings to be proud of their heritage. David's voice catches when he notes that Joyce's parents remain happily married to this day. Susan then observes an abrupt shift in David's tone: "Whatever. They had it easy. No one in America really gives a damn about the difference between Lebanese and Peruvians. For all anyone notices, her parents could have been Guatemalan or Greek. To Joyce, biracial meant being adored and well fed by two nutty but stable extended families and being exotic looking and popular in school. That's not race where I come from; that's ethnicity. In the ugly, real world, my mixed heritage is viewed entirely as an issue of race. Doesn't matter one bit that science has proven that race has no biological basis and is just a social fabrication. I love Joyce, but the bottom line is she just can't understand what I went through growing up. I didn't fit anywhere. Not with the white kids. Not with the black kids. I still don't. You know that Beatle's song, 'Nowhere Man'? That's me in a nutshell."

Susan finds herself at a loss for words, filled with associations and emotional reactions to the poignant information David just unleashed. She attempts to slow the process down a bit by exploring his feelings about even making this list, noting internally some anxiety about pushing him to talk about his feelings. To her surprise, David says that it is difficult for him, but he knows that he should work on these things. He acknowledged that he often finds himself struggling in therapy for topics to talk about, wanting to entertain Susan and keep things "light." He says that he doesn't "know how to go there." Susan notices that she feels energized by David's ability to talk about the therapeutic process, even talking about his fears of getting to topics that are more emotional. She works throughout the rest of the session to help him stay in this place—reflecting on his emotional experience of the therapy process without actually going into any vulnerable emotions. They don't talk about any of the topics on the list. At the end of the session, Susan asks David what the experience was like for him. He looks very pleased, saying that he feels that they really got to some important stuff that day. They agree that they will come back to talk about the topics on the list if he feels that they are important, but Susan reassures him that they have plenty of time to get to those things and emphasizes that she is most concerned about *him* as a person and about making sure that the work that they do together is helpful. David smiles, makes eye contact with her, and for the first time since they first met, holds out his hand to shake hers at the end of the session.

6. The Letter

David is sorting through a box of files when he finds a letter from his paternal Aunt Selma to the adoption agency. The letter is ripped in half and has yellowed with age. The letter is addressed to the "Dear Man and Woman who Adopted my Nephew David." In the letter, Aunt Selma blessed his adoptive parents for taking her nephew into their home and hearts and for trying to make a better life for him. She expressed guilt that she hadn't been able to keep him when he was living with her after his mother's death because of her own health problems and the stress of raising her own three kids. She implored his adoptive parents to allow David to maintain a relationship with his kin and said that she was sending along a box of his things. David's heart starts thumping in his chest. He has a flash of memory—playing in his aunt's backyard with his three cousins and the dog. He and his favorite older cousin, Wendell, are wrestling. Aunt Selma comes to call them inside, and Wendell gets distracted. All of a sudden, David is on top and has his cousin pinned. Wendell smiles and shoves him off, "all right, you win, you win." David remembers feeling tough and proud as he swaggers into the house.

David scans the letter again. He feels ice cold as he imagines his adoptive mother ripping up the letter. Of course, she wouldn't show it to him or tell him about it. That wouldn't have fit in with her plans for him. And he never got that box. He never knew that his aunt missed him. He flashes on an earlier memory of his father. David is around 3 or 4, and it's his birthday. His father, who wasn't usually around, had come home with a huge cake. He remembers the heat on his face from the candles and looking around at everyone singing happy birthday to him, then looking up at his father, who was leading everyone singing. His father had a big smile on his face. He was so tall, so strong, and David wanted to be just like him.

David brings the letter into Susan for her to read. "Imagine if you'd known that your aunt missed you, that she wanted to see you!" she exclaims. David is relieved: *She gets it!*

7. Completely Invisible

In their next session, David talks about the abrupt change in his life when he arrived at his adoptive parents' house. They lived in a formal home in Connecticut, with a manicured lawn and a pool. The first thing he recalls his new mother saying when he entered that house was, "First things first. Let's draw you a bath and get you out of these grimy clothes. We have nice new clothes for you to wear." His hair had been growing out in thick tight curls, and she took him to get it clipped close to his skull. "They changed me into what they wanted me to be," David explained. His mother worked with him on his language, telling him that he would never be accepted by the "good people" of their community and school if he spoke "like an uneducated hoodlum from the slums." All of a sudden, he had strict rules: he had to eat bland food; he had to dress appropriately; he had to do Saturday morning chores and home-work every day after school; he had to have his friends approved. Driven by the fear that David would be taken back to the orphanage, he worked hard to "get rid of" his personality in order to fit in and make them like him. Eventu-ally, he succeeded in "not being who I was anymore. I became someone else they needed me to me, someone who fit with the family's image."

As David is talking, Susan starts to feel very . . . white. She thinks about how his adopted parents pushed away this very tough, resilient, and alive part of David. She wonders if that part of him identifies more as being black. Susan wonders how he feels about her, as a white woman, as a Jew, as a professional. Does he look at her and see his parents? She imagines there could be ways in which David feels safer with or as if he has more in common with her than he would with a black therapist, but she cannot decide whether this is a good thing. Can Susan use her vantage point to help him identify and embrace aspects of himself that he had to push away? Or, on the other hand, to help David recognize and appreciate any redeeming qualities his adoptive parents may have had? At the very least, they certainly afforded him a huge number of opportunities in life. She wonders if, despite his anger with them, David yearns for greater emotional connection to them as well.

Remembering this time in his life, David begins to talk about how he learned to lock his feelings away. He remembers spending hours alone in his room, terribly sad, but knowing there was no space in his new family for his feelings. He had to appear perfect. Act perfect. Be perfect. And soon David *was* perfect, and the sadness went away. He tells Susan about a time, around the age of 8, when he fell off his bike, hit his head, and got a big, gushing cut above his eye. He ran home, but his mom was nowhere to be found. So he'd washed it off, found the bandages and iodine, and cleaned it out. David was so proud of himself and, in fact, knows he's always been good in a crisis because he had learned to take care of himself from an early age. Susan says, "There's such an amazing strength in you, such incredible resilience. Like, no one's helping me, so I will just take care of it myself."

David responds, "I didn't see any other options. I mean, what do you do? Do you just give up, and, I don't know, commit suicide or something?" He glances then at Susan and notices that she is looking at him with such care, maybe even admiration? He is surprised to feel a wave of emotion start to rise up. "Yeah, but I was invisible," David finds himself continuing, the tears starting to come. "All my childhood, until I met my wife, I was completely invisible. The person my parents perceived me to be was such a distortion of who I was. And they gave me plenty of feedback, telling me who they thought I was or how I should be, and I thought, isn't this amazing. You don't have a clue, do you? And yeah, I could take care of myself, but I also really wanted to be taken care of. It's hard to admit, but after that bike accident, a part of me wanted my mom to scoop me up in her arms, tell me I was going to be okay, clean me up, and give me a big bowl of ice cream."

"Yeah, you needed that," replies Susan. "What does it mean now for us to see beneath that extremely capable part of you, to see both the resilience and amazing competence, and also the pain of feeling invisible?"

David takes a deep breath, and a look of sorrow crosses his face. "It's funny," he says. "I've always thought of my childhood, once I got adopted, as being basically fine. I mean, I had everything I needed. But I don't know, maybe it wasn't so fine. They had all these rules for me, all these rules about who I had to be to keep up their image. But they never really cared to see me—to get to know *me*."

8. *Cultural Disconnect*

A few months have passed. In supervision Susan describes a recent interaction with David that caught her particularly off guard. David was exhibiting increased access to his feelings of anger and sadness. Excited by this breakthrough, Susan looked for an opportunity to explore with David what he might need to risk expressing his feelings toward someone with whom he had an ongoing relationship. Eventually, Susan asked David to consider practicing expressing his feelings by sharing any he was willing to, positive or negative, about her. After an awkward silence, David offered that he felt appreciative of Susan "hanging in there with him" in his efforts to work through his painful childhood experiences. Susan notes to her supervisor that this disclosure struck her as being genuine but incomplete, as if a "but" was being withheld. She decided to pursue this issue, asking David directly if there might be other, less positive elements of his feelings toward her that he was holding back. After some fumbling around, David told her that at times he resented her interest in his "ethnic identity," emphasizing these last two words by making quotation marks in the air with his fingers.

Susan thanked David for sharing this feeling with her and asked if he would be willing to say more. David exclaims with frustration that he is sick and tired of everyone having expectations for him based on their perceptions of his race. Growing up with his adoptive parents, he felt intense pressure to be, act, and look white. With male friends and colleagues, he often had to endure the opposite. "Then there's Joyce, who imagines that just because I'm biracial I'm supposed to be proud and assertive and confident. She's never going to be happy with me as is."

"I see," Susan replied. "How do you see me wanting you to be?" "I don't know," David muttered, "self-accepting and well integrated, maybe, but it's not really that." Susan waited, trying to reach out to David with an expression of openness and warmth. "No, with you it's more like I wonder if you find me more interesting when I talk about my struggles with being who I am than you would if I *were* just a 100% white guy. Like maybe it's exciting for you to pretend you're all down and culturally sensitive exploring identity issues with a "black man," only because in reality you're feeling pretty safe sitting in this room week after week with me, a light-skinned, mild-mannered, and for the most part white-acting man. Sometimes I bet if I looked or acted more like your mental image of a real black man you'd be scared shitless and have referred me out by now."

"Boy," Susan's supervisor replies in their next meeting, "I can't imagine what you said to that." "Neither can I, and I'm the one who said it!" "I told him, for starters, how incredibly brave I thought he was for sharing these doubts about me, and how honored I felt for him trusting me enough to do so." "That sounds like a wonderful reply," her colleague offers. "I suppose so, but then maybe I went too far, and admitted to him that on some level he might very well be right."

9. Therapeutic Rupture

Over 6 months have passed since Susan began her treatment with David. She is now rushing to get everything done in preparation for her trip to Key West next week. She has a handful of clients she is concerned about because of her vacation, including one client who struggles with suicidal thoughts and gets overcome with waves of panic and resentment whenever Susan goes away. She is pushing through a particularly busy day but is in a buoyant mood, and she can feel herself already beginning to distance herself from "work mode." David comes in stressed and dejected. He describes how his daughter was caught smoking pot and how as usual his wife blamed this on his emotional absence and spent the week berating him.

As David is talking, Susan has a moment of anxiety when she realizes that she may have neglected to forewarn David of her impending absence. She tries running through the last few sessions in her mind and is sure that she would have mentioned it at some point, but she cannot recall. She realizes that David has gone quiet, and her mind spins to come up with a response because she has now missed some of what he has been sharing. "So what are you going to do about your daughter?" she asks. David does not seem to have noticed that her attention had wandered. He is staring at the floor, slumped down into his chair. His hands are limp in his lap. "There's nothing I can do," he says, "my daughter does what she wants."

Susan sees that they only have 10 minutes left of their session. She is anxious to tell David about her absence next week, but she also feels guilty for feeling so upbeat while he is obviously so dejected. She reasons with herself that he has the money to take a vacation if he wanted to, but she quickly recognizes that she is just trying to make herself feel better. David's life is in such chaos right now, Susan cannot imagine him even thinking about a vacation. "Well, it sounds like you've had a really difficult week. Let's think a little about some things that you can do to take care of yourself this week." David continues staring at the floor and sighs. "I really can't think of anything. I'm just beaten down." Susan glances at the clock again—5 minutes. "Well, you've mentioned that sometimes just taking a mental break, exercising, or spending time with your friends can be helpful." He glances at her, "Yeah, I guess."

"Okay, so, we've just got a couple of minutes left," Susan says, "so let's look at scheduling. I think I mentioned to you a few weeks back that I'm not going to be able to meet next week, so let's look to the following week." "Oh. I must have forgotten," David replies, sounding surprised. "Are you traveling for work or going on vacation?" he asks. "Oh, a little vacation," she says, smiling. "Anywhere good?" he asks, "or can't you tell me?" "I'm just going to the beach," she says, and looks back down at her planner. They plan to meet again in 2 weeks.

When David leaves, Susan realizes that she might have sounded a little defensive, saying that she was "just going to the beach," particularly because it is February. She reflects that David seemed a little awkward when he left. She hopes he is okay, and she goes to greet her next client.

David gets into his Volvo and slams the door. He grips his steering wheel, staring at Susan's office building. He feels pressure in his chest, and his hands heat up against the leather of the steering wheel. Everything is going wrong, and he has no idea what to do about it. "Forget it," he thinks, "I'm sick of this therapy shit. I just go there every week and moan and complain. What good does it do me?" He turns over the engine and guns his car out of the parking lot, unintentionally cutting off another car. The other driver lays on his horn. David looks in his rearview mirror at the other driver, who promptly gives him the finger. David laughs and then bears the weight of his foot down hard on the accelerator, increasing the distance between himself and the other car. He momentarily accesses a welcome feeling of power and control.

10. The First Visit with David's Younger Self

Nearly a year has passed since David began therapy with Susan. They have been talking more about a younger part of him that is holding grief and sadness, and he has been able to build some empathy for this young boy. He is reflecting on a recurrent memory of himself as a young child, maybe 4 or 5, alone in the house, staring out the window at the rain, waiting for his mother to come home. He remembers feeling completely alone, frightened, and hollow inside.

Susan invites David to enter that scene as his adult self. David is not sure about this suggestion—it seems kind of whacky! But he has come to trust Susan, so he figures he will give it a shot. She explains the technique to him, and he pictures himself walking into that room, seeing the little boy just staring out of the window. "Now what?" Susan tells him he should let the boy know that he is there. David has no idea what to say. A moment passes. "Hello . . . " he begins.

NICOLE
Prologue

Nicole twirls happily as she eyes her reflection in the mirror. Not so bad, she thinks to herself with an uncharacteristic swell of confidence. The glitter lotion her friend Gracie lent her is so, well, glittery, on her arms and shoulders and matches the sparklers sewn into her skirt. Okay, so it's not a mini like many of the older girls in her middle school will probably be wearing to the dance, but it fans out when she spins around and matches nicely with the purple tank top her mom had shocked Nicole with for her birthday last month during one of her "nice mom" phases.

Her thoughts race as she heads out into the hall and down the stairs: "Will the boys actually dance or just stand around joking against the back wall like Gracie said they did at the fall dance? Will Peter be there?! Will he like how I look? Will he even notice? Anyway, who cares—it'll be fun, and my mom is actually letting me go this time now that I finally turned 13!"

Lost in reverie as she bounces off the final stair, Nicole barely registers her mother standing arms crossed in the doorway to the kitchen. "If you think I'm letting you out of the house looking like that, you've got another thing coming."

Nicole startles and turns to find the cold glare of her mother scrutinizing her up and down, a look of disgust on her face. "What do you mean, Mom, this is the shirt you bought me for my . . . "

"I didn't buy it for you to go flouncing around with your little tidbits showing and that gunk smeared over your skin like some kind of tramp!" Nicole's mother exclaims sharply.

"Bu— but, but—"

"What is it now, Nicole, have you developed a stutter to go along with all your other wonderful traits? No one expected you to inherit the brains in the family, but any dummy can see that no self-respecting boy is going to ask you to dance with that pimply face and those furry legs of yours. Now go get changed before your Jewish friend's mother gets tired of waiting for you in the car and starts charging me for wasted gas."

Her face flushed, Nicole fights back tears as she half shouts, half whines, "Mom, stop it, that's not nice! And you're the one who said I couldn't shave my legs until I turned 14! And this skirt is longer than my school uniform!"

"You wear those with leggings, Nicole. Haven't I taught you anything? Dressed like that . . . " her mother's hand sweeping the air aggressively as if trying to dispel a foul odor, "even the school chaperones are going to be getting ideas about you . . . "

"Mr. Johnson would never!" Nicole blurts out.

"Hah, Tom Johnson, he's been a dog since back in my day. Why else would he volunteer to coach the girls' soccer team? No doubt so he can loiter around the showers after practice and sneak peaks at all those sweaty, young—"

"Mom, that's terrible, he's the deacon at his church!"

"Oh, I'm sure he's a real man of God all right. You'll learn soon enough that all any man wants is to get into your pants. Just be glad your father had to work late tonight and isn't home to see you like this. God knows how disappointed in you he'd . . . "

Just then, the front door opens and Nicole's father enters the living room from the garage door, pulling off his coat and closing the door with a single sweep of his arm. Seeing Nicole, a bright smile spreads over his face. "How are my best girls today? Why, Nicole, don't you look . . . "

"Like a piece of trash, Arnold," Nicole's mother abruptly cuts him off. "Wouldn't you agree?"

The man's face reddens, and he pulls at his shirt collar. "Now Janet, I wouldn't—"

"Not another word, Arnold," the mother retorts, staring the man down until he lowers his eyes to the floor in silence. "You'd never catch Stacey looking like that, and I'll be dead before I let this one turn her little sister into a slut."

Nicole looks at her father with desperate uncertainty. "Mind your mother, honey," he mutters, not looking at either Nicole or his wife as he walks away into his study and slowly closes the door behind him.

"See, Nicole. Your father agrees. He's just too embarrassed to say so out loud. Now look what you've done. You've put him in such a state he's retreated to his fortress, and now I'm going to be sitting here by myself again all night, thanks to you."

Tears streaming from her face, Nicole races up the stairs. As she runs, her voice trails behind her in a wail. "Tu-tu tell Mrs. Lindemann I'm not feeling well and fa-fa for Gracie to go to the dance without me." Still wearing her outfit and shoes, Nicole burrows into bed. Her muffled sobs are betrayed by the small tremulous mound of her body under the covers.

Downstairs, a tight smile on her face, Nicole's mother heads toward the front door. "Obviously, Nicole," she nods to herself several times in pressured affirmation, "obviously."

1. Living in the Abyss

Nicole Vasquez is riding the train to work. Her body is drawn up into the seat. The contraction of the small muscles of her birdlike limbs, serving to avoid and ward off contact with other passengers, is as automatic a process as the shutting down of her senses. Unless Nicole were to make an intentional effort to tune in, her body has become so effective at these operations that it has virtually perfected the art of traveling to work in solitude and invisibility.

Nicole's head is spinning with the unbearableness of her life. *I can't stand it anymore!* Nicole sardonically reflects that she would be in a complete state of panic if she were not too emotionally exhausted to work up the energy.

2. Katherine's New Client

Katherine Silvester, a psychotherapist in her mid-30s, arrives at the trauma clinic where she works. Despite the demands of this position, she is proud of her work and glad to be part of an intellectually stimulating community of therapists sharing the same mission. She is especially pleased about her current supervisor, a highly sought-after person whom she had been waiting to work with for some time.

Katherine learns that she has been assigned a new client. She reviews the screening information for this case. The client's name is Nicole Vasquez. She is a 41-year-old married mother of two children: one in college and the other in high school. Mrs. Vasquez lives in the suburbs but is employed full time as a paralegal in town. The screen notes a history of childhood emotional abuse and neglect, with a question mark next to familial mental illness. The screen is positive for current marital problems, but exposure to domestic violence is denied. Past history of intermittent mental health treatment is acknowledged, with the most recent therapy having been discontinued several years prior. Presenting problems include relationship difficulties; anxious and depressed mood; sleep and appetite disturbance; hopelessness and negative self-image. The screen concludes with a statement of the client's goals for treatment: *"From the outside, people think I'm lucky: devoted husband, two great kids, nice house, stable job. Inside, I feel completely trapped in my life and can't stand it anymore. I'm convinced this mess goes way back and figured it was time I let the experts see if they can help me."*

In clinical supervision, Katherine reviews the screen and speculates about Mrs. Vasquez. She notes that Mrs. Vasquez's full-time employment is a good sign, a personal strength. She is also seemingly motivated for treatment. Katherine wonders about her marital problems and conjectures whether as a Latina woman, cultural taboos might prohibit Mrs. Vasquez from recognizing or disclosing domestic violence. Katherine leaves supervision with an eagerness to meet this client and begin their work together.

3. Nicole's Fears and Hopes about Therapy

When Nicole is provided the name of her assigned therapist by the center's intake coordinator, she immediately becomes excited and nervous. *Katherine Silvester.* The name sounds distinguished, cosmopolitan. Nicole looks her up on the Internet. She discovers a number of links: several presentations at scientific conferences and training workshops, a biographical blurb, even an article co-written by Katherine and published in a serious-sounding journal. Nicole is initially impressed but is quickly overcome with doubt. Has she been

assigned to a person with the kind of perfect life that will lead her to judge
Nicole harshly for all the bad things she has done? Or worse, is she an overly
compassionate older woman who will take pity on Nicole and mother her to
death?

These fears are quickly resolved, and substituted, when she locates several
pictures of Katherine Silvester on the Web. To Nicole's surprise, her assigned
therapist looks to be an attractive woman several years younger than herself
and similar in stature, build, and complexion. Nicole comes to suspect that
Katherine, who is referred to in multiple places on the Internet as "Ms." Silvester, not "Mrs.," is a single woman without children. Perhaps Ms. Silvester was
saved from the path Nicole's life has taken, with her freedom intact. Nicole
is struck by feelings of admiration for this therapist and envy for the life she
imagines her to lead. For the first time in a long time, she registers a glimmer
of optimism. _Maybe Katherine Silvester is someone who will finally understand_
me and help me find a way out of this misery. These musings are swiftly drowned
out by the much louder voices of Nicole's inadequacies and failures. She scolds
herself for allowing these childish fantasies to create false hope. It will only
be a matter of time before this new therapist realizes just how pathetic Nicole
really is, how unworthy of salvaging, how beyond repair.

4. The Mind's Panic, The Body's Courage

On the morning of her first appointment, Nicole's stomach is a wreck. She
decides to call and cancel. While looking for the phone number, she remembers the center's stern cancellation policy. There had been a 2-month waitlist to get this appointment, and the thought of having taken a spot from
someone else who could actually have benefited from it fills Nicole with self-
loathing. Far worse is the shame that lashes at Nicole when she realizes that
if she doesn't show, she will have wasted Ms. Silvester's time. Steeling herself,
Nicole showers, gets dressed, and rushes out the door filled with fear and anxiety. Along the way she spaces out and misses the stop. She is furious at herself
and has a flashing impulse to "forget it all," call in sick, head home, and crawl
under her bedcovers.

Moments later, Nicole finds herself running the four blocks back toward
the center, convinced she looks absurd in her work heels and oversized bag.
Her heart racing, Nicole's mind briefly clears of thinking of any kind. She
notices her body in motion: it feels strong, rhythmic, alive. For an instant
Nicole finds herself oddly exhilarated.

5. The First Session, Deconstructed

Katherine closes her door three-quarters of the way and sits at her desk,
reflecting on the initial session she just completed with Nicole Vasquez. What
an intriguing and complicated woman she turned out to be! Katherine shakes

her head and chuckles. And how off she had been in some of her assumptions, beginning with Nicole's ethnicity! Thank goodness that Laura, the center's receptionist, informed Katherine that her appointment had checked in and pointed Mrs. Vasquez out to her discreetly from the reception window. Imagine if Katherine had walked into the waiting room and had had to fumble to recover from some awkward remark she had made when the curvaceous, middle-aged Hispanic woman she had expected to find turned out to be a fair-skinned, fragile-looking Caucasian woman who could easily pass as her older cousin.

Had she been making conjectures based on ethnic stereotypes? Katherine reflects that she will have to examine this possibility with her supervisor in their next session. She wonders if her supervisor will be disappointed, or instead impressed with her willingness to critically self-examine.

Katherine assimilates the information that she has learned about Nicole Vasquez. Her paralegal job, for instance, hardly qualifies as a second career or return to work after one's kids have left the nest: it turns out that she has held this same position, in the same firm no less, for nearly two decades. Katherine had remarked that it was impressive to maintain that kind of employment longevity in this day and age. Nicole countered with a self-deprecating comment that Katherine found poignant despite its flippant delivery: "Not at all. It's just one of the many examples of my perfect track record as a lifelong underachiever."

Finally, there is the situation of Mrs. Vasquez's marital problems, and the "black hole" Nicole explained she had been lost inside for so long. Katherine mulls this explanation over. While she still is unwilling to rule out entirely the possibility of some form of domestic abuse, she concedes that she does not believe Mrs. Vasquez was lying or withholding information when she asked her about this directly. Nicole had explained in broad strokes that her family upbringing was troubled. Getting away from her family as soon as possible was a driving force in her decision to leave home at age 18 with Antonio, a Cuban man 10 years her senior, to whom she has now been married for over 20 years. Katherine reflects on Nicole's description of the "steadily creeping decline" of her marriage, how "empty and alone" she experiences herself to be, and how "trapped and controlled" she feels by the monotony of its routines.

Katherine contemplates her own life experiences in an effort to tap into the feeling states Nicole describes. She grimaces with physical recollections of a particularly painful failed relationship from her past. These feelings quickly recede, however, overtaken by far more pleasing and reassuring associations from her current, promising relationship.

Katherine recalls the imploring eye contact Nicole made when characterizing herself as having "spent the majority of my life trying to please everyone in it for as long as I can until I simply can't hold out anymore and have to escape." Katherine recalls the earnest expression of pain on Nicole's face when she admitted how simultaneously imperative and exhausting it is for her to try to please everyone all the time; how important it is for her to be seen as a "good person," to be helpful and put everyone else's needs first; and how this inevitably leads her to be taken for granted or taken advantage of in her relationships with family, friends, and work colleagues.

Katherine flashes forward to the final moments of the session, in which she asked Nicole whether these experiences ever induced feelings of anger or urges to stand up for herself. Nicole countered that she knew too well what it felt like to be the recipient of someone else's rage and that the only thing she could imagine to be more terrifying would be to be consumed by such feelings inside herself. Consequently, as a young girl she worked hard at carefully controlling her emotions and never allowing herself to feel anger, so much so that now she does not think she is even capable of getting angry. The idea of standing up for herself was equally terrifying and unthinkable. Katherine countered by asking Nicole if she had found any other outlet for all the pain she endures. This was when Nicole replied: "Well now, it's funny you should ask." Nicole acknowledged another side of herself that had been expressing itself more and more over the past year and a half, but in a highly secretive manner. Nicole referred to this as her "bad side" and explained that sometimes it helped her "sneak out of her black hole." When asked to clarify, Nicole replied in an opaque manner and then, looking up at the clock, commented somewhat brightly, "Saved by the bell! To be continued, okay?"

The timing of disclosure of this clearly significant material strikes Katherine as likely to have been intentional. She reflects on Nicole's capacity to connect interpersonally and evoke empathy from their first meeting; on her engaging, disarming, and highly protective facility with humor; and on her many layers. Katherine concludes that Mrs. Vasquez has developed a complex adaptation to her traumatic experiences, replete with resources and fraught with vulnerabilities. She decides that this nuance and richness will make for a challenging and compelling treatment process and is glad that she was assigned this particular case.

Katherine briefly considers her use of self. She feels generally satisfied with her initial attunement with this client, her capacity to remain open and curious, and her ability to respond with genuine empathy. These qualities appear to have helped engender sufficient safety for Nicole to share meaningful emotional and narrative material in their very first meeting.

6. Developing Rapport

Exiting the center after her first session, a wave of relief washes over Nicole. *That turned out so much better than I expected.* Katherine strikes her as being really smart and observant. She didn't push Nicole too hard about things she wasn't ready to talk about, which mattered to Nicole. And yet, not much seemed to be getting by Katherine either, which mattered equally to Nicole; otherwise she would end up wasting her time with another clueless do-gooder.

Nicole was especially pleased that Katherine walked back with her to the waiting area afterward and let all the other ladies in the waiting room see the two of them chatting it up with light girl-talk just like a couple of colleagues. The best part of all was the eyeroll Katherine made when Nicole explained that she was "just looking to try to talk things through," but had read an article on the Internet by a famous therapist who insisted that "the only way to help adults heal from childhood trauma was to get them to jump around and stand on their heads and other stuff"—an idea that totally stressed Nicole out. Katherine barely suppressed a laugh and said something really funny and sweet in response: "Well, if you decide you'd like stand on your head at some point down the road, I'll do my best to help you with that, but I agree that the two of us talking and getting to know each other should do just fine for now." Nicole realizes this interchange made her feel like Katherine accepted her and was treating her like a normal person. Even though Katherine would inevitably figure out that she is messed up beyond repair, it nevertheless clinched the deal for Nicole to give therapy with her a try.

7. Family History

A month has passed since Katherine began her work with Nicole. Katherine sits down to organize her thoughts in order to complete her clinical evaluation and formulate her initial treatment plan. Raised in a conservative Scotch-Irish family in the suburbs, Nicole described her mother as alternately vacant and intrusive, oscillating between neglectful and cruel. She believed that her mother suffered from some "nasty kind of off-and-on-again depression" but was too religious to seek help from anyone but her priest. When her mother would forget to pick Nicole up at school, Nicole learned to lie to her teachers to avoid calling attention to anything being wrong in her family. As far back as she could remember, her mother harped on Nicole's appearance, calling her "homely" and "fat" and warning that she was "destined to marry a loser." Despite always being a scrawny child, Nicole began restricting her eating by the time she was 8 years old. She recalled many nights after dinner when her stomach still rumbled with hunger or her eyes burned with longing for the special treats her mother would make for her siblings.

Her father was a more supportive figure during her early childhood, but his job as an auto parts salesman involved regular travel, requiring him to be away from home for long stretches at a time. Nicole recalled pleading with her father on more than one occasion not to leave; her father would always respond by fondly patting her head. He either did not understand the depth of Nicole's plight or would not allow himself to see it, or both.

Nicole was the second of three children. Her cherished younger sister, Stacey, was the adorable, freckled, outgoing "princess" of the family. Her brother, Timothy, was athletic and charming but was several years older than Nicole; he enlisted in the army and left home before she completed elementary school. Nicole described herself as ordinary and plain, a good student, quiet, obedient, and generally unnoticed—an all-around "good girl." She had explained to Katherine, though, that this characterization dramatically changed in her mid-teens when her body started to mature and she began to take an interest in clothes, makeup, music, and, most of all, boys. It was around this time that her father shifted from playing a benign if largely absent role in her life to joining in her mother's hostility toward Nicole. Whereas Nicole's mother became increasingly intrusive, listening in on her phone calls, searching through her belongings, and making derogatory comments about Nicole to her friends' mothers when she encountered them at church or the grocery store, it was her father's newfound judgment of her that most stung Nicole. One evening in 10th grade, this disapproval culminated in her father lowering his gaze and muttering the words "disgusting creature" as she left the house to go out on her first official date with a senior she knew from the high school yearbook club. Thereafter, on the rare occasions he would bother to speak to her at all, her father would not look at her, although Nicole was sure she caught glimpses of him shaking his head in disapproval as she passed by him in the house. These experiences were a source of terrible sorrow and shame for Nicole.

The one positive influence in Nicole's family was her aunt Victoria, her mother's younger sister. As a teenager, Nicole looked up to Victoria, who was single and seemed to have so much going for her. Nicole saw her as wild, fun, and full of life. When Victoria visited, she would take Nicole for rides and thrill her with stories of her escapades with her many friends and boyfriends. Nicole reminisced about Victoria nudging her fondly on numerous occasions and saying, "Us black sheep in the family gotta stick together, you know?" It was Victoria who introduced Nicole to drinking at around age 16. Shortly before Nicole turned 17, her aunt announced to the family that she had gotten engaged and was moving to Houston. The news was devastating for Nicole. Before she left, Victoria took Nicole out for a farewell dinner in New York City and surprised her by providing her with a fake ID. Victoria ordered Cosmopolitans for the both of them, which Nicole explained to Katherine back in the 1970s was a pretty new and definitely exotic drink. Katherine clearly registered how precious these memories of her time with Victoria were to Nicole.

Katherine was particularly struck by Nicole's response when she inquired what became of this relationship after her aunt moved away. Nicole sighed and said something close to, "Oh, you know, times changed. She got married and slowly became boring, fat, and old, more or less in that order. I'd see her every couple years at family weddings or funerals, and we'd send the occasional Christmas card, but the spark wasn't there anymore."

When Katherine asked if something else replaced this spark, Nicole replied, "Well Antonio did, of course." Nicole explained how she met Antonio, the assistant manager of the grocery store where she worked, at age 15. He was reasonably handsome; more importantly, he was confident, much older, and incredibly attentive to her. He "took charge," impressing her with his ability to articulate a plan for their future together.

When Nicole's mother found out that she was involved with an older "colored" man, she informed her father, who was "beside himself with rage." Her parents forced her to quit her job at the store and forbade her to see Antonio again. Although Nicole broke off the relationship, Antonio refused to accept this outcome and never ceased his clandestine efforts to maintain contact with her. On the night of Nicole's 18th birthday, in what she referred to as "an act of equal parts great courage and extreme cowardice," she packed most of her clothes into two bags and snuck out of her parents' house forever. She moved in with Antonio, got pregnant at 20, and was married shortly before the birth of their first child. Sometime after the birth of her second child, her parents relented and resumed contact with Nicole but remained emotionally distant. Nicole shared her conviction that her parents had made this decision more to salvage their public image than for any other reason.

Rising from her chair, Katherine stretches beside her desk. She senses that she is going to have her work cut out for her with this case. The traumatic nature of Nicole's early life is more subtle and diffuse, and the impact more embedded, than that of other clients she treated with more distinct, pronounced experiences of childhood physical or sexual abuse.

8. Nicole's "Bad Side"

"What gives me the spark now?" Nicole repeats. She is back at the center for the fifth or sixth time, and Katherine asks if she can follow up on some "holes" she has in her understanding of Nicole's history. *Nice choice of words,* Nicole thinks. She's impressed that Katherine apparently remembered Nicole's reference to being stuck in a black hole in her first session. Nicole realizes that she is going to tell Katherine about her "bad side" today. She tries to inhale deeply, but her chest feels tight. "Is it okay if I don't look at you while I answer your question?"

Nicole strikes Katherine in this moment as being at her most timid, and she wonders what this "bad side" that has been hovering outside the perimeter of their sessions actually looks like in Nicole. "Of course," Katherine replies, "you can look wherever you feel most comfortable, and if that changes for you midway through, that's fine, too."

Nicole thanks Katherine and launches into a thorough but swift and emotionally flat inventory of the trajectory of her marriage. She describes how the passion her husband felt early on toward Nicole was gradually redirected to his work and their children. She notes how quickly Antonio advanced in his work, becoming head manager, then regional manager, and now owner of three supermarket franchises. Katherine senses that Nicole is slowly working herself up to the crux of her current dilemma and resolves to listen with limited interruption, careful not to sidetrack Nicole from the course she appears to be on.

Nicole describes Antonio's role as the decision maker in the family; how much her children adore him; and how her kids take his side without fail in parental disputes. As if in anticipation of a lingering question in Katherine's mind, Nicole cuts her off at the pass, making eye contact with Katherine for the first time since she began speaking. "The thing is, Antonio can be very controlling around decisions, but he's never once laid a hand on me or said a cruel word to me, and in the rare moments that I work up the nerve to ask for something, he always gives in. Just in case you're wondering, he's not the problem. The problem's inside me." Katherine's instincts tell her that Nicole is speaking sincerely. Katherine nods her head slightly and waits for Nicole to continue.

Nicole proceeds to tell Katherine that she feels ineffectual in her family and life, like a house guest in her own home most of the time. Antonio is a provider, and when she embraces it, a protector, but he is emotionally distant. Lately, this has been a relief to Nicole, as she is confident that Antonio does not "see" her adequately to catch on to her recent bad behaviors. She almost wishes he would. If he got furious with her, as terrified as she would be, at least she would be feeling something from him again. For years, though, she has felt increasingly isolated and empty. This emotional distance with her husband seemed to develop gradually in conjunction with the steady decline in their sexual interest in each other over the past decade. Nicole blurts out, "When I ran off with my lean, dark, and handsome Cuban lover, I never thought I'd end up married to an overweight, boring old Mexican." She laughs and then apologizes for how offensive and inappropriate that joke must sound to Katherine. Katherine does not join in her laugh, but smiles gently and comments that it sounds like Nicole has been contending with an important change, a significant loss.

Nicole pauses and looks down at the floor. Katherine attempts to offer her words of comfort. Nicole thanks her politely, but there is no shift in her posture or affect. After a while, Katherine speaks: "Nicole, if this is a moment where you might be trying to begin to share with me how you have been coping with the painful and difficult experiences of isolation and emptiness that you've described so poignantly, how you're able to escape temporarily from the black hole you're in and find your spark, let me know how I can help you do that."

"You just did." Nicole replies. She then tells Katherine about the series of "increasingly reckless affairs" that she has engaged in over the past year and a half, the first of these with a married visiting attorney at her firm. Nicole describes him as not particularly handsome, "kind of homely, actually," but endearing in a "lost sort of way." Eventually, they began what "if someone had filmed it would have looked like a clumsy and little more than tepid affair." Internally to Nicole, however, it was like "a whirlwind: a rush of life came back to me." After he finished his business dealings at her firm, neither of them made any effort to maintain contact.

Nicole professes to Katherine that she didn't particularly miss this man once he was gone, but that he awakened a long-absent feeling inside her that she was determined to keep alive. She secretly began to direct more and more of her emotional energy and attention to thoughts of affairs. Sometimes Nicole would venture out on the Internet seeking to meet people; other times she would linger by herself at bars during her weekly "ladies' night" after all her friends had departed, waiting to see what might happen. Nicole qualifies that over the past year and a half, there have not been more than six or seven "affairs" in total, some lasting no more than a night. "They've been more like 'encounters,' really. 'One-night stands,' as they used to say in my day."

"So that's my big dark secret; a glimpse of my bad side. How disgusted are you?" Nicole asks this question in mock jest, but Katherine registers the seriousness on her face.

"I'm not finding myself feeling disgusted, Nicole," Katherine replies, "but I know this is a very relevant concern for you. I appreciate the courage it must have taken for you to share this with me. Honestly, I'm most interested in how you have been feeling about these experiences."

"Sure, make me do all the heavy lifting," Nicole replies, raising her slender arms and flexing her muscles. Nicole and Katherine share a small laugh. "Okay, fine," Nicole continues, "I'll let you off easy this one time, doc."

Nicole takes a deep breath and then proceeds to explain how the planning and anticipation of these encounters give her "a thrill, a rush, a bit of a spark." Nicole spends considerable time contemplating her next potential encounter—who it will be with, where, and how she will avoid getting caught. This makes her feel alive for days on end and allows her to "escape the black hole for long stretches." Katherine inquires how Nicole feels during the encounters themselves. Nicole replies that she is not sure how to answer, admitting that she is mostly on auto-pilot in those moments. Then she adds that her level of sexual arousal during these experiences ("regardless of how unattractive or inept they usually are") and her ability to "you know" is more heightened than it has been with her husband in years. "Immediately afterward, though, I feel awful about the whole thing, disgusted and disgusting, and resolve to end it with that person, call it quits with my whole bad side. That lasts me a good week or so, during which I throw myself into homemaking as recompense. You can pretty much track my affairs by the amount of leftovers in our fridge and the sparkle of our bathroom tiles."

Katherine checks in with Nicole, noting that they have about 15 minutes remaining in their session. Katherine wonders aloud whether Nicole would like to take some time to wind down, or else whether there was additional material that Nicole felt it was important to introduce today. Nicole looks down again and takes a few shallow breaths, her body tensing in the chair. She informs Katherine that these behaviors have been "getting more out of hand" over the past few months and that she has been feeling increasingly out of control.

Katherine asks Nicole whether she feels safe enough to share some examples of this behavior. Nicole replies, "Well, okay, but now you are really going to be disgusted and not want to work with me." She tells Katherine how two of the encounters have been with women who approached her at bars or nightclubs, and how weird it was for her that the experience itself was almost no different than her encounters with men, except that she found herself feeling more self-conscious and shame-ridden after the fact. Katherine has the sense that this disclosure was presented almost as a test, a precursor to what Nicole has been most ambivalent about sharing.

"Go on if you like, Nicole. It's okay," Katherine replies. Nicole speaks rapidly, as if she is in a race to get the words out. She discloses that after years of being unhappily on the pill, several years back she convinced her husband to have a vasectomy. A few months ago she ended up 2 weeks late for her period. In a panic she canceled work and went to two Planned Parenthoods in different cities, signed up at each under false names, lied about the date of her last sexual activity, and convinced them to prescribe her the morning-after pill. She took a double dose of the pill to ensure that she would successfully induce miscarriage. Around the same time, she contracted chlamydia and had to make elaborate excuses to her husband about not having sex for the week it took to treat it. Nicole looks at Katherine with an imploring, searching, almost desperate gesture. She leans forward, her hands gripping the arms of her chair: "The thing is, Katherine, I don't know the limits of how far I will go to feel something, and I'm starting to scare myself. That's why I forced myself to come here."

They have reached the end of their session time, and Katherine has no idea what to say to Nicole. She panics. She berates herself for letting the session time run out, for her eagerness to cover too much ground. She sees Nicole's body suspended in mid-stand, her hands clutching her chair, her facial expression imploring Katherine for some response. Katherine inhales deeply, willing her mind to go blank. Words emerge unprompted from her mouth: "I'm glad you did."

Nicole exhales slowly, then she completes her rise from the chair and heads toward the door. "Okay." She takes and releases another breath. "I guess. Thank you, Katherine."

Katherine nods slightly in acceptance. "I'll see you next week." After Nicole is gone, down the hall toward the exit, Katherine breathes a sigh of relief.

9. Misattunement and Rupture

A couple of months have passed, and Katherine is eager to make headway on the treatment plan that she and Nicole have developed. After deliberation with her supervisor, Katherine sets out to engage Nicole in enhancement of internal resources that she feels will be instrumental not only in preparing Nicole to process her traumatic experiences but also in cultivating a more positive self-image and more effectively selecting, navigating, and sustaining healthy relationships. Katherine introduces Nicole to a variety of exercises and techniques. They settle on an exercise that resonates with Nicole, utilizing it successfully to enhance the quality that Nicole wants to strengthen most to face her life: the feeling of being accepted. To the great satisfaction of both client and therapist, Nicole proves readily able to draw on positive early experiences with her maternal aunt and her more recent adult experiences with Katherine herself in order to cultivate this felt sense.

With Katherine's help, Nicole identifies the sense of being "worth something" as a second quality that she is sorely lacking. Here though, Nicole finds it significantly more difficult to locate even latent seeds of this attribute. She struggles to conjure a single moment in which she remembers having possessed a sense of self-worth. With profuse apology and obvious embarrassment, Nicole disqualifies, minimizes, or rejects every known anecdote or benchmark of personal success from her life history that Katherine attempts to offer up on her behalf.

Katherine gets creative and suggests that perhaps there is an inspirational role model from literature or history or the like who embodies this sense of being worth something that Nicole can tap into. In little more than an instant, Nicole's countenance shifts from one of puzzlement to intense concentration to sudden, welcome recognition. Nicole's face lights up and, although she remains seated, her body bursts upward in her chair. "Vivian Ward! Vivian Ward, hands down!" Katherine stares at her blankly. "Oh, sorry," Nicole replies, "Vivian Ward is Julia Roberts's character in the movie *Pretty Woman*."

Flooded with an uncharacteristic sensation of excitement, there is a lapse in Nicole's routine state of hypervigilance. She overlooks Katherine's growing expression of uncertainty as she enthusiastically elaborates on her choice. "See, first Vivian gets kicked out of this posh L.A. clothing store because the storekeeper sees her as poor white trash who couldn't possibly afford or, for that matter, deserve, to shop there, even though her new dream man just gave her a huge wad of cash. Later in the movie, though, when she's all decked out in beautiful clothes and jewelry, her hair looking terrific and her arms filled with bags of clothing from Armani and Gucci, she storms back into that store. She goes right up to the woman who shooed her away and shouts: "Big mistake!" Pleased with herself for coming up with a perfect example of what Katherine seems to be going for, Nicole looks up at her for approval.

"I'm not sure I understand," Katherine replies. "It's been awhile since I've seen that movie, but isn't Julia Roberts's character a prostitute?"

The subtle expression of disapproval and judgment on Katherine's face is crushing to Nicole. "Well, sort of, I mean, I guess that's true."

Nicole barely registers Katherine's ensuing comments that the character's worth was based on having to sell herself to a man for money. Given Nicole's own history of complicated relationships in which she feels compelled to please and win the approval of others, only to then feel trapped and compelled to act out in illicit and sometimes dangerous sexual relationships, she is not sure this example ultimately gets at what Nicole is going for. Katherine therefore suggests that the work might be better served if they were to look for another example. Nicole internally collapses. She feels more devastated than she has since beginning therapy with Katherine. She asks Katherine to suggest an alternative example, feigns agreement, and complies with being guided toward a suitable literary substitute.

Katherine ends the session with a feeling of accomplishment. She believes she managed to help Nicole avert acting out her trauma through this problematic choice and was instead able to steer her successfully toward identification with a more adaptive role model. Katherine is pleased that some tangible progress has been made. She can now begin to envision Nicole's path to recovery.

10. Sinking Back into the Abyss

Nicole leaves the session feeling shattered, freakish, alien. She spends the remainder of the day alternately mocking and comforting herself for believing things would be different this time. Thankfully, her husband is away at a convention, and so that night she meets up with a younger female coworker who sometimes functions as a semi-confidante and co-conspirator. Several drinks in, Nicole rails on the futility of psychobabble and announces to great mutual amusement that she "faked her first therapygasm." Scanning the nightclub for potential hookups, she stumbles on her way to the restroom. Returning to their table, Nicole discovers that her friend has already paid the bill, and despite Nicole's protests that she's "totally fine" and wants to "stay awhile and listen to the music," her friend insists that she drive Nicole home. That night Nicole suffers from troubled dreams that are lost from memory by morning.

Over the next week, the whole experience drifts into a place of forgetting. By the time Katherine enthusiastically praises Nicole for the important progress she made in their last session, Nicole experiences a sense of pleasure and satisfaction at receiving this generous gesture of approval. She chimes in cordially, and with the slightest effort is able to disregard a nagging physical sensation that something is wrong.

11. False Progress

By the time Katherine next brings up Nicole in clinical supervision, several weeks have passed. She reports moderate incremental progress, including this client's demonstration of a capacity to identify and enhance internal resources and coping skills. Katherine and her supervisor agree that good work is being done and move onto consideration of some of Katherine's other cases. Neither of them comments on the subtle flatness of emotion they are left with at the completion of their brief review of Nicole's case.

12. A Dissociated State Surfaces

Nicole often revisits her affairs, as she has often come to do in her work with Katherine. She explores the spark they elicit, as well as the horrible guilt and shame she experiences in their aftermath. Nicole notes that Katherine listens to her intently, asking thoughtful questions and offering useful interpretations. Emotionally, however, she notices for the first time that Katherine appears to be somewhere far away. This triggers in Nicole a terrible sense first of aloneness and then of profound emptiness. Her body is overcome with the familiar feeling of falling backward into her black hole.

Something catches in herself. Nicole abruptly asks Katherine: "So what's it like for you getting a glimpse of the person I really am?" This question startles Katherine into focus, for her thoughts had strayed from the session seconds earlier. She realizes that she had been gazing out of focus at the wall to Nicole's left. Reestablishing eye contact, Katherine takes stock of Nicole's face and observes a novel shift in her countenance and tone. She asks Nicole to explain. Nicole stands up, slaps her session payment on the desk, and gestures toward the clock while taking a step backward toward the door. She turns the handle and opens the door before looking directly at Katherine. With posture erect, eyes flashing, and an almost feral expression spreading across her mouth, Nicole fiercely responds: "Why, a disgusting creature, of course."

Katherine forcibly suppresses a shudder. Although almost exactly Katherine's height and build, Nicole has always struck Katherine as being so much smaller. In this moment, however, she perceives an energy in Nicole that Katherine had never witnessed in her before. Aggression? Sexuality? Whatever it was, it was something primal and unsettling. Nicole appears to fill the entire doorframe, dwarfing Katherine. Katherine blinks her eyes closed for one long instant. Opening them, she is relieved to find that Nicole is gone.

Leaving the center, Nicole feels first a rush of excitement and then a burning slash of intense emotion that she does not recognize, finally morphing into an immense sadness. Standing on the sidewalk, she calls in sick to work, and then she makes a series of calls, leaving no voice messages, until one of her past lovers answers and with minimal coaxing is persuaded to meet up later that morning.

Katherine spends significant time in her next clinical supervision discussing this occurrence, generating numerous suggestions for revisiting this material with Nicole in future sessions. Katherine elects to withhold one aspect of this incident from her supervisor. During this interchange, Katherine was disturbed to register in herself a fleeting but pronounced and most unwelcomed physiological arousal. Katherine is confused and somewhat embarrassed about this reaction. As a self-described "experienced trauma therapist," she has always prided herself on her ability to remain grounded with clients who struggle with dysregulation, her authentic connection with them, and her clear boundaries. She wants her work associates to think highly of her work and doesn't want her supervisor to interpret her physical response as an indication that she had a triggered or sexualized response to a client. She's too seasoned of a clinician to subject herself to the shame of a rudimentary lecture on countertransference, based on this fluke reaction. Besides, Katherine concludes, Nicole Vasquez is just one of her many cases, and she has more challenging clinical dilemmas to address today in her limited supervision time.

13. Unsettling Supervisor Feedback

Several months have passed, and Katherine is feeling increasingly stuck in her treatment of Nicole. Although she realizes cognitively that this is not helpful, Katherine has become aware that she has a strong negative reaction to Nicole's "bad" part and sees this part of Nicole as keeping her stuck by getting her into trouble over and over again. Her supervisor asks Katherine to explore whether these reactions are associated with an enactment. Katherine is surprised, as on an unspoken level she has always believed those kinds of problems were for clinicians with poor boundaries or for therapists who were uncomfortable checking in with their own feelings. Nevertheless, her supervisor persists. Katherine finds herself feeling defensive and tries to come up with something that will satisfy her supervisor.

After a period of silence, Katherine's supervisor asks her an unexpected question: "How important is it that you be seen as a good person?" Katherine is startled by the question, but then imagines that she must be exploring whether Katherine is struggling with the wish to "rescue" or "cure" her clients. Katherine relaxes and gives some response about having learned that she can't work harder than her clients or control the pace of treatment. When to Katherine's great surprise her supervisor replies that "this is not what I meant by that question," Katherine becomes visibly still, apologizes, and asks for clarification.

What Katherine hears next comes completely from left field: her supervisor wonders about limits to the depth of self-examination that Katherine is willing to undertake in their time together. Her supervisor continues, pointing out the risk of overlooking subtle but important misattunements with clients that are potentially contributing to treatment impasses. Sorting this out, the supervisor adds, sometimes requires that one first examine what personal needs one's role as a therapist are addressing.

Katherine is confused and asks how this notion relates to the present instance. Her supervisor shares the observation that her client Nicole is experiencing a fundamental struggle, or split, around the notion of being a "good person" or a "bad person." This leads her supervisor to wonder whether Katherine is experiencing any parallel process. She wonders, for example, whether Katherine's own internal pull to see herself, and to be viewed by others, as a "good person" might be contributing to a blind spot in her work with this particular client.

Katherine is beside herself. When she responds, her voice is slightly brassy, audibly different from her typically composed, careful tone: "Are you saying that you think I'm not a good person?!" Her supervisor softly replies that this was not at all the intended communication and tries to qualify and further explain herself. Katherine listens dutifully but is incapable of taking anything in. Nodding absently, and with the end of their session under 5 minutes away, she thanks her supervisor for this "helpful feedback and food for thought" and excuses herself.

14. Katherine's Awakening

Careful to remain poised as she leaves her supervisor's office, once Katherine exits the building she surprises herself by letting out a small obscenity. Her head is piercing; she wonders if she has a migraine. She is furious and feels unappreciated for all the incredibly hard work she puts in every day with such demanding clients.

When Katherine arrives home, she is greeted warmly by her fiancé, who immediately notes her uncharacteristic agitation. He is concerned and asks about her day. Katherine launches into a recount of the afternoon. She is so heated that for a long stretch she does not notice her fiancé at all. When she finally does notice him, at first she feels deeply appreciative that he has been listening so intently. Eventually, though, she becomes puzzled by his concern, as she often tries to share the challenges of her work with him and rarely is he either this attentive or this quiet. She stops talking and asks him what he is thinking.

Katherine is stunned to hear him reply that he thinks he might understand where her supervisor was coming from. Feeling her rage compound, she demands that he clarify what he means. Tentatively, he offers that sometimes she is so focused on being perfect that she loses her peripheral vision. Katherine is livid. They decide that it would be best for him to make his way to the airport by himself. Katherine spends the next several hours in miserable rumination.

The following day is Sunday. It's a dreary day, rainy and dank. Her head still aches and she feels foggy. In the late afternoon, she plops in front of the television with ice cream and popcorn. Several hours of half-hearted channel flipping later, she finds herself absentmindedly watching *Pretty Woman* on a movie classics station. During a commercial, Nicole heads to the kitchen to refill her cup of coffee. She returns just as the female protagonist, a character named Vivian Ward, is rudely thrown out of an expensive boutique. Katherine shifts into a state of sustained alertness. When Vivian Ward returns to that store for the second time, Katherine recognizes her transformed self-worth and understands that the money she received from the Richard Gere character was merely an instrument toward this end. The true catalyst was being seen, respected, and, above all, loved and accepted, regardless of the unconventional circumstances fabricated by Hollywood. Tearing up, Katherine finishes the movie. Her head is clear for the first time in days.

15. A New Therapy Chapter Begins

Three days later, Katherine greets Nicole for their weekly session. Once settled in her office, Katherine informs Nicole that she has something important to talk to her about. Nicole is panicked, certain that this opening will segue into Katherine's imminent announcement of plans to end their treatment. Nicole has no doubt that Katherine will provide a perfectly logical and compassionate rationale, underneath which will be the unspoken but definitive affirmation of Nicole's hopelessness and unsuitability for therapy.

Nicole barely stirs when Katherine begins by stating that she "owes Nicole an apology." *Sure, for believing she could make a difference in the first place,* Nicole hears herself think, her chest constricted and her body drawn upward into her chair. It is only when Katherine says that she believes there is an early piece of their work together that she got wrong that Nicole's focus shifts outward. *Now what could this be?* Working hard to keep from becoming totally hysterical, with great effort Nicole gets out the words, "Did I do something to upset you?"

"No," Katherine replies, "I'm the one that messed up, and I fear I may have steered you off course by my mistake."

Nicole remains tense. She is painfully aware from a host of betrayed friendships that admitting you messed up is a great way to soften the blow of cutting someone out of your life, particularly when the person you were cutting off happened to be Nicole Vasquez. "What are you talking about?"

Katherine replies, "For starters, let's just say I've undergone some personal experiences and careful self-reflection lately that have led me to suspect that my read of what *Pretty Woman* means to you was totally off."

"Huh?" Nicole replies, looking puzzled.

"More importantly, I don't think I've been fully seeing you and understanding what you've been going through. If that's the case, it means that I haven't been helping you to the extent that I want to be and that you deserve. I owe you a huge apology, and am committed to working on getting this right, or at least closer to right, as we go forward in our work together."

Nicole detects genuine anguish in Katherine's voice and sees that her eyes have begun to moisten. The muscles in Nicole's face soften as her body spreads back out and settles into her chair, her feet again finding the floor. Nicole exhales deeply, smiles warmly at Katherine, and rolls her eyes in a gesture that Katherine recognizes instantly as one of playful affinity and mutual understanding. Nicole notices Katherine's body spontaneously join her in those same three actions. A new chapter in their work together begins.

PART II

THE COMPONENT-BASED PSYCHOTHERAPY MODEL

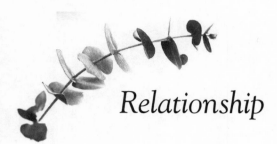

Relationship

CHAPTER 3

Client and Therapist Relational Patterns and Contextual Factors

with Margaret E. Blaustein

Think back to your earliest relationships, with those who did—or who failed to—take care of you. Think of those people who were most significant in your life. What words would you use to describe their demeanor toward you? Was one parent . . . caring? Stern? Available? Removed? Was another warm? Affectionate? Overwhelmed or overwhelming? Was there humor? Silence? Did you feel seen or dismissed?

Now think about your way of being with each of your caregivers, how you learned to manage those relationships. Were you needy? Independent? Did you feel connected or isolated? Was there comfort or tension? Vigilance or withdrawal? Notice how the descriptors of your own behaviors may match or contrast with those of your caregivers, the ways it is likely that the interactional style you developed was the one that brought you the most success in negotiating that relationship.

Margaret E. Blaustein, PhD, is the Director of the Center for Trauma Training and former Division Director for Trauma Training and Education at The Trauma Center. She has extensive experience supporting the range of care settings in integrating and building trauma-informed practices. A clinician, trainer, and consultant for nearly 20 years, Dr. Blaustein has collaborated with over 50 organizations to embed trauma-informed practices through provision of intensive training, consultation, and organizational support and has provided training to well over 10,000 providers in her career.

Consider how these relationships changed over time. Think about the relational threads that continued and those that shifted from childhood through to adulthood. Think about your new relationships—with your peers, your own adult partners, and eventually your children. What words might you use to describe each of those relationships? How have you approached others, and how have they negotiated with you? It is likely that there is continuity, in some way, across relationships and that where there are differences—where you have shifted your way of being—there has been some process to account for it.

Childhood relationships are complex and multifaceted, and they are likely the most influential factors shaping development. Although none of us is simply the sum of our early childhoods, we are surely in part a product of them. The psychology field's understanding of attachment, the biologically driven connection between children and their primary caregivers, has grown increasingly nuanced. It started with an understanding that people are hard-wired to attach—that we form long-lasting, ingrained connections with our closest caregivers that are driven in part by the need to survive but that goes far beyond that drive in function. This understanding has grown to include the myriad ways we manage and make meaning about these connections; how they shape our understanding of ourselves and our world; how they impact our development on every level, from the most observable behaviors to the invisible but influential world of our neurobiology; and how we pass these relationships on in our connections to our friends, our partners, and the next generation. And sometimes we are able to shift these relationships by reflecting on and making meaning about them, so that we are not perpetuating the cycle that may have begun long before our own childhood.

ATTACHMENT

From the first moments of life, an infant's sense of self begins to take shape within a matrix of relationships that create a unique set of experiences, for better or for worse. These experiences, co-created within infant/caregiver dyads, range from highly charged emotional moments to the humdrum rhythms that comprise the backdrop of day-to-day existence. The term "attachment" is used to describe these physiological, emotional, and behavioral interactions between a child and his or her caregivers. In better circumstances, caregivers create an ambiance of responsivity and connectedness through eye contact, touch, and intimacy, and they read the infant's cues signaling hunger, discomfort, fatigue, and the desire to play, rest, or disengage. Such "good enough" caregivers (Winnicott, 1965) rely on both conscious attentiveness and nonconscious empathic attunement to nonverbal cues from the infant. Thus, they evoke in the infant a felt-sense of being seen, understood, cared for, protected, and enjoyed. Such infants can relax into predictable rhythms of life, trusting that their basic physical needs will be met, intense emotions and distress soothed, and stimulating engagement generously offered. Such trust forms the background hum that gives rise to later exploratory urges, healthy risk-taking, and social learning that, in turn, help the child make sense of and master complex relational and identity landscapes across the lifespan.

Across the years that the attachment system has been studied, it has become clear that early caregiving interactions set the stage for almost every significant social-emotional developmental task of childhood. One of the primary functions of the attachment system is to serve as physiological regulator and therefore as the foundation for the development of more independent regulatory capacity. The newborn has almost no capacity to modulate physiological experience; other than a few rudimentary self-soothing actions (sucking, gaze aversion), the infant is entirely dependent on the adult caregiver to support optimal levels of arousal, through a balance of stimulation and soothing. Schore (2003a, 2003b) demonstrates through a comprehensive synthesis of the literature the ways in which secure attachment in infancy facilitates development of a healthy limbic system, whereas early relational trauma and neglect have detrimental effects on these same structures, leading to potentially lifelong psychobiological impacts on core regulatory systems. Interactions with caregivers also provide the filter through which we develop "emotional knowing"—the ability to accurately discriminate and understand our own and others' emotional experience and the ways this experience links with physical sensations and behaviors.

In the context of our early relationships, we also learn the building blocks of communication and how to most effectively negotiate interaction. Our caregivers respond selectively to our communicative attempts, from our earliest involuntary cries and expressions to our more purposeful words and behaviors as we develop. In one family, for instance, a quiet cry or small noise may be ignored, while a louder wail receives an instant response; in another family, the opposite may be true. The growing child in each family is therefore reinforced for—and will continue to use—different communicative methods to get his or her needs met. Our behaviors, our facial expressions, and our actions are similarly "rewarded," or not, through the responses and reactions of others. By matching these to the predictable responses of our caregivers, we learn to be effective communication partners in the context of those relationships and then generalize these methods to future partners.

Attachment Styles in Clients with Histories of Emotional Abuse and Neglect

Consider the influential effects of the early attachment relationship and the manner in which it shapes regulatory capacity, meaning-making about self and others, self-knowledge, and interpersonal skill. Also consider the ways in which these capacities are impacted for children like Nicole and David, who grow up in homes where the caregiving is less than ideal. In their drive to connect, to maintain this crucial relationship even in less than ideal circumstances, the child will develop a regulatory, relational, and communicative style that optimizes that attachment potential. The organization of our attachment style, and the resulting implications of that style, will vary according to the needs of the relationships within which they develop. We see an individual's attachment style, first established in infancy, as key to the effects of emotional abuse and neglect and central to CBP's approach to therapy.

The majority of children can be classified into one of the three primary patterns initially identified through the Ainsworth Strange Situation procedure (Ainsworth & Bell, 1970) and expanded to include a fourth pattern capturing the experience of maltreated youngsters (Crittenten, 1985). These patterns are *Secure* and three forms of Insecure attachments: *Resistant/Ambivalent*, *Anxious–Avoidant*, and *Disorganized*. These patterns of child organization have been shown to match with predictable patterns of adult caregiving behavior and to predict to differential outcomes, as it is clear that these relational patterns are enduring. A remarkable body of literature and longitudinal studies now support the long-term continuity of our early attachment organization through early childhood (Main & Cassidy, 1998) into adolescence (Waters, Hamilton, & Weinfield, 2000) and young adulthood (Waters, Merrick, Trevoux, Crowell, & Albersheim, 2000). Because early caregiver relationships lay down the initial templates for a child's relational patterns and sense of self across the lifespan (Bowlby, 1982; Lyons-Ruth & Jacobvitz, 1999), they wield a formidable and enduring formative influence. For children who have endured chronic emotional abuse or neglect, these templates assume additional damaging power as they become deeply threaded into the fibers of personality.

We rarely see adult clients with secure attachments who have significant histories of childhood emotional abuse and neglect. As posited by Bowlby (1973, 1980, 1982), early attachment relationships characterized by emotional abuse and neglect lead to alterations in sense of self ("I am bad"; "I am damaged"; "I am unlovable"), other ("People are out for themselves"; "Men are cruel"), and self-in-relationship ("I need to be in a relationship to be okay"; "I can't trust anyone"; "Other people will hurt me"). In adulthood, these relational patterns become engrained, with little to no awareness of their historic or relational roots. These emotional and behavioral grooves can give rise to endless repetitions that occur outside of conscious awareness, feeding a vicious cycle of stigma, shame, and powerlessness.

DIMENSIONS OF THE RELATIONSHIP COMPONENT

Beyond general attachment style, we can consider where our clients fall along a series of dimensions that influence the therapeutic relationship and interpersonal dynamics in the person's life: openness, expressiveness, connectedness, and power orientation (see Figure 3.1). Assessment using these four dimensions can be used to identify sources of interpersonal conflict, highlight relational strengths, and target relational goals. It is important to note that people may have different patterns of response in different situations, particularly when dissociation is a primary coping strategy (see Chapter 7).

The first dimension of the relationship component, openness, refers to the porousness of a person's boundaries with the external world, which can vary from more open to more guarded and self-protective. A person who is on the extreme open end of this dimension may have an underactive threat response system and may be vulnerable to revictimization. A person who is extremely guarded or self-protective may experience resulting isolation because his rigid boundaries prevent engagement with the outside world. Someone who maintains a balance between openness and boundaries is more likely to be able to engage safely with the world.

Second, expressiveness indicates a person's ability to communicate internal experiences, wants, and needs to others. A person who is at the very high end of the expressiveness dimension may have difficulty determining how much information to share and appropriate contexts to share personal information and desires. For instance, on the one hand, a young woman who is very high on the expressiveness dimension is late to work and impulsively shares her extensive trauma history with her new employer, in an attempt to explain her tardiness. On the other hand, people who are at the unexpressive end of the continuum may have difficulty engaging others or getting their needs met because of their difficulty sharing aspects of themselves. Difficulty recognizing and naming internal experiences, a key regulatory skill, can also impede a person's self-expression. One goal of CBP is development of the ability to identify and express internal states, while accurately "reading" interpersonal interactions and having the capacity to modulate self-expression, gradually disclosing more information as a trusting relationship develops.

With early interpersonal trauma, survivors' sense of connectedness to other people is often impacted. Some survivors feel alienated or different and

Overly Open/Vulnerable -------------------- (X – Open) ----------------------------------- Guarded

Uncontained ----------------------------- (X – Expressive) ------------------------- Unexpressive

Enmeshed -------------------------------- (X – Connected) --------------------- Alienated/Isolated

Aggressive/Self-focused ------------------ (X – Assertive) ------------ Compliant/Other-focused

FIGURE 3.1. Dimensions of the relationship component. X denotes direction of therapeutic goals.

might respond by withdrawing from other people. Others have the ability to connect but develop enmeshed relationships in which they rely on the immediate presence of another person to feel okay. As one survivor of early emotional abuse and neglect put it, "As soon as one relationship ends, I jump into another one because it helps to fill that empty hole inside of me." CBP supports the development of the capacity to allow intimacy to grow, while maintaining the boundaries needed to develop an autonomous sense of self.

The fourth relational dimension is the power orientation that persons have toward their interpersonal relationships. Some people (or more accurately, "parts" of self, as described in Chapter 7) react to being repeatedly hurt by being very self-focused on the pursuit of their own needs and desires. For example, a high-powered businessman whose father insulted and belittled him in childhood developed a style of aggressively asserting his demands in order to get his needs met, a strategy that was very successful in the workforce but that also contributed to the end of several serious relationships. On the other end of the extreme, some people have parts of themselves that avoid conflict by focusing on the other—shutting down their own desires and needs in order to comply with another person's wishes. These coping responses that helped manage traumatic threat eventually interfere with the survivors' ability to engage in mutual harmonious relationships or to feel that they exist within relationships.

In the following sections we discuss the relational stance we adopt in CBP that can contribute to a strong therapeutic relationship and can utilize interactions within the therapeutic relationship to explore and shift relational patterns.

IMPACT OF EARLY EMOTIONAL ABUSE AND NEGLECT ON ADULT RELATIONSHIPS

Various types of relationships may be impacted by people who have experienced early attachment-related trauma, including emotional abuse and neglect. When children learn to protect themselves by withdrawing from others or by approaching people in a guarded way, friendships are impacted, with some people having very few friendships and others having primarily superficial relationships or acquaintanceships. Professional relationships may be affected; for instance, despite her high educational achievements, one woman struggled with maintaining consistent employment throughout her life because of her extreme sensitivity to any criticism or negative feedback from authority figures, a reminder of her early emotional abuse from her hypercritical, overbearing mother. When people who experienced childhood maltreatment have offspring of their own, parenting can trigger posttraumatic reactions. These parents may inadvertently replay elements of their own early abuse or neglect or, desperately hoping to protect their children from the type of childhood they had, instead parent out of anxiety and hypervigilance. Intergenerational transmission of trauma is a commonly recognized phenomenon that, unfortunately subtly, or sometimes more apparently, impact many children of very well-intentioned parents. The betrayal and injury from caregivers often translates to difficulties with trust and intimacy, which can lead to avoidance of romantic relationships or to problems with emotional and sexual intimacy in these relationships. Although both Nicole and David are involved in marital relationships, they both feel alienated and misunderstood by their partners and have withdrawn into their own protective cocoons. As discussed in detail in the following sections, some people become involved in adult relationships that replay elements of their early trauma.

Attraction to Abusive or Unavailable Partners

One aspect of problematic attachment styles involves the "attraction" to emotionally abusive relationships that can evolve over time in adults with histories of chronic emotional abuse and neglect. As a profession, we tend to be reluctant to acknowledge or explore this dynamic, perhaps because of our ideologies surrounding trauma and victimization, or more practically in an effort to protect our clients or ourselves from the implied blame and likely surfacing of deep reservoirs of shame.

Most clinicians are familiar with Harry Harlow's (e.g., 1958) seminal work on attachment in primate species. Through a series of forced-choice experiments involving the social deprivation of neonatal and infant rhesus and macaque monkeys, Harlow unequivocally established that the drive for love, affection, and maternal or caregiver nurturance is at least as essential to healthy infant development as other basic needs established to be primary, such as satiation of hunger and thirst and relief from pain. For example, he discovered that these young primates would routinely sacrifice the food paired with a wire-mesh mother surrogate in favor of the perceived warmth and comfort associated with contact to a soft cloth-mother surrogate, despite the deprivation of food associated with selection of this choice of an attachment figure.

More recently, Robert Sapolsky (2009) has significantly advanced our scientific understanding of the critical and complex nature of the young organism's need to receive emotional nurturance and the hardships it will endure to maintain or restore contact with its primary caregiver. In his important research on rodent pups during the first weeks of life, Sapolsky discovered that the motivation to gain contact with its mother following separation actually serves to override the rodent pup's normative neurobiological development of capacities for threat detection and pain avoidance. Within the first 10 days of life, rodent pups learned to avoid an aversive stimulus (e.g., an electric shock) when it was portended by a paired neutral stimulus (e.g., the scent of lavender or citrus). However, a fascinating and disturbing wrinkle to this neurodevelopmental process was uncovered. When the neutral scent was paired not only with the aversive stimulus, but also with access to the pup's mother, the presence of this nurturing primary caregiver was revealed not only to disrupt rodent pups' normative danger detection and avoidance response, but also to induce over time an attraction to the aversive stimulus itself because of its paired association with the desired attachment figure.

Sapolsky's (2009) research suggests that when connection to one's primary caregiver during formative childhood experience requires a young developing organism to endure pain, pain and love can become intertwined. Sadly, we far too frequently see quite similar patterns of response in people who have experienced early emotional abuse and neglect. In most of these cases, the pain and the love stem from the very same source(s); namely, it tends to be the most important early attachment figures who represent both the desired object of affection and the principal inflicter(s) of harm. Ann Burgess, Lenore Walker, Bessel van der Kolk, and others have witnessed one dark truth about recurrent revictimization in adult trauma survivors: They have found that many of these individuals have, in essence, become addicted to this pain, drawn toward and compelled to remain with volatile, inconsistent, and at times outright abusive partners because it is primarily, if not exclusively, in the context of hurtful and even dangerous emotional connections that they find themselves able to experience poignant sensations of attraction, love, and closeness. Some people with histories of pervasive emotional abuse and neglect seem most alive and emotionally engaged when in the midst of relational conflict, heartbreak, and mistreatment. They seem pulled toward such relationships and extend far greater effort to sustain them than they show in other, less toxic relationships.

Is it only through enduring cruelty and debasement, only through clinging desperately, despite being shunned and repeatedly forgotten, that the prospect of finding love exists for these individuals? Or perhaps more accurately and insidiously, was it precisely in the context of such abusive relationships that longed-for moments of affection, nurturance, and warmth were dispensed, however inconsistently and fleetingly? Not infrequently, these dynamics unfold in the therapeutic relationship itself, with our clients simultaneously rejecting or emotionally constricting in response to our efforts to express genuine compassion or emotional connection, and magnifying and perseverating upon perceived slights or betrayals on our part. Unsteadied and activated, we find ourselves desperately fleeing from or else diving headlong into the abyss of these enactments.

In turn, a converse but thematically similar relational pattern can be seen in other complexly traumatized adult clients, particularly those whose childhoods were characterized by chronic emotional deprivation or neglect or in those who were raised by physically or emotionally absent caregivers. For many of these clients, we observe a parallel attraction to adult partners who are generally emotionally constricted or whose intermittent capacity for emotional expression and connection is routinely offset by predictable periods of disconnection. Examples of the latter include furtive relationships with individuals who are married; engagement in interminable long-distance relationships; and relationships with partners consumed by work or other obligations or who are capable of emotional connection only during episodic and controlled participation in substance abuse. We can see this pattern with Nicole, who was drawn to her husband because of his apparent distinction from her parents, when he overwhelmed her with his persistent attention. However, her marital relationship slowly transformed into a repetition of her relationship with her father, who benignly patted her head when she begged him not to leave. Similarly, it seems that Nicole seems invisible in her marriage and is engaging in high-risk behaviors, perhaps to challenge the stagnant stability of her marriage and to feel that she exists. While the limitations of these emotionally distant relationships are often an identifiable source of frustration for these clients—and the internal debate over whether to end these relationships is not uncommonly a recurrent focus of their attention in psychotherapy—many such survivors tenaciously cling to these relationships precisely because of their limitations. For adults whose formative experience of love was akin to the occasional bloom of a delicate flower amidst a vast desert, or the meager trickle of water in a dry river bed, more emotionally intense or consistently expressive intimate attachments can be experienced as overwhelming and untenable.

At either pole, the protective, trauma-driven nature of this selection of emotionally abusive or constricted romantic partners should never be underestimated. As therapists, many of us have been pulled to react too quickly to urgent pleas expressed by those parts of our clients (see Chapter 7) seeking to free themselves of these complicated relationships. These urgent appeals often activate our innate motivation to protect our clients from wrongdoing, as well as our deeply ingrained values regarding empowerment and choice. We may have been somewhat stunned and dismayed when we found ourselves the subject of unanticipated attack from other parts of these clients harboring an unshakable devotion to these very partners and the transmuted love and attachment needs they have come to represent.

Although each client has unique early experiences and has coped in very different ways, many adults who have experienced early emotional abuse and neglect share a common thread of disconnection and alienation. Although they typically desire closeness, they often feel different or damaged and struggle with forming intimate relationships while maintaining their own boundaries. The therapeutic relationship can provide a relational base from which to begin to explore and transform these issues.

REPLAYING RELATIONAL PATTERNS IN THERAPY

How do clients with insecure attachment styles typically present early in therapy? Those who are anxious–avoidant sometimes appear emotionally constrained and disengaged from their therapists, as well as others in their lives. They may, like David, approach therapy somewhat reluctantly and set time limits on the therapy. They are generally less likely to reach out for supports outside of regularly scheduled sessions, even when they are invited to do so. Intimacy in the therapy relationship can be triggering for these clients: they may become frightened and/or angry if they start to feel dependent on the therapist, and they sometimes respond by withdrawing or by acting in ways that challenge the therapeutic relationship. Because of her history of early abandonment and her resulting self-protective stance in relationships, one young woman predictably dropped out of long-term therapy when she began to feel vulnerable, returning several years later to reengage. Later in the therapy, she became increasingly able to talk about her fears and her desire to run rather than act it out.

David appears to have this type of anxious–avoidant attachment pattern. As a child, he was neglected by his biological parents, with a mother who was just a teenager herself and a father who was rarely around. David's survival instincts were strong, and he learned to shut down his own experience and to comply—to fit in with the demands around him as a chameleon changes its colors. He was afraid when his mother left him home alone to go out drinking or when she left him uncared for while she slept on the couch during the day, but this forced him to be tough. He disconnected from his feelings, particularly any hints of vulnerability and need, and wasn't able to acknowledge his desire to be cared for. David's adoption and life with his adoptive family further compounded his feelings of being unseen and "invisible." He learned to view relationships as potential threats, and he generally managed this threat through avoidance of intimacy. This pattern was repeated in his marriage and became problematic when his quiet demeanor and deference to his wife in running the household and in disciplining their daughter came to be resented as his being passive and emotionally vacant. The extent to which David internalized the need to fit in and comply was epitomized in his purchase of the Volvo—the same car his adoptive parents had that he hated so much. He brought that anxious–avoidant attachment style to his therapy with Susan, as shown by his strong tendency early in the treatment to remain disconnected from her and then by his extreme reaction to her forgetting to tell him ahead of time about her upcoming vacation. Because David's typical relational approach is designed to protect himself from precisely such surprises and disappointments, it took him quite a while to get beyond this setback with Susan.

In contrast, individuals with resistant–ambivalent attachment styles tend to be very preoccupied with their therapists and both intensely seek and resist close connections. They may try hard to please others, often seeking and sometimes needing out-of-session contact with the therapist, and be highly attuned to any real or felt nuances of disruption in the therapy relationship. The issue of how to deal with their intense need in therapy is an important one in the literature (e.g., Dalenberg, 2000; Lyons-Ruth, 2003) and is explored in more detail in Chapter 4.

The most recently identified style, disorganized attachment (Main, 1995; Main & Solomon, 1986), is one in which the intense fear of intimacy and the equally intense longing and need for connection clash. Sometimes this can manifest itself in disorganized and disoriented behavior in the therapist's presence. For example, consider the case of Nicole, whose mother was "alternately vacant and intrusive, oscillating between neglectful and emotionally cruel." Nicole's attachment relationship with her mother created a reflective lens that influenced the meaning that she made of her world, including her relationships. Nicole's different "parts," or dissociated states, led her to have varied responses in her interpersonal relationships: the relational push–pull that has been a well-documented consequence of relational trauma. We witness the corollaries of Nicole's childhood treatment in her honed "art of . . . solitude and invisibility," a state that shields her from possible emotional threat. Her self-protective stance can be seen in Nicole's somatic state as "the contraction of the small muscles of her birdlike limbs, serving to avoid and ward off contact with other[s]." Nicole sought a marriage to a man who was emotionally "safe" because of the emotional disconnection; however, this relationship leaves her with a familiar but "unbearable sense of aloneness" (Fosha, 2000), easily overwhelming her and cutting her off from authentic connection with others. She is left alone, then, in a relational "abyss." This pathogenic feeling state leads Nicole to frantically seek pseudoconnections in one-night stands, which further embed her feelings of worthlessness and stigma. Despite her strong defenses against vulnerability in relationships, Nicole's intense need for approval and support is activated in her therapy with Katherine. She then feels devastated and filled with self-loathing as a result of subtle misattunements and disappointments in her relationship with Katherine.

Nicole is unable to perceive this larger narrative that bridges different epochs in her life. Instead, we can imagine that Nicole, pretherapy, might make meaning in a much more personalized and fractured fashion: "Who would want to really get to know me—a pathetic, empty shell of a person? Even when I get a little attention from men, it never lasts. The only way to stay safe is to keep my distance from everyone." These meanings exist alongside, "I desperately need someone to be with me and take care of me. I have to get my therapist to understand that this is the only thing that is going to make me well." Nicole does not see how the seeds of aloneness and relational threat were planted in her childhood through a chronic absence of being seen and known, the pain of rejection from her father, and repeated emotional attacks from her mother. Lacking this perspective, Nicole makes sense of the resulting relational void, crushing worthlessness, and self-disgust as fundamental flaws in herself: "So that's my big dark secret; a glimpse of my bad side. How disgusted are you?" This implicit belief system feeds Nicole's affective constriction, sense of internal and external emptiness, and confusion about herself, alongside a hunger for recognition and connection.

In Nicole's case, we witness elements of an adult disorganized attachment. We see her flickering hope that leads her to call to make an initial therapy appointment, and then her experience of a flood of shame, self-loathing, and fear that make her contemplate canceling it. In adults such as Nicole, we see echoes of the inescapable paradox of disorganized attachment in childhood in which caretakers are at once *the source of fear* because of threatening or abusive behavior or of fearful, dissociative behavior (Lyons-Ruth & Jacobvitz, 1999) and *a source of comfort*, being the primary attachment figures, whose presence is imperative to the survival of the child. This child, and later adult, is thus condemned to a confusing kaleidoscope of competing needs and impulses: motivated by despair and painful need, she is pulled to an Other, but as she nears, the fear, terror, and dread of being hurt gain momentum and instigate a hasty retreat into a "safe" abyss of aloneness and helplessness. This paradox is perpetually reenacted throughout the lifespan until it can be transformed through either a therapeutic experience or a secure attachment to an intimate other. What Katherine does in the last excerpt of her therapy with Nicole is to "reach across the abyss," to find a way to bridge the horrible black hole Nicole had fallen into, thanks to Katherine's misattunement earlier in their work.

Culture, Context, and the Therapeutic Relationship

Cultural similarities and differences between clients and therapists can have a significant impact on the therapeutic relationship. As with the question of a shared trauma history or not, there are advantages and disadvantages to the therapist and client having similar or different contextual factors, whether it be sexual orientation, race and ethnicity, social class, age, religion, and so on. The therapist must be mindful of the potential advantages and pitfalls. Differences in perspective based on these issues can create barriers in the therapeutic relationship and impede progress in therapy, particularly when they are not acknowledged and discussed. For instance, a counselor was working with a young undocumented woman from El Salvador who had been trafficked into the United States. This young woman left home as an adolescent due to emotional abuse and neglect and became pregnant at age 16. She came to the United States in hopes of financially supporting her daughter, who remained in El Salvador with relatives. Despite living in poverty, she was highly motivated to send any money she made back to her daughter's caregivers in El Salvador. The counselor, a young, enthusiastic, educated Caucasian woman from an upper-middle-class family, recognized that her client had experienced extensive trauma; she encouraged this woman to set boundaries with others in her life and to engage in more self-care. This perspective was a mismatch for the young mother, whose priorities were family and basic survival, and she soon dropped out of therapy, citing conflicts.

When the therapist and client share their orientation or self-identification, and both belong to a minority group, the therapist may well be more attuned to the degree of subtle and not-so-subtle discrimination their client faces and may be more sensitive to the nuances of their experience. One potential downside of a shared orientation is that, as a result, the therapist can make assumptions about the client's experience. Once Katherine realized that Nicole was Caucasian and was born in the United States, she assumed there were no cultural or contextual issues to address, as if all people who fit that category are all the same, which is manifestly not true. Another risk of extensive client–therapist commonalities is emotional overidentification. In one such case, an African American therapist, having herself been exposed to many instances of bigotry, responded passionately when her client disclosed suffering racial discrimination in her work setting. Despite her fear of repercussions, the client then felt that she needed to speak out against her employer in order to please her therapist. Thus, regardless of whether clients and therapists have similar or different cultural and contextual factors, these issues should be actively addressed within the therapy.

David came to his first session with his outwardly "white" dress and style, and Susan did not realize he was biracial until he commented on it, and then she was thrown by it. Her reaction taps directly into David's identity confusion, of which his racial identity is one part. We don't know what this realization means to Susan, although she may share the wish many therapists have to be free of prejudice. She almost certainly has some historical experiences from growing up in a culture that at best struggles deeply with issues of racism and perhaps her own experiences of alienation as a result of growing up Jewish in a culture that is not always accepting of Jews. She likely recognizes fairly early that David's racial identity is a charged issue for him and, like most of us, is not sure what their racial differences will mean to their therapeutic relationship. In their work together, a complex issue arises related to their racial differences: David expresses resentment about Susan's apparent interest in his ethnic identity. Whether this reaction reflects David's coerced rejection of his African American heritage, or whether he is recognizing some implicit anxiety in Susan over their differences, or both, remains to be seen. Similarly, David appears to have conflicts related to his social class, including the disconnection between various phases in his life where he lived in poverty versus a very affluent setting, and the emotional implications for him of these shifts. He likely has his take on Susan and her class and how her background impacts her values and her view of him. David also seems to have some ambivalence about gender roles, including a feeling that as a man he should be strong and control his emotions, juxtaposed against his existence in a relationship where he feels emasculated and powerless. In contrast, as a therapist, Susan likely views emotional awareness as a strength instead of a weakness. Ideally, the therapy will support exploration of these issues and how they impact the therapeutic relationship and process over time.

THE THERAPIST'S ATTACHMENT STYLES
AND RELATIONAL PATTERNS

Because treatment of adults who have experienced childhood emotional abuse and neglect is inherently relational in nature, in CBP we consider the attachment styles and relational patterns of the therapist as well as those of the client. Each individual therapist's own emotional and relational challenges figure into the therapy, either as stumbling blocks or as assets to treatment, or, most often, both.

In a recent study, Nissen-Lie, Havik, Høglend, Monsen, and Ronnestad (2013) reviewed the literature, which repeatedly shows that the relational qualities of the therapist are most important in predicting the outcome of psychotherapies. In particular, warmth and high levels of interpersonal skills relate to clients highly rating the working alliance they have with their therapist and strongly predict satisfactory outcomes of psychotherapy. In this important and sophisticated 5-year study, Nissen-Lie and colleagues measured longitudinally client and therapist ratings of the working alliance and found significant variability across therapist–client pairs; not all therapists facilitate the working alliance as well as others. They took repeated measures of therapists' reports on the quality of their ongoing lives (including items such as how frequently they express their private thoughts and feelings; feel a sense of significant conflict, disappointment, or loss; and experience a sense of being genuinely cared for and supported) and then factor-analyzed those scores. Those analyses produced two robust factors: personal satisfaction with relationships and personal burdens. The therapists' personal satisfaction scores strongly predicted their own assessment of the quality of the working alliance with clients, but their reported personal burdens did not. However, what best predicted the clients' predictions of the working alliance, in a negative direction, was the therapists' ratings of their personal conflicts and burdens. Nissen-Lie and colleagues suggested that social desirability may influence therapists' ratings of their alliance, with therapists seeing through rose-colored glasses when all is going well with their lives but preferring not to see the impact when things are not going well. In this study as in others, clients were most affected by therapists' negative emotional states. They cited findings by Hersoug, Høglend, Havik, von der Lippe, and Monsen (2009) indicating that clients' rating of the working alliance is weaker for therapists who describe themselves as somewhat distant and detached in their personal relationships than for those who don't describe themselves as such. Nissen-Lie and colleagues conclude: "Even subtle signs of disinterest, rejection, aggression, or defensive behaviors may result from increased burdens in the therapists' personal life, and this may lead to deterioration in the alliance" (p. 9).

As the Nissen-Lie and colleagues (2013) study suggests, therapists with problematic attachment styles are likely to have to do considerable work in their own therapies before being able to do deep work with clients with histories of neglect and emotional abuse. We all have personal histories, and for most of us, at least sometimes, bad things have happened. Many psychotherapists working with clients who were neglected and emotionally abused have their own histories of abuse (discussed in Dalenberg, 2000; Davies & Frawley, 1994; Pearlman & Saakvitne, 1995a), which influences the treatment they offer in both helpful and problematic ways.

Sometimes even without our own attachment difficulties or trauma histories, therapists' styles are such that they cannot meet these clients where they need to be met. For instance, an experienced therapist who was new to trauma work began working with a client who had experienced early neglect and severe emotional abuse, along with episodes of physical and sexual abuse. In supervision, the therapist described her client's ongoing dysregulation and a series of enactments, or relational disruptions driven by unconscious aspects of the client and therapist (see below for an extensive exploration of enactments). In all instances, the therapist had tried to be reassuring or to focus on the positive aspects and strengths of the client, who felt her deep pain and despair were not being recognized. In supervision, the therapist was able to acknowledge that, in general, she liked to look at life positively and preferred not to go too deeply into the darker aspects. Eventually, this client was transferred to a therapist who was more comfortable with her own and others' dark sides, and so the relational disruptions essentially stopped.

No matter how well we therapists know ourselves and how much supervision we get, we are likely to be challenged at times by interactions within the therapy relationship and will inevitably make some mistakes. At the beginning of their work together, David's therapist Susan struggles with her own feelings of helplessness and hopelessness, and particularly with a lack of emotional connection with David. This is an example where Susan's history leaves her somewhat reactive to David's history. Wisely, she takes these issues to her supervisor, saying she is "apprehensive about whether she is truly qualified to take on this particular client" and feels unsettled and anxious, hoping that she is "not getting in over my head with this one." At these times, although she may be able to empathize with his emotional state, her emotional response is interfering with her ability to be helpful to David; it is becoming more about her and her anxieties and needs than about understanding and helping David.

IMPLICATIONS OF ATTACHMENT STYLES FOR TREATMENT

As discussed, our attachment relationships profoundly influence development, and our relational style is remarkably enduring over time. So where does this leave Nicole and David and the thousands upon thousands of children who grow up in homes in which their attachment relationships are characterized by absence, chaos, and criticism? Once set in motion, are negative developmental pathways set in stone? Certainly, the literature speaks to the intractable nature of our attachment approach, to the persistence and stubbornness of our often unconscious models of self and the world, and to our adaptive but often unhealthy methods for regulating our experience. And yet—there is no study of high-risk samples in which there are not some individuals who thrive despite challenging beginnings. It is likely that every therapist who works with this population has had a moment—or many—in which she marveled at the capacity of clients to maintain an air of optimism, to manage potentially overwhelming distress in a healthy way, to form lasting and meaningful relationships, and to build different futures than the ones for which they were primed.

As a relational therapy, CBP considers the therapist–client relationship as central to helping adult clients build these capacities for themselves. It is informed by what research on psychotherapy treatment outcome has taught us about the importance of the therapeutic alliance to successful interventions with clients in general, as well as with clients traumatized in childhood. Emphasis on the therapeutic relationship, including therapists' provision of empathy and warmth, establishment of boundaries and trust, and, ultimately, encouragement of clients braving emotional risks in psychotherapy, has been empirically identified as the single greatest contributor to positive treatment outcome (reviewed in Nissen-Lie et al., 2013). Similarly, in an analysis of therapist differences in a large, multisite treatment outcome study in which all study clinicians implemented the same cognitive-behavioral session protocol with chronically depressed adults, Vocisano and her colleagues (2004) discovered that clinician emphasis on the client–therapist relationship was the greatest predictor of treatment outcome, whereas other clinician-specific factors such as gender, age, or years of experience had no bearing on outcomes. Research more closely focused on adults with histories of complex childhood trauma evidences similar findings regarding the critical role of the therapeutic relationship in treatment outcome. Lending empirical support to Herman's (1992b) phasic model of complex trauma treatment, Cloitre's research on psychotherapy with women having histories of chronic child abuse identified establishment of a therapeutic alliance as an important first step toward resolution of PTSD. In effect, this research provided a predictable and compassionate holding container within which the expression of trauma-related affect could be tolerated and negative mood regulation practices could be safely undertaken (Cloitre, Stovall-McClough, Miranda, & Chemtob, 2004).

It is notable that the most well-studied method for measuring attachment in adulthood, the Adult Attachment Inventory (AAI), is based on representational process rather than experience. In other words, it is not the presence of maltreatment or challenging early relationships that define our attachment organization in adulthood; rather, it is the way in which we reflect on and make meaning about these relational experiences. It is our capacity to acknowledge and regulate our distress, to bring coherence to what may have once been chaotic or fragmented, and to pull together a past, present, and future. It is, in many ways, the development of all of those capacities that, ideally, the early attachment system would have engendered: the reflective self, the awareness of other, and the physiological regulation—capacities that many adults must build for themselves as they leave behind those early relationships and create a new attachment story.

CONCLUSION

When beginning to develop a therapeutic relationship with a survivor of early attachment-related trauma such as early emotional abuse and neglect, we should consider our client's relational patterns and how these patterns are rooted in his or her early experiences. Early assessment can include consideration of attachment style, as well as where our clients fall along four relational dimensions. We might explore how these patterns are causing difficulties in our client's life today, including misattunements, conflicts, feelings of dependency, and/or difficulties reaching out to others across what can feel like a relational abyss. CBP also requires us to pay attention to ourselves and to our own foibles and limitations in a way that many therapeutic approaches do not. We must strive to be aware of our own attachment styles and preferences and tendencies in relationships, and how our own style interacts with our client's relational patterns. We should explore how culture and other contextual factors (such as race/ethnicity, socioeconomic status, national origin, gender identity and sexual orientation, age and generation, spirituality, political viewpoints, and historical experiences) impact our worldview and that of our clients, and we should also cultivate our ability to understand how both similarities and differences impact therapeutic work with our clients in complex ways. Through the therapeutic relationship, new relational patterns can be developed; in the next chapter, we consider how the therapeutic relationship itself forms the basis of intervention with adults with early attachment-related trauma.

CHAPTER 4

Reaching across the Abyss

A Relational Approach

*I*f therapy with individuals with problematic attachment patterns hopes to influence such insidious and deeply grooved patterns of relating, the therapist must work actively and experientially within the dynamics that unfold in the therapeutic relationship (Fosha, 2000). Insight is not enough; awareness is not enough; implicit understanding of attachment guiding intervention is not enough. To effectively change relational patterns based on disorganized or insecure attachment requires a unique relational stance, a specific skill set of relational strategies, and the willingness to openly engage oneself in transformational aspects of the therapeutic relationship as a source of change.

CBP'S RELATIONAL STANCE

Therapeutic models vary in the ways therapists view their role in the therapy. Stark (2000) delineates three primary models of therapeutic action that can be defined by the role of the therapist: (1) the interpretive model, (2) the corrective-provision model, and (3) the relational model. The interpretive model emerged from classic psychoanalysis and is characterized as a one-person psychology wherein the therapist's role in therapy is as a neutral object of the client's sexual and aggressive drives. The corrective-provision model is defined as a one-and-a-half person psychology that involves the therapist as good object or good mother. The therapist in this model is an object to hold and meet the client's unmet relational needs. Finally, the contemporary relational model is a two-person psychology involving the therapist as an authentic subject whose focus is the relational engagement between the client and therapist. Stark argues that the therapist must bring her authentic self into the room, or the client may simply be analyzed but not be "found." CBP asserts that the third paradigm—a relational stance—is required to achieve shifts in attachment capacity and that the therapeutic relationship is a central tool for therapeutic change.

Many therapists come out of training with ambivalent understandings of how to deal with the intense and often conflicting needs of clients; many, even more senior therapists, may become frightened or repelled by some behaviors. The therapist may unintentionally push the client away, which leads to hyperarousal as the client tries desperately to hold on or to hypoarousal as she defensively withdraws (see Chapters 5–6). In response to earlier approaches that tended to discourage "needy" behavior in clients and emphasized responding with "neutrality," Dalenberg (2000) emphasized that survivors of childhood abuse interpret neutrality as indifference or hostility and often have difficulty taking in positive regard and quiet, nonverbal expressions of connection by their therapists. She suggests that we need to "shout" our attachment to these clients and "whisper" comments about clients' disturbing and distancing behavior. Steele, van der Hart, and Nijenhuis (2001) describe insecure attachment as an almost inevitable aspect of a chronic childhood abuse history and a period of dependency on the therapist as a necessary aspect of recovery, a "naturalistic occurrence; not only a symptom but the means by which the cure took place" (p. 5).

The requisite relational stance in CBP is committed to authenticity, emotional availability, openness to intimacy, willingness to selectively share affective self-disclosures, and, in the words of Martin Buber (1965), "a bold swinging—demanding the most intensive stirring of one's own being—into the life of the other" (p. 81). Siegel (2007) described this approach as being marked by "the quality of our availability to receive whatever the other brings to us, to sense our own participation in the interaction, and to be aware of our own awareness. We are open to bear witness, to connect, to attune to our [clients'] internal states" (p. 263). Such a stance establishes a relational culture, models and invites deep and genuine connection, and opens the door to reciprocal influence and transformation of both client and therapist. Though not using the same language, the relational psychoanalysts also emphasize the necessity of an intimate relationship between therapist and client. For example, Bromberg (in Chefetz & Bromberg, 2004, p. 425) maintains that "[f]or the deepest growth to take place, patients need to allow themselves to be a 'mess'; within our relationship, and in order for me to truly know them, I had to become a part of the mess in a way that I could experience internally." Fosha's accelerated experiential dynamic psychotherapy (AEDP) (e.g., Fosha, 2000; Fosha, Paivio, Gleiser, & Ford, 2009) draws from psychological theory and neuroscience in its emphasis on the therapeutic relationship as a mechanism for change and its recommendation of specific therapeutic activities that foster trust and confidence in people whose lives have taught them mistrust and doubt in self and others.

Maintaining a stance of openness and engagement often leads therapists to have a strong connection with many clients; in its most intense form, this connection can include feelings of love. In some cases, feelings of love between the client and therapist are a sign of an enactment (see further description later in this chapter). For instance, a client who was abandoned by her biological parents and grew up within the foster care system may dissociate from her intense longing for love and connection. When she experiences a sense of being seen and cared for by her therapist, a young part of her can experience love and gratitude as the therapeutic relationship taps into this unmet need. The therapist may feel drawn in by this younger part of the client, perhaps with a desire to take care of him or her. Similarly, some clients experience confused sexual feelings toward their therapists. In some cases, these sexualized feelings may be held by a young part of the self who has difficulty distinguishing sexuality from intimacy, power, or security. Sometimes, however, these loving feelings do not feel problematic or enactment based and may instead facilitate the therapy (Pearlman & Saakvitne, 1995a). The decision about whether and how to convey these feelings is dependent on careful consideration of the meaning of the communication to all parts of the client and therapist. Although in some cases, it may be appropriate to communicate openly about these feelings because, as Pearlman and Saakvitne (1995a) note, the word *love* often connotes sexual love to parts of the self, terms like "deep caring," "commitment," "strong affection," or "deep fondness" are often used instead and suffice. Even when these feelings are not directly voiced, therapists' strong positive feelings and attachments to particular clients are often "caught" by the client and can contribute to a strong therapeutic alliance.

Present-Moment Relational Attunement, with Contextual Meta-Awareness

For those who have grown up feeling "unseen" and invalidated, the experience of having a witness can be transformative. Empathic attunement occurs when the therapist notices and opens him- or herself up to connecting with all parts of the client (see Chapter 7). It moves beyond simple listening to include an awareness of the client's posture, emotional expression, eye contact, movements, intonation, and other nonverbal cues. Attention is paid to moment-to-moment microshifts in affective, cognitive, or somatic states. The matching of nonverbal rhythms of speech, prosody, and affective arousal are essential allies in applying relational skills with sensitive timing and execution. Brief or not-so-brief therapeutic disruptions or ruptures may occur when therapists become distracted, focusing on issues in their personal lives or something as simple as a phone call that they need to remember to make when the session is over. Therapists may also be pulled out of the present by concerns about themselves in the treatment: "I have no idea how to respond to that"; "Do I sound like I don't know what I'm talking about?"; or as David's therapist Susan thought, "Am I getting in over my head?" We need to be aware of these brief departures so that we can bring ourselves back to a fully present state in the therapeutic interaction. In addition to being aware of multiple aspects of the client's verbal and nonverbal communications in any therapeutic interaction, empathic attunement also requires that therapists work to maintain mindfulness of their own shifting internal states and use this internal experience to further inform themselves about their clients. For instance, Susan is immediately aware of her own emotional disconnection from David and "wonders whether she might be getting an initial glimpse into one aspect of David's dynamic with his wife."

While immersed in what Stern (2004) has termed "the present moment" experience with a client, the therapist must take a relational stance that also moves beyond this in-the-moment experience to include attention to the larger contextual frame. Figure 4.1 depicts the balance between the therapist's present-moment engagement and this "meta-awareness" and how this balance is supported through supervision. For instance, if a client asks for a hug, we need to be aware of not only the verbal request and nonverbal communications from the client and our immediate responses to the request, but also of the larger context. What is the client's experience with touch? What is the client's cultural background, and how does that culture view touch in various contexts? Is there a history of confusing physical and sexual contact? What would a hug mean to this client at this point? Has there been physical contact within the therapy relationship previously? Why is the request coming up now? And, just as importantly, what does this request elicit in us? Does this request evoke fear, ambivalence, or other conflictual emotion? Are there more buried cultural issues stimulated by the request? Are there unresolved questions about our personal boundaries and professional role? Are we prepared for this line of questioning, or does it take us by surprise, and in doing so does it provoke a subtle nonverbal gesture on our part (a contraction in our chair, a hint of apprehension on our face) that serves to affirm our client's belief in his or her fundamental defectiveness, repulsiveness, and unworthiness of love and care from others? Holding these two perspectives simultaneously is a challenging undertaking: the therapist ideally is present and immersed in the current relational moment and, at the same time, maintains a larger perspective on the present moment within the larger backdrop of the client's contextual environment and relational processes over time.

RELATIONAL BALANCE IN CBP

CBP involves a constant process of balancing, both internally and relationally. Several domains impact the relationship between therapist and client, as

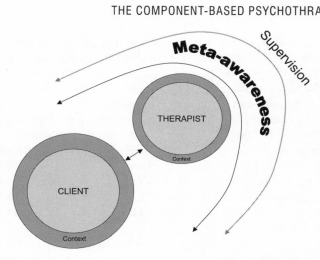

FIGURE 4.1. Present-moment engagement and meta-awareness in the therapeutic relationship.

well as the therapist's and client's own internal experiences, including boundaries, self-disclosure, level of action, "holding" experiences, and meeting clients' needs.

Connection and Maintaining Boundaries

While being open and engaged are essential to CBP's relational approach, structure and consistent, predictable boundaries are also key elements of creating relational safety, particularly for clients who have experienced boundary violations and volatile relationships with caregivers. In CBP, the therapist works to build consistency and predictability by establishing clear boundaries around issues such as protecting the therapy time (including attendance and starting and stopping sessions on time), establishing clear financial agreements, limiting touch, maintaining confidentiality, getting adequate supervision, and making sure self-disclosure is always done in the service of the client. Further supporting this structure, individualized patterns and rituals may be co-created within each therapy relationship. For instance, a man who had historically been very disconnected from his body had recently discovered trauma-sensitive yoga as a means of becoming more self-aware. He and his therapist developed a pattern of beginning and ending each session with a few minutes of chair-based yoga to support emotional containment of the session.

Boundaries in therapy are intended to provide structure and safety, rather than rigid rules, and more flexibility may be needed at certain times or with particular clients. For instance, one young woman had a pattern of showing up late or not coming in when she was relationally triggered in the therapy.

Instead of focusing on her attendance, her therapist invited her to consider this pattern and to wonder together what might have happened before she began pulling away. In another case, a woman who had never been able to feel safe in any apartment or house bought a house and was finally able to create a feeling of "home" for herself and her friends. Although she did not regularly go to clients' homes, the therapist accepted the client's invitation to her house-warming party, recognizing the importance of this transition in their work together; her presence at this event contributed to the client's growing trust in her therapist. Thus, in order to give clients room to learn and grow, these boundaries need to be based on active collaborative decision making specific to each client–therapist dyad and should be adapted based on the changing needs of the therapy over time.

Level of Self-Disclosure

Clinicians vary greatly in their use of personal disclosures about themselves, such as describing aspects of one's personal life or where one is going on vacation. There is a long history of rules about these kinds of self-disclosures, certainly including, if not beginning with, Freud and his injunction that the therapist must be a "blank slate" to the client in order for the transference to develop. However, contrary to these official tenets, analysts' and their patients' lives were often entwined (Malcolm, 1981). Feminist therapists in the 1970s (e.g., Greenspan, 1983; Miller, 1976) began to openly challenge such psycho-analytic rules as "neutrality" and not answer clients' questions about themselves, arguing that these practices increased the already steep difference in power between client and analyst. Instead, they advocated for engaging in a real and mature relationship with the client in sessions, in which it is acceptable for therapists to share aspects of their lives and relevant feelings with clients, as long as what they say is in the service of the clients' healing, rather than serving their own psychological needs. Dalenberg (2000) found that clients generally described therapist self-disclosures as helpful, particularly when they asked for information. CBP holds closer to the feminist perspective and asserts that it is important to have a genuine and relatively mutual relationship, which can involve self-disclosure in the service of helping the client grow and heal. We should be thoughtful about what, when, and why we disclose, weighing the needs of particular clients and being careful that disclosures do not burden clients or interject material irrelevant to their own process.

Early learned lessons about boundaries, sometimes unconscious, can play a role in what is comfortable for each person, including the therapist as well as the client. Negotiating differences in interpersonal styles can be an important aspect of relational therapy. For instance, one client with a particularly painful history of emotional abuse and neglect was able to express her discomfort with the more transparent style of her therapist, whose approach included occasionally offering personal anecdotes. Over their longer-term therapy, this woman and her therapist were able to negotiate a balance around boundaries and self-disclosure, which provided the client with a greater sense of safety but also allowed her the opportunity to gently expand her comfort zone around intimacy in relationships.

The use of personal self-disclosures is a different issue than therapists' affective disclosures regarding the therapeutic relationship. As discussed in the later section on enactments, CBP emphasizes the importance of therapists' sharing their relational experience when working with a client, including acknowledging their own (often initially unconscious) contributions to misattunements and ruptures in the therapy relationship. In this type of affective disclosure, the important question is pacing—when and how much information to share—rather than whether or not to disclose, a question that is more relevant to therapists' disclosures of personal information.

Therapist's and Client's Level of Action

In CBP, there must also be a balance between the level of action of the therapist and client. A common mistake of early career therapists, and not infrequently of more experienced ones as well, is to try to "help," or do too much, to encourage a client to "feel better," or to try to "fix" a distressing situation or emotion. In some situations, the client might just need a witness—someone to be present with them as they sit with a difficult feeling or sensation. When Nicole is distressed by her feelings about herself, Katherine "attempts to offer Nicole words of comfort. Nicole thanks her politely, but there is no shift in her posture or affect." At this point, Katherine must recognize that Nicole is not ready to move away from the distressing affect. Instead, she is struggling to share darker elements of herself. Katherine shows Nicole that she sees her struggle: "Nicole, if this is a moment where you might be trying to begin to share with me how you have been coping with the painful and difficult experiences of isolation and emptiness that you've described so poignantly, how you're able to escape temporarily from the black hole you're in and find your spark, let me know how I can help you do that." This invitation opens the door for Nicole, who replies, "You just did."

An active therapist should be engaged and participatory but must also be aware of the client's need for space to learn to notice her distress, put words to her experiences, and tolerate distressing feelings and somatic states. The therapist often needs to stay out of the way by allowing a narrative to unfold without being directed. When Nicole tells her therapist that, although her husband is controlling, "he's not the problem. The problem is inside me," Katherine "nods her head slightly and waits for Nicole to continue." Recognizing that Nicole is moving closer to the heart of the matter, she allows her the space and time to share her story. Similarly, there is also an important role for silence in therapy, which allows a greater level of right-brain processing of internal states by not requiring that the client try to immediately translate his or her experience into language. Sometimes, however, especially early in therapy, it is too anxiety-arousing for clients to be asked to fill empty spaces without support from their therapist. For example, one woman would freeze when she came into session, filled with anxiety about what to say. After some discussions, her therapist learned to help her with the question, "What are you feeling right now?" which helped her to orient to her body and emotions and provided the containment that allowed her to begin. The therapist also offered a structure that invited moments of silence and reflection. For instance, she might say, "It seems like a feeling is welling up right now. Do you want to take a few minutes just to notice that?"

Extent to Which the Therapist "Holds" the Client's Feelings and Experiences

In CBP, balance is also required in the extent to which the therapist "holds" emotions, memories, and hope for the client, in contrast to asking them to begin to hold their own experiences and memories. When clients are unable to tolerate the intensity of certain experiences or feelings, they may dissociate, with these experiences or feelings being held by a part of themselves (see Chapter 7). Remembering what clients have shared, often when they don't remember, is one important way that therapists can help to build continuity and connection for their clients. A therapist may, for example, maintain awareness of what he has learned about his client's life experiences when the client begins to repeat a common relational pattern. Another therapist may remember what has happened from session to session, despite her client's sense of disorientation.

It is not uncommon for a therapist to experience strong emotional reactions from which a client is dissociated. For instance, one therapist found herself feeling enraged with the father of a young transgender client for severe emotional and physical abuse, while the client expressed only gratitude toward her father for making her stronger. With supervision, this therapist realized that the intensity of her reaction was linked to her client's dissociated pain and anger toward her father.

When despairing parts of clients are dominant, and when being hopeful is perceived as dangerous by many parts of the self, one role for the therapist is quietly or implicitly to hold the hope for them, without asking them to hold it. For example, a therapist might say to such a despairing client that she can understand his despair and how difficult it is to feel, even though she doesn't have similar feelings about his future. The timing of when to begin to gently encourage clients to take ownership of their own feelings can be complex. When a therapist recognizes that she seems to be "holding" a client's feelings, she may share her reaction and gently inquire whether part of the client may be experiencing this feeling. If the client is adamant that no part of him has that feeling, the therapist should not insist but should instead become more consciously aware of these reactions in herself and revisit the conversation with her client at a later time to see if the client is able to tolerate this reflection.

Degree to Which the Therapist Seeks to Meet the Client's Needs

Some clients want and/or need a great deal of support from their therapists at various points in their therapy, and therapists' comfort with such needs and requests can differ based on temperament, training, and life situation, to name a few factors. From the perspective of CBP, such dependence is neither surprising nor necessarily problematic. It is, of course, important for clients to continue to make use of their attachment figures in the world outside of therapy to get support, and therapy should support clients in sustaining good relationships and developing new supportive ones. However, many people with histories of emotional abuse and neglect come to treatment without adequate support and sometimes without any supportive connections at all. At times, clients might need increased concrete supports. For instance, a young woman showing signs of hypomania was placed on a mood stabilizer, but she became increasingly emotionally dysregulated, had confused thinking, and asked her therapist to help her figure out what to do. Her therapist supported her by providing containment and co-regulation but also helped her to call forth additional resources and to communicate clearly with her medical providers. This concrete assistance helped her to stabilize and to access more resourced parts of herself.

It is important to be aware of how a client's relational style impacts the concrete and emotional needs that she conveys. On one hand, a client's progress may be stalled when a part of her is fearful that if she becomes too independent, the therapist will not continue to care for her or will abandon her. On the other hand, clients with an avoidant attachment style may convey such a strong sense of autonomy and rejection of help that a therapist may back away rather than gently challenge this style. Many people who were maltreated during childhood have a strong ambivalence about their emotional needs, where one part of them desires connection, while another part is fearful of feelings of dependency.

For many clients with early emotional abuse and neglect, younger parts of the client want to be taken care of as they never were during childhood. The therapeutic relationship fills a vital role here, providing a safe, consistent, authentic, and caring relationship. At the same time, as therapists, we need to be clear about our own limitations around our availability in order to take care of ourselves and our need for time with family and friends, recreation, exercise, and the like. How much accessibility we can offer depends on our stage in life, health and energy, personal styles, and demands on our time, among other things. It is important to note that there is nothing wrong or pathological about the client's needs; these needs are a normal result of growing up in an unsupportive or abusive environment. Although therapists often struggle with this issue, it is also important to recognize that there is nothing wrong or selfish about a therapist not being able to provide everything the client needs.

Because the therapist cannot satisfy all of the client's unmet emotional needs, it is important to actively negotiate the structure of the therapy so that it works for both client and therapist. This often involves helping the client find additional resources for support, such as a therapy group or yoga class, and helping them develop friendships that are healthy and can provide support. It can also involve conversations about the therapist's own need for self-care, so that the therapist can continue to be available to the client in their work together. For instance, the therapist may say something like: "There is nothing wrong or abnormal with your need for more support, and right now it is exceeding my comfort level. We need to find a way for you to manage these distressing periods that does not require quite as much out-of-session contact as we are now having." Clients—and often therapists—dread these conversations, but they can be very constructive, beyond dealing with the immediate issue. Some clients respond by saying, "Part of me is saying I will never call/email you again!" to which the therapist might say, "I can understand that part of you feeling that way, but I think it would be unfortunate for our work because sometimes these calls and emails seem to be very helpful to you. Let's see how it goes." Sometimes a month may go by without such extra-session contacts, and then one will occur again, usually more disciplined and restrained or shorter. The therapist responds comfortably and supportively. A new step in the relationship has been achieved in which both client and therapist can honor and respect each other's needs.

EXPLORING ENACTMENTS

Imagine that, after becoming sidetracked by concerns about David's daughter, Susan notices a moment of disconnection with David. She says, "I noticed that you just looked down when I wondered whether your daughter might be feeling out of control because of the lack of rules in the house. I'm curious how it felt to you when I said that?" David looks interested but is not able to respond verbally. Susan makes a tentative attempt to put language to David's nonverbal communication, pondering, "I wonder if it felt like I was blaming you when I said that?" David makes eye contact, with a wrinkling of his forehead and a slight tearing in his eyes. Susan goes on, "It's really important that you're able to open up about what's going on without feeling judged, huh?"

In this hypothetical example, Susan is able to notice and immediately repair a brief disruption, or an enactment. These types of interactions are inevitable, given the early attachment experiences of these clients and the fact that trauma therapy often stirs up old and painful experiences that have been held outside of the client's conscious awareness. CBP views enactments as providing important therapeutic opportunities for reworking relational patterns. In considering enactments, we are indebted to McCann and Pearlman (1990) who, although they use different terminology, present a rich discussion of how therapist responses can trigger clients and how the therapist might deal with these events.

What Are Enactments?

Relational strategies often include a more explicit focus on the therapeutic relationship, incorporating a strong experiential component into the work. Children whose caregivers are busy, absent, belittling, intrusive, and/or otherwise hurtful have difficulty understanding what is happening to them or expressing their emotions about it. Instead, their emotional response is confused, jumbled, and often dissociated. The pull of desire for nurturance and love is at war with their need to withdraw to safety. As adults, they may have had years of practice pushing the hurt and anger aside or blaming themselves or others. Recognition of how entrenched emotional patterns crop up in the therapeutic relationship is central to CBP, as is recognition of new, healthier patterns being co-created.

Enactments, dissociated or partially dissociated interactions between client and therapist, are a point of intersection between the relationship (this section) and parts components of CBP (see Chapters 7–8). In an enactment, an exchange within the therapy is triggering to a part of the client or therapist, leading them to respond in a way that set off some part of the other, and so on in a cyclical fashion until the enactment is interrupted and ideally recognized and repaired. In the moment, the therapist may notice feeling suddenly confused, helpless, or silenced, as may the client; each may wonder how they arrived at this point of hurt, frustration, desperation, or alienation within the relationship.

The concept of enactments is borrowed from modern relational psychoanalytic thinking, which has moved away from the traditional psychoanalytic concepts of transference and countertransference originally described by Freud (described at length in Pearlman & Saakvitne, 1995a). These old psychoanalytic terms apply to the unconscious and irrational feelings the client has for the therapist and then to the often unconscious and sometimes irrational feelings the therapist has in response to the client's transference, which was an illustrious step toward understanding the interactive nature of relational psychotherapy. However, in our view, the term "enactment" seems to better capture the intersubjective reality that is created between therapists and clients in these exchanges.

Leaders in the attachment field have formulated enactments as nonconscious, procedural ways of relating to another, built on early attachment relationships (Bowlby, 1973, 1980, 1982; Howell, 2005; Lyons-Ruth, 1999). Both therapists and clients have nonconscious and nonverbalized ways of relating to others, including protective and defensive maneuvers related to their early attachment figures' own ways of protecting themselves. Bromberg (1998, 2009) has focused his entire distinguished career on integrating trauma theory and therapy with modern relational psychoanalysis. He describes enactment as the process in which a dissociative part of the therapist or the client evokes a dissociative part in the other. In these dissociative places, therapists and clients do something that involves a part of each seeing in the other something that comes from their own psyche, and that matches in their mutual dissociative states, "an intrapsychic phenomenon that is played out interpersonally" (2009, p. 647). According to Bromberg and others (e.g., Chefetz & Bromberg, 2004), deep change in clients occurs primarily through the processing of enactments. bad/good.

Utilizing Enactments in Therapy

As we have described, CBP emphasizes the importance of the therapist's meta-awareness, of the larger context and the relational "story behind the story." Because of entrenched trauma-driven relational patterns, often multiple opportunities arise to work through enactments in therapeutic work with adults who have experienced early emotional abuse or neglect. In order to utilize these enactments as therapeutic moments, the therapist tracks and verbalizes moment-to-moment fluctuations in the relational field of connection and disconnection. Working with enactments requires therapist affective self-disclosure in which the therapist thoughtfully shares elements of her own emotional experience within a therapeutic encounter (Fosha & Slowiaczek, 1997). Without such attention to therapeutic self-examination, we are bound to slip unaware into enactment and for that moment become one of the many historical Others the client carries, reinforcing previously held beliefs about relationships. In contrast, through repeated achievement of mindful, attuned, therapeutic encounters in which our clients feel seen and validated, and in which we can reflect on and share our own internal process, we begin to create a relational narrative (and with it new neural pathways) that is different from the interpersonal patterns they have learned to expect.

In a subtle example of an enactment that was identified and repaired within a relatively short time, a long-term client came to the session indicating strong feelings, which was not atypical of him. His therapist had just looked at his notes from the previous session and been reminded that there was something he wanted to raise with the client early in the session. Ignoring the client's strong emotions, he asked about this previous issue. The client had trouble responding to the question and after a few minutes said, uncomfortably, "I'm still struggling with the feelings I had when I walked in." The therapist, realizing that he had dismissed the client's evident distress, apologized and now asked about it. The client was immediately able to talk with coherence and affect about a difficult phone conversation he had just had. The therapist quickly reviewed in his own mind why he had ignored his client's feelings, which was unusual for him, and realized that a part of him was tired and was avoidant of the dark feelings this client often brought to therapy. The therapist realized he had to be mindful of those feelings through the session, and the two of them were able to reconnect.

In a more blatant enactment in long-term therapy, Erin came into a session furious with her 13-year-old daughter. While this was not new, at the beginning of the session she was entirely in an enraged state as she described this "worthless, selfish, hateful" girl. The therapist was aware of her own tendency to overidentify with clients' children as a result of her history of childhood mistreatment. However, she was caught off guard by Erin's unmodulated rage and found herself instantly responding with feelings of bitterness and resentment. The therapist did not know why but tried to keep her intense anger from spilling over into the work. Of course, it did, though not blatantly. Finally, the therapist was able to acknowledge that something important was happening between them and that she felt angry and did not know why or what to do about it at the moment. Erin shared that she had perceived this anger, which felt awful. They sat together with this mutual acknowledgment, eventually able to reflect on it verbally. In a much more connected way, Erin's therapist expressed feeling bad about her reaction and said that she would talk to her peer supervision group about it. At that point, right at the end of the session, Erin began to sob and cried for about 5 minutes.

Through consultation, the therapist realized that a younger part of herself had been triggered and had mistaken a part of Erin for the whole. Furthermore, she saw that whole as a terrible, abusive mother rather than a young part of a mother who actually was doing quite a good job, given all things, with her daughter. When the therapist shared that she had been responding from a part of herself, Erin asked, "Does that mean we can't go any further?" The therapist acknowledged it as a valid question but said no, now that she was aware of it and actively working with her therapist on this issue, they would be able to continue. And they did. That was a full-blown enactment, with both client and therapist fully involved. The process of repair took a number of sessions but led to a deepening of their relationship, as they saw each other in new ways.

Approach- or Avoidance-Oriented Enactments

Relational enactments can be seen as approach-oriented, avoidance-oriented, or both. The approach-oriented interactions are attempts to seek out a relationship and sometimes involve boundary confusion. One example is a client who attempts to take care of her therapist, as in, "How are you feeling this week? I was worried about you last week. Your voice sounded scratchy. You should really be taking extra vitamin C." This protective stance toward a therapist can extend to a concern about the therapist's emotional state, leaving clients reluctant to share "too much" because of concerns about overwhelming their therapist. Attempts to please are not uncommon among people who have experienced early interpersonal trauma. As a child, Nicole was "quiet, obedient, and generally unnoticed—an all-around 'good girl'." We see reflections of this childhood state in Nicole's approach to her therapist, when she attempts to please Katherine and then looks to her for approval.

Some clients experience anxious ruminations about their therapists, such as, "Did she think I stayed too long?" or "Did he feel offended that I paid by credit card this week instead of check?" There can also be role and boundary confusion, such as when a client feels a desire to have a friendship or romantic relationship with the therapist. These desires suggest a need for intimate connection with an Other, which may be expressed as a wish for a sexual relationship with the therapist but often actually comes from much younger parts who long for intimacy and, because of their early history, do not know other ways of expressing it. When there is a deep internal sense of emptiness or isolation, it may be difficult to somatically, cognitively, or emotionally experience this sense of connection, leading clients to seek greater and greater amounts of contact. Clients may seek out multiple meetings per week, call or email extensively, or express high levels of distress, all in an attempt to feel connected to their therapist. From the therapist's standpoint, approach-oriented enactments can involve constantly thinking about a particular client, having a desire to take care of or to save a client, or allowing boundaries to become too porous.

In a common example of avoidance-oriented enactments, the client's way of being in the world is to keep things pleasant and free of conflict or confrontation. Perhaps his early experience taught him that he had to comply to be accepted. He is often very pleasant to sit with and may be subtly or overtly complimentary to the therapist. He wants to be close, but he is fearful of showing all the parts of himself, leaving him in a chronic state of alienation because he is not known or seen by the Other. The therapist, herself reluctant to "make waves" in these nice exchanges and possibly herself preferring pleasant conversation to confrontation, goes along with the client's implicit request to "keep things nice." Therapies like this can proceed for a long time, but likely nothing much of use is happening. Sometimes supervisors can note the lack of substantial work and help the therapist see that some respectful confrontations are important, and indeed necessary, for the work to move to a deeper level.

Avoidance-oriented enactments involve creating distance or withdrawing from a relationship, which Pearlman and Saakvitne (1995a) describe as defensive maneuvers. A client may discount therapy as a useful experience, such as when David questioned why he was even attending therapy in the first place. Clients may be unwilling to consider relational issues in the therapy, as in, "I am just here for a service. This is a business transaction. I pay you, and you have to listen to me." Some clients will attend therapy sporadically or cancel meetings when they are dealing with difficult material or when they need more distance in the therapeutic relationship. People may also consciously or unconsciously use excessive verbalizations and storytelling to create distance from relatedness or deeper emotional experiencing. From the therapist's perspective, she may notice herself losing track of what a client is saying, feeling shut down, dreading an approaching therapy session, or feeling emotionally distant or judgmental about a client. These are signs that an enactment is occurring.

Enactments Reflecting Ambivalence

Some enactments reflect a push–pull in the relational field. For instance, expressions of anger and disappointment can reflect both the need for closeness and the fear of it. "You weren't there for me" may mean both "I don't trust you" and "I want you to be there for me." On one hand, expressions of suicidal ideation can also have complex relational meanings. Suicidal ideation may reflect hopelessness and an intention to withdraw from a relationship with self and Other and from life. On the other hand, expressions of suicidal ideation can be attempts to seek connection: "I need you to see that I am in excruciating pain." While, ideally, the therapist would be able to listen to his client's feelings of distress in a grounded, centered way, and then help the client to increase safety if needed, this is not always the response to such a high-stakes scenario. In mutual enactments, the therapist may respond to expressions of suicidal ideation through intense anxiety and an attempt to "solve" the problem, often by engaging in a suicide risk assessment and relying on hospitalization. Of course, risk assessment is extremely important at times, and connecting clients with a higher level of care is vital when needed, but sometimes these strategies are applied rigidly and more out of fears of liability and following rules and procedures than out of true risk of harm. Alternatively, some therapists may respond to their anxiety through rejection and withdrawal, rationalizing that "she says this all the time."

When the Therapist Initiates the Enactment

Susan initiated an enactment when she forgot to tell David ahead of time about her upcoming vacation and then tried to minimize the effects of this oversight on him. When Susan returned from her week away, David did return but was very reticent, expressing little emotion and avoiding eye contact. Part of Susan wanted to pretend nothing had happened, but supervision had helped her to become clear that she needed to raise the issue. When she initially brings it up, David doesn't meet her gaze and mumbles something about it not having been important. He says he has been wondering if the therapy is actually useful to him. Susan tells him she was thinking about him and that particular session while on her vacation and thinks she really blew it when she forgot to tell him ahead of time. She says she knows it possibly caused parts of him considerable distress, and she is sorry. Susan also asks if he would like to hear what she now understands was going on in her mind that led her to forget. He sits forward in his chair; he wants to know.

Susan tells David that during the week when she was telling clients she would be away, she had a vague sense of dread about telling him. She was aware that she and the therapy had become more important to him over the 6 months of their meetings, and she was feeling protective of him, but she also was afraid of disappointing him. So parts of her were stirred up in ways that led her to "forget" that she had not informed him. Susan then asked, "What is that like for you to hear?" David tells her he is greatly relieved to hear it; he has never encountered anyone in his life who was willing to take responsibility for doing something hurtful to him. He is then able to tell her just how difficult the week was for him, how unimportant he felt he was to her. She commiserates, and they then discuss other times he has felt alone and abandoned.

Therapeutic enactments offer particularly fertile ground for reworking repeated relational experiences. In their seminal work on infant development, Tronick and Weinberg (1997) reveal that, within primary attachment relationships, the key to healthy child development is the caregivers' ability to repair errors they make in interactions with their babies, rather than their ability to achieve constant attunement. As trauma-focused therapists treating adult survivors of chronic emotional abuse and neglect, we serve a belated but not dissimilar function. The therapeutic relationship can be a practice ground for reworking enactments of past injuries by addressing them "in the moment" and co-creating different outcomes. This current-day emotional experience can help clients to build empathy for the child that they were as well as the part of themselves that still feels like a hurt child. The therapeutic relationship is a safe place for exploring these vulnerable emotions of hurt, rage, and despair.

These encounters are not always easy for the therapist. In order to establish new relational patterns, the therapist must be able to acknowledge and explore their own missteps in the therapeutic relationship. We are fallible and should not expect to be perfect therapists. The good news is that interactive errors offer the possibility of working through conflict in connection and the opportunity to safely grapple with relational issues.

Ongoing Enactments

Clients who relentlessly project large amounts of their dark feelings and thoughts onto their therapists create a kind of ongoing enactment. This process is what some analysts call projective identification (e.g., Sands, 1997; Schore, 2003b), a term that has come to have many different meanings and implications (e.g., Ogden, 1979). In this type of ongoing enactment, a client perceives in her therapist the dissociated characteristics she cannot tolerate experiencing in herself. From the very beginning of therapy, she may display deep, angry, and critical views of the therapist, which seem to occur regardless of the personality or style of the actual therapist. Because many survivors of child maltreatment are acutely attuned to subtle psychological shifts in their therapist, their attacks are often directed toward vulnerable aspects of the therapist, whether it be their appearance, their inexperience as a therapist, their manifest anxiety, their perceived poor performance as a therapist, or some other characteristics about which the therapist is sensitive. Such repeated intense negative attacks are often difficult for the therapist to withstand without becoming defensive, angry, frightened, avoidant, and/or in some way retaliatory. When the therapist is repeatedly or chronically triggered within the therapy relationship in this way, it becomes a mutual enactment.

In such situations, therapists' sharing their own experience of the relationship can sometimes lead to increased dysregulation and conflict. In these enactments, the clients are filled with such dark and difficult feelings that they cannot bear to hold them within themselves, but need someone nearby to hold these feelings for them and to tolerate being seen in this way by the client, without retaliating. This is not an easy therapeutic task because being attacked and criticized in these ways evokes a variety of negative feelings in the therapist, who must find a way to hold the feelings, with support from supervisors or colleagues. If a therapist can do this long enough for the client to be able to begin to tolerate seeing that these feelings and characteristics are, in fact, their own, then these therapies can survive and flourish.

SUPERVISION AND THE RELATIONSHIP COMPONENT OF CBP

Because of CBP's emphasis on the often complex interpersonal dynamics within the therapist/client dyad as a means of therapeutic change, supervision is essential to support and reflect on this relational process (see Figure 4.1). Ideally, the supervisory relationship will parallel efforts of the therapeutic relationship to build safety, mutual respect, transparency, consistency, predictability, attunement, and clear boundaries. Open discussions about each person's past supervisory experiences, current hopes for supervision, therapy experience, training and conceptualizations of treatment, expectations about boundaries, and growing edges may help to establish safety in the supervisory relationship. Depending on the setting, there may be tension between supportive and evaluative roles of the supervisor, which should be openly explored. CBP supervision should provide a "holding" environment that supports the therapist in tolerating very intense traumatic content, emotional expression, and interpersonal dynamics. CBP supervisors refine the art of conveying insights and corrective feedback in ways that are uniquely accessible to each supervisee, often through a reflective process that draws on the supervisor's experience but also invites the therapist to collaboratively explore the issue. A supervisor may highlight a parallel process of an interaction between herself and her supervisee in order to inform dynamics that are occurring in the therapeutic relationship or in the client's other relationships. Through these means, supervision provides a place to reflect on therapeutic issues such as pacing and the capacity of the therapeutic bond to safely hold intense experience, intimacy, boundaries within the therapeutic relationship, and enactments.

Various therapeutic enactments can lead to ruptures within the therapy relationship (Chu, 2001), and supervision can be used to explore these interactions and the therapist's unconscious processes that may be contributing to the enactment. Table 4.1 offers some examples of comments and questions in supervision that may help to identify and/or explore enactments in the therapy. A clearer recognition and understanding of the unconscious dynamics within the interaction can support the therapist's ability to regulate and to intentionally share aspects of her experience of an interaction, such as, "I felt really pained when you treated me as though I could never understand." In one instance, a therapist was becoming increasingly frustrated as her client asked repeatedly to change their appointment time, but was trying to contain her emotions. This resulted in her unintentionally disengaging from her client. After reflecting on this process in supervision, she was able to share her reaction with her client: "I felt frustrated when you asked me to rearrange my schedule again. I was feeling worried that I was valuing our work together more than you were, and I noticed that I was starting to pull back a little. I wonder if I created some distance between us by not letting you know how I was experiencing this." In a more complicated example that acknowledges dissociated parts of both client and therapist, one therapist shared her complex reaction to an encounter: "I feel a little upset because you promised a young part of you that you would discuss her pain after you finished telling me about the doctor's appointment, and then you decided not to. There is a part of me that feels very protective of that young part of you that has been unheard" (see Chapters 7 and 8).

Three-Way Enactments

Nicole has a history of identifying potential "rescuers" in her life who ultimately disappoint her. She recalled pleading with her supportive, though often absent, father not to leave for business trips. During her teen years, Nicole's aunt rescued her from the fear, sorrow, and shame in her childhood household. However, after her aunt moved away, their relationship changed and "the spark wasn't there anymore." Filling this void, Nicole's husband Antonio initially excited and impressed her when he "took charge" of planning for their future together. However, her husband's passion for her was gradually redirected toward his work and their children, leaving her feeling abandoned

TABLE 4.1. Use of Supervision for Identifying and Addressing Enactments

Enactment/rupture	Triggered/dissociated response	Reflection in supervision
Inattention	You don't care about me	Was your attention drawn to something else, or were you reacting to something happening in the room?
Absences	Abandonment	How did you feel when [your client] got angry about you going away? Thoughts? Body reactions?
Lack of consistency or follow-through (missed appointments, didn't call when you said you would)	I can't trust you	What was happening with you in between when you said that you would call [your client] later that day and when you got her crisis call? How did you react when [your client] _____?
Lack of attunement (got it wrong)	You don't understand me, I'm unseen/invisible	What were you noticing in [your client] at the time? Is there anything, looking back on it, that you think you might have missed?
Trying to "fix" it; solution-oriented	You don't want to hear it; I'm not okay/you don't accept me	What is it like for you to sit with [your client's] distress/feelings of helplessness?
Attention to protocol (e.g., safety, paperwork) versus client	You don't care about me/you're covering yourself	Did you feel a conflict in between [your client] and following the protocol?
Involvement of systems (CPS, law enforcement)	You're controlling me	How did you feel as you were making the decision to involve the system? How did you include [your client] in this process? How did you react when she got angry?
Feeling stagnant, disconnection	Helplessness/hopelessness/This isn't working	It seems like you're feeling some of the same feelings she is.
Strong emotional reaction	I don't want pity/It's not safe to feel this	What do think happened when she shut down after you got teary?
Overidentification (we're the same)	I need to act like _____ to be accepted/okay	[Your client] always seems to act in ways that make you comfortable/feel good. I wonder if there are any other parts of her that she isn't showing.
Pull to rescue	I need you to survive.	I'm noticing that you often feel pulled to intervene when she's struggling with something.

again. There was no resolution to these perceived abandonments by her rescuers. A similar dynamic is reenacted in her therapy relationship.

As Nicole enters therapy with Katherine, she is initially apprehensive but experiences a wave of relief when she feels that Katherine quickly understands and accepts her. We may wonder if she also experiences Katherine as a "good mother" or as a person who might be able to "rescue" her from herself. Nicole develops a sense of hopefulness about the therapeutic relationship and begins to open up about her "big dark secret" self. However, after a couple of months, when Nicole uses the main character of *Pretty Woman* as a resource and "looks up at [Katherine] for approval," Katherine instead rejects her chosen internal resource, resulting in a therapeutic rupture. Nicole "internally collapses" and feels "devastated." She no longer experiences Katherine as a rescuer or even as a helper. Instead, Katherine is, at best, a helpless bystander who is unable to help a person who is so "shattered, freakish, alien." At worst, she experiences Katherine as a perpetrator or as a repetition of her "bad mother" and is crushed by "the subtle expression of disapproval and judgment on Katherine's face." This episode ultimately "triggers in Nicole a terrible sense first of aloneness and then of profound emptiness." If Nicole left therapy at this moment, her relational experience in therapy would be a simple repetition of past relational experiences, reinforcing her perception that "people hurt you" and that "I am bad and unlovable."

In this example, there is a three-way avoidance-oriented enactment between Nicole, Katherine, and Katherine's supervisor. As she later realizes, Katherine's rejection of this figure parallels her implicit rejection of Nicole's "bad side," which conflicts with Katherine's need to feel successful as a therapist. Nicole's part of the enactment is to avoid talking about her feelings and to back away from Katherine and from the therapy by avoiding all difficult or intense topics. Katherine responds by not acknowledging or raising the potentially difficult question about what was happening in the therapy, despite it seeming to be stuck. We can speculate that Nicole's emotional withdrawal and implicit shift in her perception of Katherine may have further threatened Katherine's self-perception as a good therapist; her avoidance of raising these issues may be driven by the need to be perceived in a positive light by her supervisor. In a parallel process, Katherine's supervisor was also part of the enactment when she waited quite a long time before she shared her thoughts and feelings about Katherine's style that were related to the enactment.

Once the supervisor broached this difficult issue, it opened up the system's ability to recognize and shift the enactment. Through supervision, Katherine is able to understand how her own need to see herself as "good"— a good person, good partner, good therapist—may have interfered with her ability to fully see and understand Nicole. Her ability to acknowledge this misstep to Nicole offers an opportunity to change the "ending" of their relational encounter. For Nicole, the meaning of this interaction shifts from "people hurt you" to "sometimes I will feel hurt in relationships, but that doesn't necessarily mean that the relationship is damaged or that it is over." This enactment also offered the opportunity for Katherine to grow as a therapist and a person, in her ability to acknowledge and accept her own foibles and to have more authentic relationships.

THERAPEUTIC RELATIONSHIP OVER TIME

As is evident from the discussion thus far, an essential characteristic of therapist–client relationships is that they change over time. Although this work rarely proceeds in a linear manner, ideally, the relationship deepens over time; the client is able to share more dissociated material and can work on it without major periods of dysregulation; the client begins to take more responsibility for the work and the relationship; and the client begins to see the therapist more as an actual person and less as a fantasy figure based on projection. How long this change takes depends greatly on the client, the therapist, and the quality of their relationship. Some clients can do an important piece of work in three or four sessions, as can happen in a consultation or an evaluation, many in a year or less, and some in a few years. Others may continue to struggle, although they may well see some improvement in their lives and a reduction in symptoms. Clients' internal and external resources to support the work, as well as their motivation for this kind of endeavor, vary widely and make a great deal of difference in their healing process.

Long-term therapies in particular, but also shorter treatments, can be greatly impacted by events in clients' or therapists' lives. For example, if either has a baby, gets married or divorced, becomes ill, or suddenly needs to care for an ailing family member, there can be a significant effect on the relationship. In many cases, ruptures and repairs over the course of the therapeutic relationship provide much fodder for progress in CBP.

CONCLUSION

When using the CBP model, a relational stance is central. We must work to cultivate a general relational approach that promotes authenticity, openness to intimacy, warmth, empathetic attunement, and a willingness to selectively disclose. A particularly challenging skill is the ability to simultaneously be immersed in the present-moment experience, with full attention to the nuances of our own and our client's experience and the interactions between us, while also "holding" the larger context. This larger context may include our client's historical life experiences, our own worldview and "hot" buttons, and the course of the therapy over time. In negotiating the therapeutic relationship, we must strive for a balance between achieving connection and maintaining boundaries, in our level of self-disclosure, in negotiation of intimacy and strong feelings between us and our clients, in our level of action as compared to those of our clients, in how much we "hold" our clients' feelings versus asking them to hold them, and in the degree to which we seek to meet our clients' needs.

As we become increasingly aware of (at least partially) dissociated reactions in ourselves and our clients that are driving difficult or complicated interactions in the therapy, we can begin to gently name and explore the roots of these interactions. By actively exploring enactments, we can interrupt a pattern of traumatic reenactment for our clients, creating a new pattern through open acknowledgment and repair of relational ruptures. This process supports the development of relational capacity in adults who have experienced early attachment trauma, building tolerance for interpersonal tension, the ability to communicate about internal experience and interpersonal connections, and more effective skills for reengagement in a relationship following a rupture.

Table 4.2 summarizes the major foci of CBP within the relationship component for the client, therapist, and supervisor, including experiential elements of treatment that occur within the therapeutic relationship. In the next section, we explore the regulation component of CBP, highlighting the importance of regulation in trauma work and describing a variety of regulatory tools that can be applied within the CBP approach.

TABLE 4.2. Intervention Strategies for the Relationship Component of CBP

Client
- Establishing a relational stance; maintaining empathic attunement
- Offering a consistent, predictable, safe relationship
- Building awareness of attachment style and implications for relational patterns
- Developing relational skills, such as communication, attunement, assertiveness, problem solving, and boundary setting; practicing in the context of the therapeutic relationship to generalize to other relationships
- Learning through therapeutic ruptures and repairs

Therapist
- Maintaining present-moment relational attunement and engagement while concurrently developing meta-awareness of the client's and therapist's individual processes and interaction patterns
- Developing balance in regard to boundaries, self-disclosure, level of action, "holding" experiences, and meeting clients' needs
- Understanding our own attachment style(s) and relational patterns and how these impact the therapeutic process
- Exploring the ways in which cultural and other contextual factors influence worldviews of the client and therapist and impact the therapeutic process

Supervisor
- Providing a holding environment for the therapist and the therapy itself
- Reflecting on parallel processes (between client's relationships, the therapeutic relationship, and the supervisory relationship)

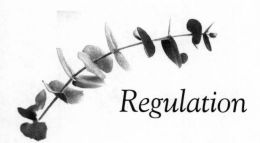

Regulation

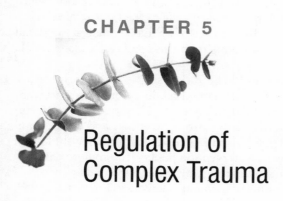

CHAPTER 5

Regulation of Complex Trauma

Nicole's early descriptions to Katherine emphasize her limited ability both to manage her lifelong experiences of pain and to regulate her drive toward impulsive, guilt-ridden affairs. As Katherine thinks about the work they will be doing together, she is very mindful that helping Nicole learn to regulate her various difficult feelings will be one of their first tasks. In this chapter, we discuss the essential role of regulation in CBP.

IMPORTANCE OF SELF-REGULATION IN TRAUMA TREATMENT

Perhaps the greatest legacy of Judith Herman's (1992b) seminal book, *Trauma and Recovery*, was its contribution to clinicians' understanding of the pivotal role of emotion regulation in treatment with adult survivors of childhood relational violence, neglect, and betrayal. Virtually all treatment development and outcome research on the complexity of adaptation to trauma in adults has stemmed directly from her initial delineation—and the field's subsequent elaboration and expansion (van der Kolk et al., 1996b)—of primary phases of intervention with this highly impacted and exquisitely vulnerable group of trauma survivors. A full two decades later, the body of systematic clinical research in support of these formative conceptual models has finally attained the level of evidence needed for both the World Health Organization and the International Society for Traumatic Stress Studies (ISTSS) to formally recognize CPTSD as a veritable and distinct diagnosis. The World Health Organization has done so in its forthcoming update to the International Classification of Diseases (ICD-11), whereas the ISTSS has promulgated official guidelines for treatment of adults suffering from this condition (Cloitre et al., 2012).

At the heart of these advances has been the establishment of the necessity for treatment with complexly traumatized adults to enhance survivors' capacity for self-regulation: namely, their ability to identify, tolerate, modulate, and express states of internal arousal and perception and their consequent behavioral impulses. This recognition represents a major shift from prior conceptualizations of trauma intervention predicated on more narrowly focused, brief treatment protocols that embark more immediately on exposure, desensitization, and processing of traumatic memories (Brom et al., 1989; Foa, Rothbaum, Riggs, & Murdock, 1991). Rather, this paradigm shift has led to an understanding that effective treatment of CPTSD must typically place initial and often greatest emphasis on the cultivation of key functional capacities for self-regulation, as well as the bolstering of emotional, relational, and psychological competencies.

Marylene Cloitre's contributions have been at the core of the small but important body of empirical literature examining the role of emotion regulation in the treatment of complex trauma. In her research, Cloitre succeeded in verifying the intricate relationship among therapeutic alliance, affect regulation, and reduction of PTSD in adult survivors of complex trauma (Cloitre et al., 2004). Specifically, she found that negative mood regulation mediates the relationship between therapeutic alliance and reduction of PTSD in adults with histories of complex childhood trauma. What precisely do these findings mean for clinical practice with complexly traumatized adults? In Chapter 3, we underscored Cloitre's observation that the strength of the therapeutic relationship is predictive of the ultimate success of trauma processing for adult women with histories of complex childhood trauma. Unpacking her findings further here, we see that the relation between therapeutic alliance and trauma symptom reduction is at least partially mediated by gains in the survivor's capacity to regulate negative mood. Translating these findings into the language of clinical practice, we learn that the act of establishing a strong therapeutic alliance is a necessary, but not sufficient, condition in the treatment of complexly traumatized adults. Specifically, the therapeutic relationship appears to function as a vital containing structure for these highly vulnerable individuals within which the capacity for self-regulation can finally be safely cultivated, felt, and put into practice. Moreover, these capacities must take root before clients with histories of chronic and complex childhood deprivation and maltreatment can tolerate and make use of other aspects of trauma-focused treatment, such as memory processing, meaning-making, or life narrative development, which are commonly referred to collectively as "Phase 2" of trauma intervention (Cloitre et al., 2013; Herman, 1992b).

Building on this formative research, other studies have demonstrated the relative merits of interventions for complex trauma survivors that focus on aspects of emotional awareness and regulation, such as mindfulness and affect management, prior to or instead of prolonged exposure or memory processing (Ford, Steinberg, & Zhang, 2011; Zlotnick et al., 1997). Most notably, in the only published randomized controlled trial consisting of a head-to-head comparison of a regulation-focused versus exposure-based treatment for adult complex trauma survivors, Cloitre and colleagues (2010) found that adult women with histories of complex child sexual abuse responded best to a phase-based sequence of regulation-focused treatment followed by exposure therapy. They responded second best to treatment involving regulation skill-building alone and worst to intervention consisting exclusively of exposure-focused therapy. It is perhaps not surprising, then, that in a subsequent international expert survey on best practices in complex trauma intervention for which an equal number of classic PTSD researchers as complex trauma scholars (including two of the authors of this book) were selected to participate as content-matter experts, emotion-focused and affect-regulation strategies were the only forms of intervention that received across-the-board, first-line ratings in effectiveness, safety, and acceptability (Cloitre et al., 2011).

This compelling body of research and expert consensus raises important questions about what emotion regulation work can and should "look like" in adults with childhood histories of severe emotional neglect and/or emotional abuse. For instance, are the management and modulation of distressing or dysregulated affect the principal or sole self-regulation needs for adults with histories of exposure to chronic childhood emotional abuse and neglect? And are the regulatory needs of this too-often-overlooked but quite large subpopulation of trauma survivors the same as those of adults impacted by other forms of complex childhood trauma? To begin to address these questions, we must first return to an earlier time in the lives of these clients.

DEVELOPMENTAL ORIGINS OF SELF-REGULATION

Self-regulatory capacity develops through safe, consistent attachment relationships with caregivers who possess their own self-regulation capacity and skills. In a healthy early attachment relationship, when an infant expresses distress, the caregiver typically responds in a manner that ultimately meets the child's need (for food, a clean diaper, warmth, or contact), soothing the child and helping her to return to a calm, regulated state. To understand this process on a deeper level, we must recognize that this early transmission of regulating behaviors and responses is not a one-way process from caregiver to infant. Rather, in adequate caregiving, it occurs in a reciprocal, fluid, "living" manner. An infant becomes soothed as much by her sensation of her mother's state of physiological equilibrium as by the calming sounds and containing physical contact her mother undertakes in response to her child's communications of distress. In turn, the caregiver herself attains a deepened sense of physiological calm in response to the sensation of her child's shift to a more regulated state.

Developmental psychologist Alan Fogel (1993) originated the term *coregulation* to capture this "continuous unfolding of individual action that is susceptible to being continuously modified by the continuously changing actions of the partner." Taking place across neurophysiological, sensory, and behavioral levels, this dyadic mirroring and adjustment of affective and physiological experience has been discovered to be at the heart of the infant's development of self-regulatory capacity and central to the formation of one's earliest attachment structures, sense of self, and capacity to communicate (Rizzolatti & Sinigaglia, 2008). Notably, this nurturing response hardly needs to be perfect; it simply needs to be "good enough" for the developing child within the evolving context of his or her environment, experiences, and needs (Winnicott, 1965).

As a result of these formative coregulatory experiences, over time children begin to develop their own regulatory skills. They learn to more purposefully "ask" for their needs to be met. As they physically develop, they begin to be able to meet some of their own needs. They learn how to tolerate frustration and other uncomfortable feelings and how to soothe themselves.

In contrast, children reared in an environment of prolonged or severe emotional neglect or emotional abuse may not develop these skills. Children who grow up with insufficient love and support, or who are exposed to emotional aggression and distortions of reality in their primary caretakers, typically do not develop adequate attachment relationships or internalize their own healthy regulatory skills. They often live with a sense of uncertainty, helplessness, and panic. Because many children have limited coping skills for managing their response to this kind of experience, they may attempt to contain their experiences through rigid or constricted responses, including dissociation. David, in trying to change his whole persona to fit into a world in which he feels that he is wrong and bad, creates a "self" that appears to be in control and perfect. Any aspects of himself that do not fit into this new self-construction are rejected and alienated, that is, dissociated. This rigidity of response can lead to a sense of being stuck. There is something that deeply troubles him, but David is unaware of what is wrong because he has expelled it from his consciousness.

TYPES OF DYSREGULATION

Dysregulation, which we see as resulting from dissociation, can occur across numerous areas of experience, each of which impacts the other. Most commonly, when mental health professionals refer to "dysregulation," they are

speaking about affect dysregulation or dissociation. A person with affect
dysregulation may be emotionally volatile or reactive, experiencing extreme
emotional swings. Or he may live in an anxiety-prone state, having difficulty
feeling calm or relaxed. Another person may feel chronically sad and be
unable to access feelings of hopefulness. Another way that dysregulation can
be expressed is through disconnection with aspects of their own experience.
This person may feel emotionally numb and so will shut down. Nicole has
several of these characteristics.

Emotion regulation has undoubtedly received the greatest attention in
regard to the problem of dysregulation and the striving to enhance the self-
regulatory capacity of trauma survivors. Moreover, in many cases self-regulation has been written about, conceptualized, and experientially approached
as if it were synonymous with *emotion regulation*. This narrower perspective
overlooks the many other forms of self-regulation that are routinely derailed
by chronic exposure to complex childhood trauma (Courtois & Ford, 2013).
A variety of manifestations of dysregulation are identified within the ISTSS
expert survey, including affective, behavioral, and attentional dysregulation
(Cloitre et al., 2011).

Aside from emotional dysregulation, a person may have difficulty regulating physiological or somatic states, biorhythms, thoughts, and behaviors.
Somatic dysregulation can include states of hyperarousal (rapid heart rate, shallow breathing, muscle tension) or hypoarousal (lack of energy, listlessness).
Some people experience physiological reactions that are linked in some way to
their earlier experience of trauma. For instance, a woman whose mother died
in a car accident when she was a child noticed that she felt a familiar light-
headedness, constriction in her throat, and pit in her stomach every time her
new boyfriend would leave her apartment—the same physical reactions she
had when she learned that her mother was gone. These "body memories" can
occur without conscious awareness of the link to earlier trauma. Impairments
in sleep, appetite, and energy are reflections of dysregulated biorhythms. The
human body is designed to operate in a natural rhythm that ensures survival,
with regular cycles of hunger, fatigue, and so on. Instead, for people with dysregulated biorhythms, their body's urges tend to get stuck in a loop. For one
person, this might include an inability to fall asleep; while for another, it may
involve never feeling satiated after eating. Chronic physiological dysregulation and dissociation can lead to medical complications such as high blood
pressure, ulcers, and other stress-related conditions. A sense of disconnection
from one's body can also be considered a sign of physiological dysregulation.

Many of the behavioral "disorders" commonly associated with trauma
are, in fact, attempts to cope with overwhelming internal experience, often in
response to perceived external pressure, threat, or demand. Most often, they
are associated with issues of control. *Behavioral dysregulation* can manifest
both in efforts to overcontrol one's internal experience, as well as in attempts
to relinquish responsibility or control. These expressions of dysregulation can

evolve over time into chronic behavioral problems and disorders. For example, eating disorders, substance abuse disorders, self-harming behaviors, compulsive behavior (hoarding food, excessive order/cleanliness, sexually compulsive activity), depression, and anxiety are often the outgrowths of adaptation to early life adversity, trauma, and attachment disruption.

Finally, other forms of dysregulation associated with exposure to complex childhood trauma, if perhaps more subtle or in the background, are just as important to consider in terms of their lasting impact on the functioning and internal world of adult survivors. Early emotional abuse and neglect also affect children's developing worldview and their ideational approach to themselves, relationships, and the world. Beyond having "shattered assumptions" (Janoff-Bulman, 1992), these children never had the opportunity to develop healthy assumptions about the world. Instead, their early development leads to trauma-related assumptions, such as the idea that "I am bad" or "other people are not safe." These aspects of self- and social appraisal are highly vulnerable to attributional or *cognitive dysregulation* in these adult survivors. In fact, as we explore in the next chapter, vulnerability to recurrent dysregulation in the context of relational interaction may be the single greatest challenge in working with these clients.

DIMENSIONS OF THE REGULATION COMPONENT

The ways in which these types of dysregulation can present in adults with histories of chronic childhood emotional abuse and neglect vary across several dimensions, impacting how we intervene. Figure 5.1 describes four dimensions for the regulation component: arousal level, consistency in regulatory state, directionality of expressions of distress, and degree of control.

The first dimension, arousal level, indicates whether a survivor tends to be highly activated (hyperaroused), more shut down (hypoaroused), or somewhere in between. This dimension includes multiple aspects of experience, including affect, somatic states, cognitions/attributions, and behaviors. A person who is hyperaroused tends toward more anxious, distressed, or angry affect; sympathetic nervous system activation; activating attributions; and impulsive fight-or-flight behaviors. In contrast, a person who is hypoaroused tends toward depressive affect or emotional numbing; parasympathetic nervous system activation; attributions of helplessness and hopelessness; and avoidant or compliant behaviors.

Regarding consistency in regulatory state, some people experience more volatility in their states, whereas others have a more fixed presentation, with stability in their mood, somatic states, thoughts, and behaviors. Those who have a more fixed presentation are not necessarily well regulated: They may have difficulty adapting to the needs of the environment, or they may have a more stable, trait-like hyper- or hypoaroused presentation. People who have

Hypoaroused ---------------------------- (X - Alert/Calm) ----------------------------- Hyperaroused

Volatile -------------------------------------- (X - Flexible) --- Fixed

Internalizing ----------------- (X - Adaptable Expressions of Distress) -------------- Externalizing

Controlled --------------------------- (X - Active Acceptance) ------------------------ Uncontrolled

FIGURE 5.1. Dimensions of the regulation component. X denotes direction of therapeutic goals.

more volatile states tend to vacillate between hyper- and hypoarousal and have difficulty maintaining stability in their lives. In the middle of this continuum is a more flexible regulatory system that is able to adapt to the needs of the environment, while maintaining some level of homeostasis.

The directionality of expressions of distress dimension refers to the way in which distress is manifested and whether its expressions tend to be internally or externally directed. (Notably, we are not using this terminology to refer to locus of control.) People who are more internalizing are more likely to experience distress through self-focused emotional states such as anxiety and depression, somatic complaints, and cognitive attributions such as self-blame. In contrast, externalizing refers more to other-directed emotions such as anger and behavioral expressions of distress such as aggression, substance abuse, or self-injurious behavior. At the same time, people whose distress is more externalized may disconnect from internal awareness, including somatic disconnection or emotional numbing. The goal of the therapist here is to help clients feel a mix of emotions, as appropriate to the situation, rather than maintain a rigid style at one end or the other.

The final regulatory dimension, degree of control, refers to a person's approach to self-regulation. A person who is highly controlled attempts to dictate his or her own regulatory states. This might occur through attempts to restrain, deny, or alter their emotions, somatic states, thoughts, or behaviors. In contrast, an undercontrolled approach is a more passive stance toward regulation, giving free rein to regulatory states. In a more balanced approach, some people are able to both accept their current state (even if it is unpleasant or dysregulated) and actively work to regulate, what we call "active acceptance."

SAFETY CONCERNS AND HIGH-RISK BEHAVIORS

One of the hallmarks of trauma, included in the DSM-5's diagnostic description of PTSD, is impulsive or high-risk behavior. When a person is highly dysregulated, safety is a primary ongoing clinical consideration. In their review article on the relationship between childhood trauma (sexual abuse, in this case) and adult self-injury and suicidality, Ford and Gómez (2015) found that emotional dysregulation was an important mediator of this relationship. Dissociated anger and rage can emerge as aggressive behavior toward others. Self-hatred or despair can be expressed through self-injury, substance abuse, or suicidal gestures or attempts. Relational dysregulation can lead to involvement in risky sexual behavior or violent relationships. These high-risk behaviors are almost always intended to reduce or eliminate the intense and sometimes intolerable internal pain the client is feeling in the moment. For instance, self-harming behaviors and substance use tend to induce dissociative states that often do bring immediate relief from pain. These risk behaviors then can become addictive because of their capacity to reduce intolerable emotions, despite the client's cognitive awareness of the problems they cause.

In addressing safety concerns, CBP emphasizes a balance between reflective awareness and action on the part of the clinician. In cases of more imminent risk, the therapist may need to intervene at the contextual level to ensure an environment that supports the client's physical safety, such as a psychiatric hospitalization or detoxification facility. The purpose in these situations is to create external stopgap measures to prevent impulsive lethal behaviors until the client becomes more regulated. Even in these cases, the relationship component is essential in attempting to make a collaborative plan with the client, empowering the client to make choices to stay safe. In other cases, the "action" of the therapist will focus more on regulatory efforts and efforts to engage parts of the client who wants to remain safe. As discussed in Chapter 6, these types of safety concerns can create dysregulation in the therapist. Regardless of our behavioral response, if we are able to cultivate our capacity to tolerate the reactions that high-risk behaviors often create in ourselves, we have greater potential to serve increasingly as coregulator of the client's intense distress, which leads to these high-risk behaviors (Courtois & Ford, 2013).

PSYCHOPHARMACOLOGY AND REGULATION

While it is beyond the scope of this book to explore the issue of psychopharmacology in treatment of adults with histories of early emotional abuse and neglect, we want to highlight the fact that psychiatric medications can play an important regulatory role in treatment (Ursano et al., 2010). Psychopharmacology is typically considered a second-line or adjunctive treatment for traumatic stress (Foa et al., 2010). Medication can provide relief from incapacitating depression, increasing the client's energy and motivation for change. It may be important when a client's thought processes are impacted, leading to impairments in reality testing. It can play a role in supporting executive functions when a person's difficulties with attention and concentration interfere with his or her day-to-day functioning. It can help to regulate biorhythms when a person is unable to reestablish regular sleep patterns through behavioral means. Globally, the role of psychopharmacology in trauma treatment is to decrease the dysregulation to a level at which the person is able to practice other coping strategies for managing it.

There are, of course, potential countertherapeutic impacts for some individuals. Some people go down a rabbit hole of complex medication regimens, with debilitating side effects interfering with the ability to accurately assess or treat underlying issues. Others overrely on external agents for change, with medication leading people to feel disempowered to create change through other means. Complicating this picture is the physiological dependence associated with some medications, creating, for instance, an increase in anxiety or sleep disturbance when these medications are decreased or removed. Benzodiazepine dependency is a specific, documented problem in the treatment of traumatic stress, anxiety disorders, and related conditions (Guina et al., 2015), so caution is needed with the use of this class of medications. Overmedication causes some people to experience emotional numbing and to lose access to self-connection. Some people with high medication sensitivity or fragmented self-states have unpredictable or variable responses to medications. Thus, psychopharmacologists working with this population should be well versed in the impact of complex trauma and should utilize a team approach, operating in close coordination with the therapist or other mental health providers.

DEVELOPMENT OF REGULATORY CAPACITY IN TRAUMA TREATMENT

In the session during which Nicole tells Katherine about her affairs, Katherine takes time near the end of the session to ask Nicole how she is doing. Nicole looks at Katherine with an imploring, searching, almost desperate gesture and says, "The thing is, Katherine, I don't know the limits of how far I will go to feel something, and I'm starting to scare myself. That's why I forced myself to come here." Katherine struggles for a few moments with what to say to help Nicole leave in a more regulated and centered place. She then says, "I'm glad you did," and Nicole visibly relaxes. In this instance, Katherine helps Nicole regulate.

Regulation is a cornerstone of trauma treatment. In trauma treatment, building regulatory capacity refers to the development of skills to move from a state of imbalance to balance. These skills include building awareness of internal states, developing greater tolerance for internal states and for intimacy in relationships while establishing clear boundaries, developing the ability to communicate about one's internal states to others, making links between aspects of internal experience, and transforming inner experience.

Many survivors of emotional abuse and neglect lack awareness of their internal states. Accordingly, a major treatment goal is to increase awareness of internal experience. We work to make the unconscious conscious. When something is out of awareness, it is more likely to feel—and to be—out of control. When it becomes known, there is suddenly an option to do something about it. We may choose to draw attention to somatic, affective, cognitive, or behavioral elements of experience. Each of these realms of regulation offers different points of access to exploration of internal experience, allowing us to adapt regulatory work to the unique needs of different clients (see Figure 5.2). An emergency medical technician (EMT) named Frank has entered therapy for the first time at the age of 42. He notices that, when he feels afraid, he immediately disconnects from his body and goes numb. He is barely aware of a fleeting thought, "I can't do it," before going into problem-solving mode where he jumps into action. Frank's career as an EMT has left him in "action" mode all of the time. He stays busy, frequently puts himself in dangerous situations, and is rarely aware of his feelings, causing relationship problems. As Frank begins to build connections among elements of his experience, he starts to become aware of chronic underlying feelings of fear and a somatic sense of being "frozen" in the face of this fear. This somatic and affective awareness forms the foundation for Frank to explore what is driving his reckless behavior and the emotional distance in his relationships.

Implicit in this increased awareness is a second clinical objective, the development of greater tolerance for experiencing a range of internal states.

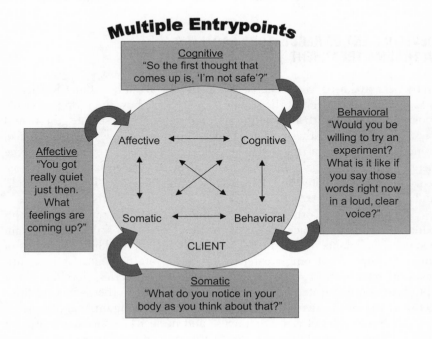

FIGURE 5.2. Intervening across regulatory realms.

In CBP, the therapist and client work together to develop a noticing self who can be curious about strong feelings or sensations without becoming dysregulated. We may gently encourage a client to "stay with" a particular experience, building tolerance for discomfort and distress. Through this intervention, we are helping clients to face their fears and to "sit" with anxiety, sadness, rage, or despair. Often, when they do, they see it's not as scary as they had anticipated. They learn that experiencing upsetting feelings does not mean that they will fall apart, go crazy, or be unable to function. Along with this increased toler-ance, over time, the window of tolerance (see next section) slowly expands, so that the client is able to acknowledge and "stay with" a fuller range of distressing emotions, somatic states, or thoughts for a greater length of time. One young woman had grown up in the foster care system, largely in survival mode as she bounced from one failed placement to the next. She had continuing upheaval and repeated losses in her life but noted that she felt unable to cry. When she finally entered long-term therapy in adulthood, she was initially overwhelmed by the realization of "what could have been," but over time, as she experienced feeling "held" and cared about by her therapist, she was slowly able to experience grief about her childhood and found herself able to cry about it.

Through relational treatment, adults who experienced childhood emotional abuse and neglect will ideally develop increasing tolerance for relational connection, including intimacy as well as conflict in relationships. The therapeutic relationship offers an experiential world in which the client and therapist must negotiate the emotional aspects of relatedness, developing both intimacy and boundaries. In an interaction between the relationship and regulation components, and often through an exploration of enactments, this relational practice-ground can help increase the client's capacity and tolerance for closeness in relationship without fusing and for distance in relationship without rupturing.

Another clinical objective that involves the regulation and relationship components is communication to others about internal states. The ability to put words to inner experience is essential here, including sharing intense thoughts and feelings while remaining within one's window of tolerance. The therapist may work with a client to expand their vocabulary to describe these internal states and ways to represent verbally the intensity of the feeling. This is a challenge particularly for clients for whom their parents or primary caretakers communicated their feelings indirectly (for instance, by providing praise or lavish gifts to a sibling but not to the client) or whose caregivers lacked awareness of, or language for, their own emotions (as may happen when the caregiver has his or her own trauma history and struggles with dissociation). Communication about internal states can also be quite difficult for people who were punished for emotional expression as children, who grew up in families where certain feelings (such as anger) were taboo, or whose internal experience was denied (e.g., "That's silly, of course you don't feel that way!").

The development of regulatory capacity involves an increase in the ability to make linkages between various aspects of experience. For instance, a therapeutic intervention may begin with an identification of somatic states that are then linked to an underlying cognition and affective state. In a session several months into treatment, Susan and David are discussing what David has called his "ethnic identity," which he puts in finger quotes. Although he is talking calmly and with his usual reserve, Susan notices that he is gripping the arms of his chair. She wonders if he's noticed this reaction, which he hasn't. As they bring attention to this behavioral sign of dysregulation, David becomes aware of a similar clenched feeling in his stomach. They are eventually able to link these somatic and behavioral reactions with a deep resentment of others' assumptions about the meaning of his race. He realizes that he is feeling mistrustful of Susan and is worried that she is judging him in some way. It is a perfect opportunity to use what is happening between them in the session to deepen their relationship and help him understand one way he keeps his emotions outside of his awareness. Eventually, they will explore how David's anger links back to his original trauma and includes his feeling of not being seen and valued or accepted for who he is.

Finally, trauma treatment for adult survivors of childhood emotional abuse and neglect can lead to a transformation of inner experience. As in the case of David, by acknowledging and tolerating the "knowing" of these rejected experiences, with the support of his therapist, a door is being opened for actual change in the parts holding the traumatic memories (see Chapters 7–8). David's coping system will gradually become more fluid and flexible, creating an opportunity for new experiences, such as understanding that Susan, in addition to staying mindful about his ethnicity and how it might have affected his life experiences, is also very much aware of and responsive to him as an individual and values him for that. This transformation of experience can occur cognitively, somatically, emotionally, and behaviorally. The thought of "I am bad" may shift over time to "I have good intentions" and later to "I'm a good person to whom bad things have happened." Somatically, his body may become "unfrozen," and he may feel more relaxed and at home in his body. Instead of being tightly constricted around emotional experience, David may allow himself to notice and sit with his sadness and loss. This increased access to his internal experience may enable him to be more present and authentic in his relationships.

Window of Tolerance

Psychiatrist Daniel Siegel (1999) introduced the idea of the "window of tolerance," by which he was referring to the range of internal states that are acceptable/bearable/endurable to a person's conscious experience. Each person has his own "window," with some people feeling more comfortable sitting with a larger range of emotions, somatic states, and ideation. Pat Ogden's application of Siegel's window of tolerance in clinical intervention has had a pivotal influence on our understanding of complexly traumatized adults' manifold expressions of affect dysregulation (Ogden et al., 2006).

Many people who have experienced early trauma have a dramatically narrowed window of tolerance. That is, they have developed a phobic response to intense emotion or experience. This may include an avoidance of negative emotion, such as sadness or anger. But it can also include an avoidance of strong positive emotions, such as love or joy or hope. When someone's arousal level increases beyond his or her window of tolerance, the person shows signs of "hyperarousal." Hyperarousal is one of the key symptom categories within the diagnosis of PTSD and can include reactions such as concentration problems, sleep disturbance, startle response, and hypervigilance. A survivor can show signs of being hyperaroused through her body's responses in the moment. For instance, imagine that Lin, a young professional Chinese American woman, is talking to her therapist Sam about a distressing interaction with a coworker; because of her discomfort in talking about sexuality in general, particularly with a male, and because of her embarrassment and shame about the encounter, she avoids mentioning that her coworker groped her. As Sam asks questions, the muscles in Lin's back, neck, and shoulders begin to tense up. She crosses her legs, and one leg swings rapidly back and forth. She folds her arms tightly across her chest and clenches her jaw. As Lin's arousal level continues to increase, her breathing begins to become more rapid and shallow. She notices sweat on her palms and feels her heart pounding in her chest.

When a person with limited self-regulation skills moves outside of her window of tolerance into a hyperaroused state, she often tends to cope in the simplest possible way—to shut it down. There is a sudden disconnection from this painful, overwhelming experience and a collapse into a hypoaroused state. Porges's (2011) polyvagal theory has implicated the dorsal vagal nerve as a physiological basis for this dissociative response. Feeling out of control and unable to tolerate her level of arousal, Lin suddenly shifts into another state or part. Her body goes still as she stares off into space. She is suddenly unable to feel anything, and her mind is blank. Her arms and legs feel numb.

When we notice that clients are outside their "window of tolerance," we typically move our focus from distress tolerance to regulation. Early in treatment, we will often walk a client through the use of regulation tools (see Chapter 6 for a cautionary statement about this approach). This is co-regulation, when we use our own reactions and awareness of a client's apparent reactions to highlight the need for regulation and provide an in-the-moment, coached regulatory experience. Instead of just objectively teaching self-regulation skills and expecting that our clients will use them on their own outside of session, we encourage our clients to learn by doing in a supportive environment.

As an example, we return to Frank, the EMT. Frank has begun to work on noticing his internal states, using a parts perspective (see Chapters 7–8). He recognizes that the "Crisis Manager" part of himself has been blocking a more fearful part of himself. His therapist guided him to ask the "Crisis Manager" to relax his controls, creating a sense of quiet and stillness so that he can see what happens when he is not in crisis mode. Frank has tried this technique several times and has felt a cold, numb, heavy feeling in his arms and legs, and then "nothing." Now, he notices a feeling of being "dead" inside. Suddenly, he begins to feel panicky. His heart is racing, he feels dizzy, and there is a choking sensation in his throat. His therapist asks him to just notice what happens. Frank begins to see flashes of his father throwing his mother up against a wall and then putting his hands around her throat. He is a 6-year-old boy, standing in the doorway, frozen. He begins to pant and then gasp: he is outside his window of tolerance. Frank's therapist guides him to bring his attention to his breathing and asks him to breathe in and out with her count. As his breath slows, she asks him to bring his hands to his chest and diaphragm, to feel his breath becoming deeper and more relaxed. She checks in about how Frank is feeling, and he says, "Dizzy; everything is blurry. I feel out of it." She asks him to put his feet on the ground, to notice his legs on the chair. She guides him through seated leg lifts, a body-oriented technique drawn from yoga that allows him to feel the strength in his abdomen. Frank begins to joke about keeping in shape. He shows her a push-up in his chair. He shares that he feels "back to normal." They talk about pacing and how they might utilize some regulation tools to slow down the process when he begins to feel signs of panic.

TOOLS FOR REGULATION

A range of treatment techniques have been developed for therapists to teach clients to use in calming themselves first in the session and then outside of therapy as well. We only briefly describe them here since there are many places clinicians can find detailed descriptions (see Briere & Scott, 2012, for an exhaustive review). Briere and Scott (2012) suggest an organization of regulation techniques into two functional categories: those utilized to help diminish acutely dysregulating emotions and symptoms, and those used to help clients build capacities for regulating their chronically difficult internal states. In the first category, they emphasize use of *grounding techniques*— techniques that invite the client to draw attention to aspects of his or her immediate surroundings. Doing so can help clients shift focus from perseveration on past traumatic experiences and/or associated states of dysregulation and dissociation within which individuals often become stuck toward more mindful, present-focused awareness of current experiences and sensations. For more chronic dysregulation, they particularly recommend the following types of regulation strategies: relaxation and breath control; learning to notice and identify particular emotions; noticing and countering thoughts that come before hard and intrusive emotional experiences; learning to identify environmental triggers that lead to such states; and learning not to engage in former tension-reduction procedures, such as drug use and self-harm.

A second category of regulation techniques that we frequently utilize in CBP with adult survivors of childhood emotional abuse and neglect uses *imagery* to develop *containment skills*. For example, we might guide clients to imagine a container that might hold their difficult feelings when they are not able to otherwise manage or explore them. Expressive therapists at our Center might invite the client first to create a container out of art materials for holding such thoughts and feelings, and then to write them down on a card and put them into the box. Other regulation strategies commonly incorporated into CBP include *sensory* and *emotion-focused* regulation techniques; a wide variety of diaphragmatic and controlled *breathing* techniques; *relaxation* and *stress-inoculation* techniques including biofeedback, progressive muscle relaxation, and exercise; as well as *distress-tolerance* and *distraction-focused* techniques. Technique-driven interventions of particular usefulness in promoting regulatory capacity in our clients include sensorimotor psychotherapy (SP; Ogden et al., 2006) and AEDP (Fosha, 2000). Both interventions are noteworthy for the wealth of clinical and anecdotal observations of their effectiveness and innovation in gently and systematically pursuing incremental advances in the recognition, tracking, labeling, and shifting of long-standing, troubling, and often well-defended affective, physiological, and behavioral states in highly vulnerable, complexly traumatized adults.

CBP emphasizes that regulatory techniques, though potentially helpful and instrumental, are not typically sufficient with clients suffering from complex trauma, particularly for people with histories of chronic childhood emotional abuse and neglect. In our experience, these strategies tend not to work unless they are embedded within a containing therapeutic relationship and are gently and incrementally introduced with the client's permission, understanding, and acceptance. If Susan simply suggested to David that he do one of these exercises, without first talking with him about his appearing to be upset, he would likely have reactions to it, not be fully or even partly in agreement with doing it, or possibly reject it out of hand as silly or inconsequential against the scope of his problems. Instead, Susan might explore with David what his dysregulation means conceptually (e.g., that a part or parts of himself are dysregulated, and it's hard for anyone to learn when they are activated in that way); explain that there are a variety of techniques to help people calm down; inquire if he might be interested in trying one; and then maybe describe briefly some of the possibilities. If Susan had not provided such psychoeducation and allowed him to make a choice about trying something, and David ultimately, albeit ambivalently, had agreed to attempt the recommended technique, it would have been set up not to work or to work only marginally at best.

Likewise, if the therapist is dysregulated at the time, lacking confidence in the strategy or ambivalent about introducing techniques at this juncture in their work, it would be highly unlikely that she could use any technique to help her client get regulated. As we explore at length in the next chapter, in CBP we consider the successful engagement in regulation strategies with our clients to entail a dyadic process between client and therapist and to be contingent on establishing and sustaining an empathic, containing therapeutic partnership.

More common trauma triggers associated with regulation techniques, such as the reactivity of some abuse survivors to controlled-breathing techniques, should always be anticipated, and contingent responses and adjustments should be thoughtfully considered in advance of regulation work with complexly traumatized adults. The inevitability of more idiosyncratic reactions derived from particular trauma experiences need also be recognized. For example, in our efforts to introduce yoga to our adult clients, our Center learned early on the importance of slow pacing of the class, loose-fitting dress, and subdued vocal tone of the instructor, avoidance of unsolicited physical assists, and careful introduction of more innately vulnerable postures (Emerson & Hopper, 2011). However, it took us longer to discover that our assumption that chair-based yoga would provide a gentle introduction to regulation was not a universal truth. For a subset of clients—most notably those who as young children were left stranded due to chronic neglect in playpens or jumper seats, or those who were sadistically forced to remain for long periods of time locked into high chairs as punishment—the mindful attention to one's body in a chair could become a direct catalyst for traumatic reenactment.

Another challenge frequently encountered in treatment with adults complexly impacted by chronic childhood emotional abuse and neglect involves the prescriptive nature of most regulation techniques, tools, and approaches. Some clients will require and gladly accept structured ideas, protocols, and sequences for assisting them in better recognizing, tolerating, and modulating their arousal states. However, this responsiveness to external prompts about how to self-regulate is not always the case. For many of our clients, such seemingly innocuous directives as inviting them to imagine a pleasant nature scene or to direct their attention and efforts to the tension and release of a certain muscle group can be experienced as a repetition of historically invasive infliction of someone else's worldview, values, interests, or language onto their experience, stripping away personal agency and selfhood in the process. Actively involving them in the generative process of regulation strategies is essential, whether this entails drawing on their own metaphors, symbols, and resonant experiences in the elaboration and installation of soothing imagery and other internal coping resources or using invitational language to explore or decline participation in a trauma-sensitive yoga pose.

For example, after several failed efforts to utilize traditional regulation techniques or generic coping resources, Rachel, a highly creative, dissociative client, was able to co-create a personally resonant, effective grounding exercise with her therapist based on her experience of chronically feeling alone and disoriented, like "one girl" alone in "10 universes." "One Girl Ten Universes" became the stem for a guided imagery sequence that incorporated elements of parts work (see Chapters 7–8) with a focus on increasing regulation. In this imagery sequence, a young, bereft, overwhelmed part of Rachel would wander through varying depictions of immense geography and adversity until she came into contact with a second, slightly older, and more resourced part of self, the connection with which would in turn immediately shrink the 10 universes through which they traversed down to nine galaxies. Discovery of a third, older-still child part, then a fourth, a fifth, and so on, brought incremental confidence and access to resources and with it continual reduction in the vastness of the landscape (e.g., eight solar systems, seven planets, six continents, five countries, four states, three counties, etc.). This guided imagery sequence culminated in the arrival at "home" of an array of integrated self-representations spanning from infancy into adulthood. From a starting place of isolation, overwhelm, and despair, Rachel ultimately found herself empowered, anchored, and sheltered in a cohesive, meaningful, and safe place of her design.

Research Basis for Tools of Regulation?

An important meta-analytic study conducted by Stephen Benish and colleagues (2008) demonstrated that all trauma-focused treatments for which randomized controlled research trials had been conducted (to date, these had all been memory processing/exposure-based treatments for classic PTSD, largely in response to acute adult-onset traumatic events) performed equally well and superior only to non-trauma-focused treatment-as-usual, waitlist, placebo, or other nondirective approaches (Benish, Imel, & Wampold, 2008). It will be some time before a sufficient number of stabilization-phase and regulation-focused interventions are subjected to a similar level of controlled outcome research, largely because of the immense challenges of obtaining research funding to study innovative treatments that fall outside the currently prevailing cognitive-behavioral therapy paradigm. (For more information on this issue, see Bessel van der Kolk's newest book, *The Body Keeps the Score* [2014].) When this eventually happens, we expect to find similar results. Namely, the various approaches to affect and behavioral regulation that have been developed or adapted for adults impacted by chronic childhood trauma will quite likely be discovered to be more or less equivalently effective when randomized across large groups of diverse trauma survivors.

Of course, neither Benish's meta-analysis nor the studies on which it was based undertook to assess the differential benefit of particular intervention models matched to clients' readiness, interests, and strengths or to their clinicians' training, comfort level, and unique talents. In the rare instances in mental health research in which client and clinician readiness, aptitude, and preference can be taken into account, the value of certain approaches for particular individuals, circumstances, and contexts becomes as clear as we know them to be in clinical practice (e.g., see Norcross, Krebs, & Prochaska, 2011).

Innovative Tools for Regulation

As trauma therapists, we are involved in a continual process of exploration, development, and refinement of various approaches to advancing the regulatory capacity of our clients. We recognize the important role of established behaviorally oriented techniques and skills that integrate mindfulness with the cultivation of coping skills, such as dialectical behavior therapy (DBT; Linehan, 1993), in the treatment of complexly traumatized adults. In fact, for the past 15 years, we have offered ongoing DBT-based coping skill groups for our adult clients at our Trauma Center clinic.

Nevertheless, we have struggled with the limits of otherwise very good behavioral and skill-based approaches to sufficiently address the self-regulation needs of many of the adult clients we serve. One major limitation shared by many of these interventions is their reliance on a client's capacity to access and focus on higher-order cognitive functions in order to advance trauma recovery, particularly development of self-regulatory capacity. The frequent ineffectiveness of such approaches is perhaps best understood from the vantage point of neuroscience research demonstrating the shutdown or reduced activity of higher cortical functions in the face of overwhelming experience or, subsequently, when trauma-related arousal states are activated by memories or reminders (for a review, see Shin, Rauch, & Pitman, 2006). This same body of research has also unequivocally demonstrated that trauma-related sequelae are primarily held in more primitive parts of the human brain. These findings have led to insufficiently tested but conceptually sound theorizing that resolution of these symptoms is in turn predicated upon engaging these same parts of the brain in the intervention process in order to disrupt and reset maladaptive patterns of neurophysiological reactivity. These limitations typically become more pronounced in direct proportion to the intensity and complexity of the trauma exposure and associated adaptation over the lifespan.

Research at the Trauma Center has shown that a trauma-processing protocol utilizing eye movement desensitization and reprocessing (EMDR) was most consistently effective for adults with adult-onset trauma, while much more variable for those with childhood-onset trauma. Some resolved their PTSD, some showed modest improvement, some remained unchanged, and some worsened (van der Kolk et al., 2007). In contrast, while no one was "cured" of their PTSD in the medication condition (fluoxetine), virtually all showed moderate symptom improvement irrespective of trauma onset. These findings further support recognition that implementation of monophasic, memory processing, or desensitization-focused treatment models is generally inadequate in treating adults with childhood-onset trauma, and that integration of emotion-regulation components of intervention is vital to ultimate treatment success. In this vein, those participants in our study who had already achieved sufficient emotional stabilization and regulatory capacity prior to the study were ready to benefit from rapid introduction of the exposure-based EMDR protocol. These adults without childhood trauma had, by and large, the fortune of developing and internalizing normative capacities for self-regulation that mitigated the broader impact on self-image, relationships, and emotional well-being of the traumatic experiences they encountered in adulthood. In contrast, acquisition of these vital capacities was more variable in participants who experienced childhood-onset trauma, likely as a complicated function of the nature, extent, onset, and duration of their childhood trauma; their innate internal resources, temperament, and resiliency; the social supports, resources, and subsequent adversities they encountered throughout their life trajectory; and the degree to which gains in self-regulatory capacity had been made in therapy or other self-care or recovery-based pursuits prior to the study.

It is critically important to note that the limited body of research to date on regulation-based intervention for adults suffering from complex trauma has been most extensively applied to and found to be most effective with adults with more primarily hyperaroused, reactive symptom profiles and behavioral difficulties. In contrast, virtually no research has been done on elucidating best practices to reach and help improve the regulatory capacity of our most vulnerable clients—those with predominantly dissociative, avoidant, or hypoaroused clinical presentations and patterns of reactivity in response to trauma triggers. The challenges to effective treatment with more emotionally "shut-down" or avoidant trauma survivors has been generally established (see, e.g., Dunmore, Clark, & Ehlers, 2001). These findings are consistent with emerging neuroscientific research on the variability in physiological expressions of trauma reactivity. Most notably in this research, we and our colleagues have begun to demonstrate that a significant subset of trauma survivors responds to triggered activation of traumatic memories and affects states not with the traditionally sympathetic nervous system–driven hyperarousal response, but rather with a parasympathetic nervous system–driven hypoarousal and distancing response (Hopper, Spinazzola, Simpson, & van der Kolk, 2006; Lanius, Hopper, & Menon, 2003).

 Adults who experienced early emotional abuse and neglect, perhaps particularly those with avoidant or shut-down presentations, may be initially anxious or uncomfortable with novel treatment approaches and may have difficulty accessing innovative, embodied approaches to intervention. Thus, the therapist is tasked with careful attunement to the client's state and careful pacing to address his or her unique regulatory needs. Adding further complexity to this equation, many survivors of childhood physical or emotional neglect have also fallen prey to associated or ensuing emotional, physical, or sexual maltreatment, exploitation, or violence in childhood or adulthood. Thus, even those adult complex trauma clients with predominantly hypoaroused, dissociative, or avoidant clinical presentations have typically also developed more reactive, hyperaroused, or aggressive survival-based adaptations as a result of their cumulative life experiences. These latter coping manifestations are particularly susceptible to being activated in the context of psychotherapy seeking to engage trauma-related material. Thus, we encounter the magnified challenge of struggling to identify viable avenues to engage regulatory capacity in "shut-down" adult survivors of psychological maltreatment without activating dormant eruptions of affective, physiological distress, and associated behavioral disruption.

As we explore in greater detail (see Chapters 7–8), these dormant affective and neurophysiological states associated with the most desperate fight-or-flight survival adaptations of complexly traumatized adults are often held by fragmented self-states of dissociative parts intricately tied to formative traumatic experience. For example, many of the clients we serve have found ways to survive and endure in the midst of chronic suffering by overreliance on one or more forms of dissociative coping or other strategies of suppression of intolerable memories or affective and physiological arousal states associated with the trauma. Common strategies for this kind of suppression include self-destructive behaviors, social isolation, restriction or compulsive excess of food intake, sexual and other addictions, and substance abuse and dependency, including excessive reliance on or misuse of prescription medications. For many such clients, regulation skills and techniques predicated on cognitively oriented discussion of trauma-related symptoms, triggers, and difficulties often fall short. Many of these clients are highly reluctant to talk about their experience. When they are required to engage in discussion of trauma-related material, they do so in a highly disembodied state in which the emotions and arousal states being targeted for change are hopelessly out of reach.

Accordingly, CBP incorporates a variety of somatically and neurophysiologically based approaches to affect regulation. We have been influenced by the work of colleagues emphasizing body-oriented treatment (e.g., Levine, 1997; Ogden & Fisher, 2015). Some of the somatic approaches utilized in CBP are primarily nonverbal and movement or mindfulness based, such as sensory motor approaches, trauma-sensitive yoga, controlled breathing, and bio- or neurofeedback. CBP also endeavors to access limbic experience through displaced, symbolic, or ritual-based forms of self-expression, such as improvisational theater and expressive arts–based interventions. Finally, CBP also incorporates tools for developing regulatory capacity that have emerged from more established trauma-focused treatment approaches such as EMDR, but with greater reliance on the cultivation and installation of internal coping resources using techniques such as guided imagery and the use of metaphor (e.g., see Korn & Leeds, 2002; Omaha, 2004). Findings from our Center's ongoing program of clinical research speak to the promising utility of each of these avenues for regulation with otherwise highly treatment-resistant adults with histories of chronic childhood trauma (Finn, Warner, Price, & Spinazzola, 2017; Kaiser, Gillette, & Spinazzola, 2010; Price et al., 2017; Rhodes, Spinazzola & van der Kolk, 2016; van der Kolk et al., 2007, 2014, 2016; Warner, Spinazzola, Westcott, Gunn, & Hodgdon, 2014; West, Liang, & Spinazzola, 2016).

CONCLUSION

In CBP, it is important to understand the empirical basis for emphasis on self-regulation in effective treatment of adults with complex trauma, including the developmental origins of self-regulatory capacity and the ways these capacities become thwarted in response to early disruption to secure attachment. Early assessment of the regulation component of CBP can include several dimensions, including arousal level, consistency in regulatory state, manifestations of distress, and degree of control. As we work with our clients on regulation, we can utilize both traditional approaches and innovative, emerging strategies, including those individually codeveloped with each client. While building regulatory skills, it is essential to maintain awareness of the pivotal role of the therapeutic relationship in successful engagement in interventions designed to build regulatory capacity. In the chapter to follow, we explore the relational dilemma of regulation and the role of the therapeutic relationship in successful regulation and pacing in CBP.

CHAPTER 6

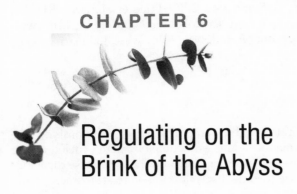

Regulating on the
Brink of the Abyss

As Nicole laments, adult survivors of chronic childhood emotional abuse and neglect often find themselves caught within a "black hole." For our most profoundly impacted clients, this black hole defines their very experience of being. In a seminal book on traumatic stress, Bessel van der Kolk and Alexander McFarlane (1996) introduced the metaphor of the *black hole of trauma* to characterize the consuming fixation evidenced by many complex trauma survivors with past memories, events, and ways of functioning.

In the two decades since van der Kolk introduced the metaphor, continuing exploration of the complexities of trauma adaptation has uncovered additional dimensions of trauma's black hole. We have come to recognize in our clients not only the preoccupation with the experiences of their traumatic past, but also the sense of emptiness that accompanies a lack of awareness of and connection to self. We have felt the immense gravitational pull of many of our clients' simultaneous insatiable yearning for, hypersensitivity to, and terror of interpersonal connection, nurturance, and intimacy—the "abyss" within relationships. The inner torment and self-abasement engendered by the toxicity and ambivalence surrounding unmet fundamental attachment needs is perhaps the harshest and most enduring legacy of chronic emotional deprivation in early childhood. Moreover, it provides the most compelling interpretation of emerging research that increasingly links exposure to chronic emotional abuse and neglect with the most pervasive and lasting consequences of all forms of childhood traumatization (Spinazzola et al., 2014).

Lacking consistent and nurturing mirroring and reflection, children who are emotionally abused and neglected do not have the opportunity to begin to know themselves. Instead, they are forced to adapt their behavior to the demands around them in an effort to survive. For many children, this means discounting their own internal cues. A child who is afraid but is not comforted learns to ignore the fear. A child for whom expression of anger results in aggression and belittlement learns to suppress any expression of anger. By continuously ignoring, controlling, or disconnecting from their internal states, children who are emotionally abused or neglected miss out on the opportunity to develop a sense of who they are, what they feel, and what they want. As adults, many of these people are left with a core absence, a feeling of "Who am I?" or even "I don't exist." This black hole of selfhood creates challenges for a therapist who jumps too quickly to regulating responses. How can you control what you don't know? For many people who have coped in this way, any brief foray into awareness of internal states can lead to an iron-fisted "shutdown" of feeling. As further discussed in the Parts section, this "shutdown" may be carried out by a part of self that has long served a protective function.

In approaching stabilization-phase work with these clients, clinicians who are newer to trauma work are frequently dismayed as they encounter successive rejection after rejection of each new approach to regulation that they introduce to their clients. Initially enthusiastic about applying innovative new mind–body regulation techniques with their clients, these clinicians often face a steady incremental decline in confidence and enthusiasm and rise in trepidation as their efforts are met with resistance, failure, or outright rejection. This response naturally leads many conscientious, intelligent, and determined clinicians to strive harder to find the "right" regulation techniques for each of their clients. This seductive trap can pull clinicians, and sometimes their supervisors, into the whirling gyre of the emotional voids in which many of our clients are trapped. In other moments, often with the very same clients, clinicians may experience a helplessness and hopelessness that evokes an urge to retreat and flee in the face of this abyss. Katherine and Susan's work with Nicole and David vividly portray the oscillating pulls and tensions of this process.

Many of our clients suffer from chronic dysregulation of affect, impulses, physiology, and self-appraisal that is exacerbated by relationship with others due to survivors' intertwined longing and conditioned reactivity to intimate connection. Therefore, attempts by clinicians to focus excessively on behavioral-regulation techniques with these clients are often premature and can backfire woefully. These efforts commonly overlook that the primary source of ongoing dysregulation in the moment of therapeutic interaction is the very presence of the clinician him- or herself. In these instances, prevalent in work with adult survivors of chronic childhood neglect and psychological abuse, an essential first step in advancing the client's self-regulatory capacity is often to attend to relational regulation through the clinician's intensive, ongoing monitoring of his or her own regulatory capacity and use of self in the treatment and his or her function, intentionally and incidentally, as object of or catalyst for (dys)regulation.

CLINICIANS' REGULATORY CAPACITY AND CO-REGULATION
Therapist as Barometer and Pressure Gauge

Owing largely to the contributions of feminism, women's and gender studies, and the relational therapy movements of the 1960s and 1970s, clinical practitioners became much more sophisticated about how to approach the treatment of adult survivors of child sexual abuse in a manner sensitive to recognizing, minimizing, and mitigating inadvertent triggers. Adult survivors of emotional abuse and neglect require the same, or perhaps even greater, thoughtfulness, deliberation, and attention on the part of the clinician about how these clients are engaged, the tools that are used, and the space that is arranged. Far more important in this regard than the setup of the office or the array of skill-building objects and techniques used are the subtler, nonspecific characteristics of the clinician's physical presence. These include their demeanor and nonverbal communication and engagement, ranging from their judicious decision making about whether, how, and when to use humor, confrontation, or interpretation in sessions to their tone of voice, posture, physical proximity, or physical contact and their modulation in response to shifts in the client's regulatory state. In our work, we have time and again observed that these special and relational elements of treatment are critical factors in regard to bolstering or undermining the regulatory capacity of adult survivors of chronic childhood neglect and psychological abuse.

CBP emphasizes the primacy of the therapist's own regulatory capacity and embodied presence in this work over the array of regulation tools, skills, and strategies that they seek to impart. Just as with successfully co-regulated infants, we are increasingly attuned to the reality that how we are in the room with our most vulnerable, dysregulated clients is the greatest determinant of our capacity to successfully co-regulate our clients. Therapists who try too hard can get sucked into the vortex of enactments with their clients (see Chapter 4) in which there is a reciprocal failure to soothe and be soothed, no matter how much effort, nurturance, and care is expended. Our prized regulatory tools are rendered useless within this black hole we now share. Likewise, when our clients feel us pull away in frustration, fear, hopelessness, or at times even disgust in response to the desperate intensity of their unmet needs, the meaningless, irrelevance, if not offensiveness, of whatever regulation technique we offer next becomes sharply palpable in the room.

In contrast, if we can endeavor—through patience, supervision, the support of our colleagues, and for some of us, faith—to find a way to remain present in the room and to hold our ground, neither drawn into nor repelled from the void, it is through these moments that we can cast a tiny beacon of hope for our clients. Likely they will not be able to find their way out of the hole in that session or the next; sometimes it might even take weeks, months, or years. Regardless, the key to early co-regulation with these clients appears to lie more in their experience of our abiding presence; of our effort to sustain patience, understanding, and acceptance of their plight; of our fight not to fall into or retreat from this abyss and to draw ourselves out or back when we do; and, above all, of our refusal to yield in our belief that in some future moment we will together bridge this divide, forming the base from which we can work to build regulatory capacity.

What do regulation skills look like, then, at the edge of this black hole? We can think about the therapist's role in these interactions as a "barometer" of the "pressure" in the session room. As such, we strive to attune equally to the degree of emotional intensity or constriction being expressed, embodied, or suppressed by the client as well as the therapist (whether in response to traumatic memories or triggers). At times, these strong reactions are expressions of a relational enactment that has been activated in that moment or has been unfolding over time between client and therapist. In other instances, they can manifest in response to external demands, pressures, or stressors that either the client or therapist has brought with him or her into the session. CBP suggests that the ability to connect empathically with complexly traumatized clients is in large part a function of the clinician's corresponding relative success in maintaining this level of intra- and interpersonal attunement in the moment.

In turn, our capacity to function as a "pressure gauge" to regulate our own emotional intensity and engagement in these moments can often serve as the catalyst for clinical growth. For instance, following an early therapeutic rupture, a therapist named Marco found himself suffering through several sessions of a "cold war" with Victoria, a highly intelligent client. Although his "barometer" of the pressure in the room was functioning quite well, leaving him in considerable discomfort, Marco was less aware of the ways in which his own dysregulation was contributing to this pressure. In an effort to move the work forward and resolve this uncomfortable situation, which was characterized by a loss of trust and involved protracted periods of uncomfortable silences often spanning multiple sessions, Marco tried to repair this rupture by cognitively processing what had transpired. Victoria perceived these interactions as an increasingly aversive "debate" predicated on denial of her experience. Not surprisingly, the harder and more fervently Marco worked to amend the therapeutic rupture in this manner, the more he fell short, infuriating Victoria and increasing his own sense of frustration and hopelessness. Pulled into this enactment, Marco was flailing helplessly and was in effect blindly lashing out, worsening relational wounds that had been left open and now made vulnerable by the initial therapeutic rupture.

It was not until several sessions later, after sitting through a solid 20 minutes of uncomfortable silence, that something finally quieted within Marco and he found himself able to appraise this dynamic from a more detached, empathic, curious vantage point (a feat that is often more easily achieved within a good reflective supervision session than in the midst of an emotionally intense, conflictual therapy session). From this place, he immediately recognized that both he and Victoria were stuck, despite their excessively logical and overly sophisticated capacity for verbal discourse, and were reacting from young states of functioning. They both felt wounded and were attempting to cope with this situation by alternately confronting and retreating from each other in response to the impossibility of finding adult words to resolve overwhelming experience held by these more primitive aspects of self. Experiencing this realization in an embodied, authentic manner, Marco spontaneously began softly humming a nonspecific melody reminiscent of a young child's nursery rhyme. Almost immediately he felt the pressure in the room lessen and observed nonverbal softening of Victoria's affect, an opening of her tightly constricted posture, and a shifting of her completely closed down interpersonal engagement to a tentatively curious stance. Almost no talking ensued, but by the end of the session Marco and Victoria attained an unspoken, shared recognition (confirmed and put to words in a subsequent session) that an abysmal divide had been bridged. Extensive work remained in what became a long-term therapy case, but the process of building regulatory capacity within a containing relational frame had begun.

Each clinician has her own window of tolerance (see Chapter 5) and set of regulatory skills that she often unconsciously weaves into the fabric of the therapeutic process. If a clinician is outside of her window of tolerance during a therapeutic interaction, she will not be able to work effectively. Priya, an experienced clinician, walked into a session with Chantelle after having just learned that there was a fire in her own home. With her thoughts swirling around the potential damage and losses, she was not able to be mentally or emotionally present with Chantelle. She quickly realized that and followed her usual practice of being open with her clients about her state in the session. She and Chantelle were able to discuss options and decided to reschedule their session for later in the week. Chantelle was appreciative of Priya's transparency and found her trust in her increasing. Because of the relational element of the therapeutic model we are describing, our own emotional process is a central tool in therapy. We can't impart skills while we ourselves are agitated, distracted, or shut down.

In an even more complicated scenario, Barney has just disclosed to his therapist Joanne that he cheated on his girlfriend and that he is angry about his girlfriend's "neediness" and nagging. Joanne finds herself suddenly enraged with him. As he is talking, she finds that she can no longer hear his voice. Instead, all she can think about is her father's abandonment of her family when she was young and her daughter's husband, who recently left her daughter for another woman. Although Joanne cognitively recognizes that she is overreacting, she feels resentful and sees Barney as just "another rotten man."

This reaction, and Barney's frustration with Joanne's apparent distractedness, is another example of an enactment (see Chapter 4). From the perspective of regulation, Joanne has rocketed outside of her window of tolerance. She is not able to maintain a curious, mindful stance about her reaction. Instead, she is caught *in* her reaction, miles away from Barney, of whom she is fond, and what he is bringing into the therapy.

Trauma is ubiquitous, and many clinicians have their own histories of exposure to trauma. It is a common recommendation in graduate training programs and in the mental health field that therapists need to deal with their own "stuff" in order to provide quality therapy. But why is this so? One reason is that a clinician who has not confronted her own demons may be coping through a restricted window of tolerance. In the preceding example, Joanne herself lacks self-regulatory capacity when she becomes overwhelmed, so she has arranged her life so that it is calm and secure. She has not dealt with her own childhood experience of abandonment, and her daughter's recent marital issues have triggered these early losses. Joanne is therefore quite vulnerable to becoming dysregulated in the face of reminders in her clinical work. Although he does not fully understand what is happening, Barney, like many trauma survivors, is highly attuned to interpersonal signals of disapproval, rejection, or withdrawal and "reads" Joanne, despite her best efforts to cover up her reaction. Joanne needs to do her own trauma work to acknowledge her own losses and their impact, to increase her window of tolerance, and to be able to engage more fully in her therapeutic work.

Regulation in the Face of Clients' Suicidality or Self-Harm

Imagine that Nicole comes into a session and tells Katherine that she feels empty, hopeless, and would rather be dead. What's more, she says that she always feels this way but has been unable to tell her. As an evolving trauma therapist, Katherine has developed increasing capacity to manage various dark and hard feelings. In a moment such as this, however, like many therapists, Katherine might find herself shaken off balance by her client's unexpected admittance of acute suicidal despair and become visibly anxious herself in the session. This could lead Katherine to offer a reactive response that, despite its intention to ward Nicole away from this line of thinking, instead serves to magnify her client's sense of hopelessness.

For example, Katherine might respond in this imagined scenario by imploring to Nicole that she "shouldn't be thinking that way" because she is important, and her children would be "lost" without her. This response is unintentionally experienced by Nicole as shaming and judgmental. Now Katherine and Nicole could find themselves swallowed up into the abyss, both feeling helpless and anxious. Katherine might think to herself, "I'm so ineffective. I can't even keep her from thinking about killing herself." In response to her own inner distress activated by this relational enactment, Katherine might find herself quickly trying to resolve the discussion by eliciting agreement from Nicole that she won't act on her thoughts and then changing the subject, perhaps unconsciously. Nicole, reading Katherine's misattunement and discomfort, might half-heartedly contract for safety and let the topic go. This avoidance is reinforced for both women by an ensuing experience of emotional relief from the interpersonal tension that had built up in the room. In clinical interactions such as these, the therapist's dysregulated emotional response becomes the focus and catalyst for the direction of the session, leaving little room for the client's darker emotions.

Fortunately, the Katherine featured in our vignette has regular access to a trauma-focused clinical supervisor and is able to talk about difficulties that come up in the work she is doing. In an imagined scenario such as this, Katherine would hopefully bring this matter to her supervisor, who could then support Katherine in exploring her own reactions to this interaction. Katherine's supervisor may address her self-blame and assure her that she is hardly the only clinician who has panicked or felt helpless at the mention of suicide by a client. Together, Katherine and her supervisor consider ways to talk with Nicole about what happened in the session, inviting her to share more about her experience. Katherine and her supervisor may consider potential benefits of Katherine beginning (or resuming) therapy herself and the impact that this might have on her clinical work with Nicole. Katherine' supervisor can be a resource for her in thinking this decision through and, if appropriate, in helping her identify potential clinicians. The recommendation of personal therapy for therapists who are newer, less experienced in treating trauma, or facing new challenges in their work is common; in addition to the personal benefits, this opportunity for increased self-reflection often jump-starts new insights and opportunities in clinical work with clients.

Instead of avoidance, some therapists use active problem solving to manage their dysregulation in the face of clients' self-harming behaviors or suicidal ideation. For instance, a college student named Manuel has hidden his self-injurious behavior for several years. In despair, he finally goes to see Roger, a therapist at his university's clinic. Roger sees bandages on Manuel's arms. With prodding, Manuel admits that he cut himself severely the night before and ended up passing out; he shows Roger the injuries. He says that his parents were always cold and judgmental, but when he finally came out to them as being gay the year before, they told him they wished he had never been born and cut him out of their lives. Manuel expresses that, since that point, he has thought about killing himself every day and that he sometimes cuts himself to get relief from the pain. Another student in the clinic had recently committed suicide, and Roger is unable to tolerate the anxiety that he feels on hearing this story and seeing the deep cuts near Manuel's wrists. He calls in an emergency response team to further assess Manuel's risk for suicide. Instead of being supported in being able to acknowledge and communicate some very difficult feelings, Manuel retracts back into himself and puts on his calm, friendly face. He leaves the clinic feeling angry and frustrated, thinking that he narrowly escaped being locked up.

Although Manuel's risk is high, and Roger's response may have been "appropriate" from an external perspective, the process (his anxiety hijacking the therapeutic process) and the outcome (aspects of the client's emotional experience and parts of self were shut down further) increased the client's mistrust of therapy. In contrast, if this therapist had been able to invite his client to share more about his suicidal feelings and impulses and his self-injurious behavior, they would likely have been able to work together to plan a response that maintained the client's safety while increasing his sense of agency and choice. Even when safety ultimately necessitates difficult decisions such as an involuntary psychiatric hospitalization, the therapeutic relationship is ultimately more likely to survive, and the client is more likely to benefit, when any action steps are preceded by this type of more deliberate, thoughtful, and collaborative process.

With chronic safety concerns, such as ongoing serious suicidal ideation and impulses, repeated self-injurious behavior (e.g., severe cutting or burning, and dangerous dissociative behavior (such as a fragmented part of the client going into dangerous parts of the city late at night to pick up men), there is an essential role for distress tolerance and affect regulation, both for the therapist and the client. It is usually not possible to repeatedly hospitalize clients who are engaged in such behaviors, and a strict focus on containing the behavior is inadequate because it does not tap into the underlying drivers of the impulse or behavior. Therapists working with these clients have to have strong tolerance for sitting with clients who are at risk without themselves panicking or being constantly worried in and out of session. Supervision and consultation are often essential in these cases for balancing risk management with exploration and regulation of affective states. One important role is for the therapist to, over time, keep talking about these issues both calmly and empathically to explore ways that very distressed self-states, or parts of self (see Chapters 7–8), can be heard and comforted. Gradually over (sometimes a long) time, the client can learn to self-regulate around these behaviors.

REGULATION IN THE CLIENT–THERAPIST RELATIONSHIP

When considering the regulatory capacity of the relationship between the client and clinician, we can move beyond the client and therapist's windows of tolerance to consider a new construct that we are introducing in this book, namely, the *window of engagement*. By this term we mean the range of arousal states within which there can be an authentic, present-moment connection between the therapist and client. It is based on the windows of tolerance of the therapist and client and the match between the two. In particular, the window of engagement is dependent on the therapist's ability to meet the client where he is and to sit with the client in his dark places (including hypo- and hyperaroused states), without becoming "triggered" himself. The therapist's challenge is to be able to experience what the client is experiencing, to acknowledge this experience (whether or not the client is self-aware in this way), and to remain regulated while doing so.

Clinicians may have a healthy window of tolerance for their own emotional states but that does not mean that they are necessarily able to tolerate the extremes of hypo- and hyperarousal experienced by their clients. As therapists, our window of engagement needs to be as wide as that of our clients; otherwise, we will be handicapped in the work. If our window of engagement is too narrow, we will either become dysregulated if we move outside of our window of tolerance in order to become attuned to our clients, or we will remain stuck within the parameters of our own window of tolerance, risking the client's feeling that he has been abandoned again.

Let's first consider a therapist who is regulated but maintains this self-regulation by moving outside of the window of engagement. In the above example, in response to the client's disclosure of his feelings of hopelessness and his expressed desire that his life should end, another therapist can remain very calm and respond in a supportive way. She acts very much, in some ways, as you might hope a therapist would, but her internal response is dismissive. In an effort to protect herself against getting triggered and overwhelmed, she moves outside the window of engagement by focusing on her own self-care and reminding herself that "we can't work harder than our clients," "it is not in our control if they hurt themselves," and "we have to stay grounded." Yet, in so doing, despite her verbal messages of support, the therapist is sending nonverbal messages to the client that she is not as emotionally engaged as she had been moments before. The client, being highly attuned to his therapist's emotional states with regard to him, perceives this shift as a rejection. In this case, the therapist is regulated but misattuned. Despite the fact that the client may feel he can open up, his progress in therapy is met by an emotional retreat by his therapist. With supervision and therapy, we would hope the therapist would recognize her emotional retreat instead of getting locked into an ongoing enactment of the emotional rejection that the client received from his mother during childhood.

Some clinicians may have a restricted range on just one end of their window of tolerance, which also truncates their window of engagement. Amanda, an experienced female therapist, has difficulty tolerating hyperarousal, particularly anger. She is very comfortable sitting with lonely, sad clients who have low energy and struggle with motivation to change. She has a large caseload of clients suffering from depression. But when the husband of one of her clients comes into a therapy session with his wife and becomes agitated, yelling that his wife is going to die and that therapy isn't doing anything, Amanda freezes. Her mind goes blank. She is panicked and just wants to leave. She sits mutely while the husband yells, until he gets up and storms out the door.

Amanda does not invite further contact with her client's husband and avoids discussing the session with her client, instead discounting her client's husband as a potential source of support because of his "dysregulation."

Now imagine Leroy, a young, energetic therapist who has no problem with hyperarousal but has difficulty with hypoarousal and disengagement. As an African American man who grew up in a rather poor neighborhood with significant gang activity, Leroy has sought out therapeutic work with urban adolescents who are high energy and high risk. Leroy has unending ideas about how to harness that energy and direct it in more adaptive ways. He draws kids in with his humor and approaches them as a "buddy." His colleagues are amazed at how he is able to get kids who have been gang-involved off the streets and into a studio, recording rap songs about their lives. But when one of his clients becomes severely depressed and gives up on life after his brother is shot, Leroy doesn't know what to do. His energy spins higher and higher, trying to rally this teenager to keep going. He comes up with ideas about his client becoming a youth leader and speaking out about gang violence—becoming stronger and more motivated because of this experience. But his client just sinks lower and lower. After failing repeatedly to impact this young man, Leroy becomes frustrated and resentful. The client feels that he is disappointing Leroy and stops coming in for therapy.

Another problematic therapeutic issue occurs when the therapist and client have a shared window of engagement and are attuned, but neither is regulated. The young male therapist Leroy may maintain himself in a high-energy state in order to avoid his own sense of hopelessness and despair, which always seems to be waiting in the wings. He seeks out adolescent male clients who are coping in a similar way. Because of the restricted range of affect that both client and therapist allow themselves, the therapeutic process becomes a collusion in which no change occurs. Instead, therapist and client are supporting each other in their avoidance, in the name of therapy. Similarly, consider a therapist who is able to engage with her client in hopeless places because she feels hopeless herself. This therapy also becomes stagnant, a repetition of sadness and despair, with no glimmer of hope or change. The therapist may become "captured" by the client's emotional presentation, or the client may model himself after the therapist's emotional state in an attempt to please or connect. In these situations, the therapist is not able to use him- or herself as a tool to help the client to co-regulate.

We see these tensions play out between Nicole and Katherine. The misalignments between Katherine's otherwise well-adjusted and healthy personal window of tolerance, and Nicole's oscillating states of dysregulation, set off a series of mutual enactments. We encounter this, for example, in Katherine's failure to observe signs of Nicole's dramatic shift in affective state in response to Katherine's "blind spot" around Nicole's positive self-identification with the protagonist in *Pretty Woman*. Nicole leaves the encounter reeling with heightened feelings of shame, hopelessness, and impulses to engage in habitual

self-destructive coping. In turn, we observe a subtle and gradual but undeniable drift in Katherine's emotional engagement in her work with Nicole.
At a subsequent juncture in treatment, Nicole's abrupt manifestation of an
emotionally charged, negatively attributed, sexualized part of self engenders
in Katherine an unexpected parallel sensation of physiological arousal that
startles her and is experienced with revulsion. Katherine subsequently withholds disclosure of this personal reaction in supervision, seeking to distance
herself from it and inevitably from Nicole. We understand this decision as a
self-protective gesture, likely not fully conscious, aimed at safeguarding Katherine against the somatic dysregulation the incident occasioned as well as
against the threat it posed to her view of self as an empathic, well-boundaried
psychotherapist (we explore this latter concept in Chapter 10).

In CBP, we strive to attend carefully to and maintain awareness of our
own shifting affective and somatic states in relation and response to those of
our clients. These moments of synchrony and asynchrony between our own
and our clients' windows of tolerance provide vital sources of information and
potential inroads to treatment progress. In supervision with therapists like
Katherine, we undertake to support their becoming more aware of and better
able to weather the alignments and misalignments between their clients' and
their own windows of tolerance, toward the goal of expanding the window of
engagement. As in this instance with Nicole, not uncommonly this involves
helping clinicians to reflect on how strong, and at times negative, emotions
and sensations generated in themselves in the context of this challenging work
function as windows into the worlds of their clients. As therapists serving adult
survivors of emotional abuse and neglect, we must continually work to stay
regulated in these moments, particularly when our own window of tolerance
is being "stretched" to accommodate those of our clients. For this to occur—
instead of disengagement through clinician withdrawal or reactivity—we must
cultivate patience and compassion toward ourselves as much as toward our
clients, as well as grant ourselves permission to experience and sit with "dark,"
troubling, and at times ego dystonic affects and impulses. When we are successfully able to accomplish this, it often results in enhancing our clients' own
capacities for self-regulation through the powerfully co-regulating, deepening
therapeutic relationship that is being fostered by these interactions.

So when we are working with adults impacted by complex trauma, how
do we know whether we are in this window of engagement? One way we can
answer this question during a clinical interaction is to assess carefully whether
we are simultaneously experiencing a quiet, grounded empathy in conjunction with reflective curiosity. Although we can certainly experience affective
attunement and mirroring with our clients while flailing alongside them in an
enactment in which we are personally consumed by a shared sense of despair
or panic, it is highly unlikely that we remain self-possessed, grounded, and
within our own window of affect tolerance in these moments. In turn, reflective curiosity is a form of metacognition that by nature requires us to maintain

some perceptual vantage point outside of our intimate interaction with our client. Its absence indicates that we have either been drawn too far into the black hole to maintain an objective perspective and "see things as they truly are," or else that we have retreated too far from our client's suffering to a place too cold in its disengagement for our good thinking to be of use. Whenever we recognize that either of these states of being is missing in an interaction with a client (often not identified until after the fact through supervision), we typically come to realize that we have been outside our window of engagement, regardless of how compassionate we may have been feeling or how rational our thinking may have appeared to be at the time. In contrast, in those therapeutic moments in which we can attain this convergence of empathy and reflection, even and especially when our client is in a hyper- or hypoaroused state, we cast open this window of engagement and with it the possibility that we can aid our clients through co-regulation in expanding their capacity for self-regulation.

Because of the affective intensity, which is common in work with adults with attachment-related trauma, therapists frequently have their own strong responses to this work. Mirroring the therapeutic process, supervision assists therapists in bringing awareness to their own emotional reactions such as helplessness, hopelessness, or triggered reactions. For instance, a supervisor might reflect on a therapist's tendency to overrely on regulatory tools to manage his own discomfort when he is faced with a client who is phobic about overwhelming emotion. In CBP, supervision helps to support regulation within an expanding window of tolerance and window of engagement. It supports therapists' ability to sit in dark places with their clients, to tolerate anxiety about high-risk behaviors, and to use their own regulatory responses to inform the work. Within the regulation component, supervision also has the essential role of bringing awareness to patterns (overworking, emotional porousness, disengagement, blurred boundaries, lack of proactive self-care) that may be problematic, or resulting consequences such as burnout, ethical violations, or vicarious trauma.

REGULATION WITH DISSOCIATIVE CLIENTS

To complicate things further, the development of regulatory capacity generally requires an understanding of dissociated aspects of self (see Chapters 7–8). While a person can become profoundly dysregulated across all domains of functioning, expressions of dysregulation are rarely reflective of fully integrated, cohesive experiences. Instead, dysregulation is often held and expressed by parts of self; these expressions are often associated with vulnerable parts of self that are holding unresolved traumatic affect. These parts of self often proactively or reactively protect and defend against perceived threats to the self. In this case, the therapeutic focus initially may be to help regulate these parts in order to restore equilibrium, enabling the return of frontal/executive function capacity, information processing, and higher-order decision making and planning.

What we conceptualize as "younger" parts—by which we mean parts that develop when the individual was a young child (see Chapter 7)—often require different, developmentally "younger" regulation tools and approaches. Skills and techniques that work to help a complexly traumatized adult *sustain* regulatory capacity "at baseline" may be insufficient to help him to restore a healthy state of regulation in the midst of the aftermath of exposure to salient triggers. Similarly, approaches to regulation that have been found to be effective when working with clients in more "adult" states of functioning may fail to be effective, and at times even evoke strong negative reactions in these same clients when younger or more primitive states of coping have been activated. Clinicians undertaking to work with this population should bear that carefully in mind and plan accordingly. For example, even those clinicians who do not enroll children into their practice should consider stocking their offices with a broad range of potential coping tools, including items such as stuffed animals, dolls, children's books, crayons, putty, small musical instruments, and "fiddle" items that may otherwise be traditionally thought of as more suitable contents of a child therapy practice. Conversely, symbolic objects, figurines, or works of art that are routinely considered acceptable and even richly evocative contents in the office of the traditional psychodynamic clinician or aspiring sand-tray therapist should be carefully evaluated for their potential to function as destabilizing triggers for complexly traumatized adults with developmentally younger self-states or parts.

The need to comfort, soothe, or attend to the safety of younger parts often emerges as a critical precursor to the successful pursuit of more present-focused, "adult" initiatives in the treatment of adults complexly impacted by chronic emotional neglect and emotional abuse. Important clinical target areas for this population routinely include exploration and resolution of current challenges to such domains of life as relational intimacy, sexuality, vocation, identity, autonomy, self-worth, and personal meaning. For many of these clients, these areas of focus in therapy are minefields that entail high risk of triggering trauma-related sequelae, the experience of which is intolerable to some younger parts of self. Moreover, precisely because of this risk, it is not uncommon for more dissociative clients to find their efforts at adult growth and progress undermined or sabotaged by terrified parts of self desperately determined to avert perceived danger, if not annihilation, should the individual dare to traverse one of these minefields.

In consequence, we have come to learn that successful engagement in these lines of treatment requires careful prior planning, preparation, and intervention directed toward the emotional regulation of frightened or vulnerable parts of self, particularly younger or "child" parts engendered from early traumatic experiences. This work often includes the identification, creation, or co-creation of "safe spaces" for child parts to inhabit and be cared for and shielded from more adult-oriented clinical material and responsibilities inappropriate for child parts to participate in or shoulder. Examples of such topics are manifold and include efforts to circumvent, confront, or dismantle historical landmines associated with the pursuit of risk or change in the service of self-growth in areas of adult life, such as sexual activity or emotional intimacy; financial or vocational success; independence and autonomy; assertiveness and conflict resolution; access to present-focused experiences of pleasure or joy; and the judicious tempering of chronically rigid or extreme protective defenses. These safe spaces can be cultivated utilizing various guided imagery with clients, or else through the more sophisticated approach to engagement of dissociative parts we introduce in Chapter 8, which describes our approach to parts work. Other practitioners may also find incorporation of mindfulness, meditation, or self-hypnotic approaches helpful in this regard.

Finally, the importance of regulation through co-regulation with younger, more fragile parts of self should be underscored. For many clients, the successful establishment of safe spaces where child parts can feel supported and protected while adult issues are addressed in treatment often necessitates the inclusion in these spaces of caring or protective adult representations. While the clinician can, of course, make suggestions based on her knowledge of the client, both the need for insertion of adult caregivers into these safe spaces and the specific identity of these adult representations should always stem from the client. As is discussed in more detail in Chapter 8, whenever possible, we seek to involve adult representations of the client in efforts to regulate child parts of self. In some instances, clients will also request participation of representations of the therapist in the soothing and protection of child parts, particularly when the therapeutic alliance represents one of the few or only past or current relationships with adults the client has experienced as trustworthy, boundaried, and safe. In other instances, clients may draw on positive adult representations from earlier life experience (e.g., a benign or helpful relative or teacher), popular culture (e.g., Oprah Winfrey, Mr. Rogers), or fiction (e.g., Batman, a squad of G.I. Joes). Some clients, particularly those for whom human relationships have consistently been fraught with peril or strife, may choose more symbolic representations as protectors (e.g., a real or fictional protective animal such as the Lion from *The Lion, The Witch and the Wardrobe* or a protective dog, wolf, or elephant; a force field; a protective tree or geological formation). These and other options and scenarios speak to the complexity and layers of regulation work with dissociative adult survivors of chronic emotional neglect and abuse.

CONNECTIONS AMONG REGULATION, RELATIONSHIP, AND NARRATIVE

In the opening of this book, we highlighted one of the central myths that has become almost ubiquitous in the subfield of complex traumatic stress, namely, the myth that the "stabilization" or regulation "phase" or component of trauma intervention should or must be substantially completed before safe and effective narrative processing can begin. On the one hand, as previously noted, these important best-practice guidelines arose out of recognition that for many complex trauma survivors, delving too quickly into narrative work in general, and traumatic memory processing in particular, can, and frequently does, have deleterious consequences for clients who are not ready or able to tolerate that aspect of the work. These guidelines have emerged from a wealth of clinical wisdom, as well as a solid empirical base of evidence. On the other hand, although this careful pacing should be an ongoing consideration in complex trauma treatment, we also need to be alert to the potential negative consequences of misapplying these guidelines, which can lead us to shy away from trauma processing or other narrative work because we aren't "done" with stabilization.

Problems within the therapist's window of tolerance or within the shared window of engagement can significantly impact the therapeutic process over time, including choices regarding the focus of therapy and the timing and pacing of therapy. It is not uncommon for us to make clinical decisions that are unintentionally colored by our own apprehensions and fears about processing traumatic memories and the potential dysregulation it may lead to in our clients. If we do not consistently work to increase our awareness of our own implicit desire to retrospectively protect our clients from their own horrific experiences and distress, we may end up colluding with and unintentionally reinforcing our client's often implicit self-protective avoidance of this vital element of the work. In the forthcoming section on narrative (Chapters 9–10), we explore more deeply these and other issues surrounding clinicians' readiness to undertake the narrative component of trauma intervention.

Occasionally, clear evidence of this disconnect between client and clinician around readiness to shift from regulation-focused techniques to engagement of specific trauma material is revealed through the too-seldom practice of careful review of recorded sessions. During one such opportunity at our Center afforded through the context of a highly systematized, federally funded treatment outcome study for adults suffering from chronic PTSD, several noteworthy expressions of these complicating clinician factors emerged. In one example, a male clinician who was relatively new to trauma work had been carefully trained on a systematic trauma intervention protocol. Despite this training, his quite experienced female supervisor noticed that he was exhibiting a pattern of progression from emotion regulation work into narrative processing, as per study protocol, quickly followed by manifestations of personal emotional distress and consequent abrupt discontinuation of in-process narrative work and resumption of regulation techniques. This pattern was observed during review of study sessions to transpire relatively consistently when study participants evidenced a spike in the intensity of their expression of vulnerable emotions such as fear, grief, and rage when recounting memories of past trauma. The clinician may have been nervous or uncertain of what his clients' difficult emotions and memories would bring up in him, leading him to shut down the processing. He may have been out of his own window of tolerance, or he may have been trying to protect himself from exceeding his window of tolerance. Alternatively, he may have sensed parts in himself and/ or his clients that were fearful or cautionary about approaching memories. After the brief attempt at processing, he and his clients may have each pushed away the parts of themselves that had built confidence in the clients' abilities to acknowledge their emotions and confront some difficult memories. The clinician may have ended up colluding with the clients' avoidance by focusing back on safety and stabilization.

Through session reviews, this clinician's supervisor was able to help him recognize how his own protective but reactive response to his clients' emotional states was a misread of their otherwise healthy emotional engagement of their traumatic material. This reaction was unintentionally undermining their process by augmenting whatever doubts they may have harbored regarding their capacity to face their traumatic experiences, inducing an elevation of the clients' defensive and avoidant coping. The supervisor used this information as an opportunity to help the clinician to differentiate normative, expected, and even adaptive elevations of affective response when processing traumatic material in an emotionally engaged, nondissociative manner from indications of extreme affective dysregulation necessitating discontinuation of narrative work and redoubling of stabilization efforts. Through this support and guidance, the clinician became highly effective in his capacity to tolerate the emotional responses of complexly traumatized clients and to guide them through processing of their traumatic memories and experiences.

With clients for whom the principal source of their complex trauma adaptation derives from childhood histories of emotional abuse and neglect, as exemplified in the two central vignettes of this book, the interconnections and tensions among regulation, relationship, and narrative work are often even more embedded and insidious. CBP does not address the components in discrete stages, but attends to the interrelationship between components throughout the therapy process. Like David and Nicole, many of these clients find that their emotional dysregulation is intimately connected with negative attributions of self or schemas of relationship that arose from their formative experiences of attachment disruption, inconsistency, betrayal, and disappointment. Accordingly, clinicians operating under the assumption that they are supposed to help move their clients clearly out of the gravitational pull of the abyss before engaging in narrative work can find themselves waiting forever to begin narrative work, orbiting in an endless regulation phase of intervention. We contend that in working with this subpopulation of complexly traumatized adults, a more accurate and realistic guiding strategy is to seek and attune to moments in the treatment in which the client has emerged from the center of their abyss of dysregulation and disconnection to its outer edge, and when registering this movement, endeavoring, deftly and in modest increments, to integrate narrative components into the work. Ultimately, it is in these intermittent, often fleeting, moments in which present-focused sensory experience, emotional connection, embodied movement, agentic action, and future vision become possible.

CONCLUSION

There are numerous challenges in undertaking the regulation component of work in treatment of adults with histories of pervasive childhood emotional and relational deprivation and disconnection. The metaphor of the "black hole of trauma" can be used to conceptualize the abyss of unmet attachment needs that many of our clients face, which interferes with the development of regulatory capacity. A central part of this work involves assisting our clients in building their regulatory capacity, including awareness of, tolerance for, communication about, and ability to modulate internal states. Traditional and innovative, tailored tools can be used to support this work. Because of the intimacy of the therapeutic relationship, we, as therapists, can be a catalyst for both regulation and dysregulation for our clients. Therefore, CBP emphasizes our own regulatory capacity as therapists and the use of ourselves as coregulators. When we use our self as a "barometer," we attune to dysregulation in our clients, ourselves, and in the room between us; when we operate as a "pressure gauge," we focus on regulating ourselves to initiate a ripple effect on the therapeutic process. We need to strive to remain within the "window of engagement," the convergence of client–clinician regulatory capacity that promotes therapeutic change. As shown in Table 6.1, supervision is essential as we reflect on the interconnected balance between the relationship and regulation components of CBP, assisting us in cultivating work within a carefully paced expansion of the window of engagement and supporting us in taking care of ourselves in this work. In the next section, we introduce increasing complexity to the CBP approach as we consider the impact of dissociative processes on our clients who have experienced early relational trauma and explore implications for the therapeutic process.

TABLE 6.1. Intervention Strategies for the Regulation Component of CBP

Client

- Building awareness of, tolerance for, linkages among, skills to regulate, and ability to express aspects of experience, including affect, cognition, somatic states, and behaviors
- Teaching affective, cognitive, somatic, or behavioral tools for regulation
  □ Applying standard tools/utilizing existing tools (grounding, imagery, breathing, mind–body tools, neurofeedback, yoga)
  □ Working with client to tailor tools (modifying standard tools or creating new tools by drawing from experience, using client-specific metaphors)
- Matching regulatory tool to type of dysregulation (affective, cognitive, somatic, behavioral)
- Expanding window of tolerance

Regulation × Relationship

- Using the therapeutic relationship for containment, reflection/self-awareness, and co-regulation (therapist as barometer and pressure gauge)
- Progressing in the regulatory role of the therapeutic relationship—from providing containment, to supporting exploration, to encouraging client's internalization of skills
- Developing regulatory tools that emerge organically from the therapeutic relationship
- Working through the therapeutic relationship as a dysregulating force (intimacy as dysregulating)

Therapist

- Managing our own reactivity, including affective (such as anxiety, resentment, frustration, boredom, numbing), somatic (sympathetic activation, fatigue, intrusive triggered somatic symptoms), cognitive (wanting to "fix" it, helplessness, hopelessness), and behavioral reactivity (such as overengagement or distancing mechanisms)
- Expanding our window of tolerance

Regulation × Relationship

- Maintaining an optimal window of engagement
- Recognizing our own reactivity to clients
- Understanding the impact of our tendencies regarding pacing (colluding with avoidance or pressure to "do" more in treatment)

Supervisor

- Use of reflection to increase awareness of regulatory processes of client, clinician, supervisor, and their interactions
- Supporting therapist's regulatory processes and proactive self-care; addressing vicarious trauma responses

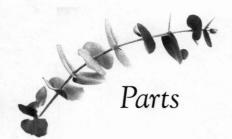

Parts

CHAPTER 7

Fragmentation of Self and Dissociative Parts

After Katherine questions Nicole's choice of Julia Roberts's character in *Pretty Woman* as an internal resource, Nicole maintains her pleasant and friendly facade but in fact is feeling shattered. In this enactment, Nicole has shifted into a dissociative state in reaction to her therapist's misattunement, a fragmented part of her that feels freakish and alien. This part of her holds her early traumatic exposure of being judged and rejected by those who should have cared for her the most.

Dissociation is not a new concept, nor is the idea that traumatic experience can lead to disconnection in one's sense of self (Ferenczi, 1980/1933; Janet, 1889; Sullivan, 1953). Many theorists and clinicians have built upon these early conceptualizations in the modern era (e.g., Richard Kluft, Kathy Steele, Paul Dell, Ellert Nijenhuis, and Frank Putnam, among others), and our thinking has been heavily influenced by their work (for a historical review of the field, please see Dell & O'Neil, 2009; Howell, 2005). In CBP, we view dissociation as a commonly used coping mechanism that can be quite adaptive. It can prevent us from being overwhelmed by the sheer quantity of information available to us, and it can protect us from the intensity of unbearable emotional, cognitive, or somatic experiences. However, dissociation becomes problematic when it is uncontrollable or is used to the exclusion of other forms of coping. Nonpathological examples of dissociation include daydreaming while engaged in a menial, repetitive task or eliciting an assertive or self-confident part of self while giving a presentation. A problematic example is a person who acknowledges fighting with his wife but doesn't grasp the intensity of the conflict and cannot recall all of his behaviors during the fight. A more extreme example of pathological dissociation is a client who, in session, has no memory of what she just told you or who you are.

In the regulation section of this book, we addressed dissociation as a regulatory tool. In this section, we focus more on fragmentation in self-states, what we call "parts." Similar to Putnam's (1994) conceptualization of the impact of dissociation on sense of self, we consider fragmentation to be a process that keeps different mental states and body experiences from linking with one another, which can but does not necessarily create new and highly discrete states. In this chapter, we address the impact of attachment-based trauma on parts of self, and in the next, we describe CBP's approach for working with parts, including the role of the therapeutic relationship in exploration and acceptance of dissociated aspects of self.

DIMENSIONS OF DISSOCIATION

In CBP, we can assess a person's dissociative process across a series of dimensions: cohesiveness, engagement, embodiment, and level of resources (see Figure 7.1). We approach this work under the basic premise that everyone has different parts of self that are more or less interconnected. Consider, for instance, the part of you that is your "work self," versus who you are with your family of origin, versus the part of you that engages with other people at a party or other social event. Cohesive parts of self are able to work together rather fluidly, as a person shifts according to the demands of the situation. For instance, an executive may have a part of self with a strong drive toward success but notices when that drive begins to interfere with his home life. He is then able to draw on a softer side of himself to reorient more toward his relationships. In this example, the executive's "work self" and "family self" are relatively cohesive and are able to work together to maintain homeostasis. However, early trauma can lead to a disconnection among these parts of self. In a person who is less cohesive, these parts may operate in conflict with each other, viewing other parts as weak, untrustworthy, or dangerous. For instance, a person with a dominant part of self who believes that "it is not safe to be angry" might experience irritation or resentment but disconnects from these reactions, discounting the impulse to express anger as "ridiculous." As these dissociated emotions proliferate, the silenced part may become embittered or begin to simmer with rage. At the least cohesive end of this continuum of fragmentation, parts of self may not have knowledge of each other and instead will operate in isolation, with little to no communication within the larger system. Generally, more severe early abuse and neglect is associated with more fragmentation in parts of self. Clients who have been diagnosed with dissociative identity disorder (DID) would be at the more fragmented end of

Fragmented -- (X) Cohesive
Disengaged (from Environment) -- (X) Engaged
Disembodied -- (X) Embodied
Underresourced --- (X) Resourced

FIGURE 7.1. Dimensions of dissociation. X denotes therapeutic goals.

this continuum. However, it is important to note that CBP considers "parts" language and conceptualization to be helpful with many survivors of early relational trauma, including many people who would not meet the criteria for DID or another dissociative disorder in DSM-5.

The continuum of engagement refers to awareness of and connection with the external world. The most engaged clients are attuned to their external environment, using all of the five primary senses to interact with the environment. Moving toward the disengaged end of the continuum, some people have a tendency to separate from awareness of their surroundings in stressful situations. They may "space out" or have trouble tracking a conversation. At the farthest end of this continuum, some people are generally disconnected from the external environment and from other people. This can impact memory, narrative, and continuity of experience. For instance, some of our clients have described living for many years in a fog and having limited to no memories of this time period. It is important to note that, for more fragmented clients, different parts of self often fall at different points along dimensions of the CBP components, complicating assessment and treatment planning with these clients. For instance, considering the continuum of engagement, Nicole has a hypervigilant part that is highly engaged with the environment but is anxious and fearful. However, she also has a self-protective part that disengages from the world around her in an attempt to regulate.

The third dimension, degree of embodiment, refers to the ability to connect to one's body and internal sensations. While external awareness relies on the use of the five primary senses, embodiment draws on a host of other senses such as proprioception (the sense of one's body in space), equilibrioception (sense of balance), thermoception and nocioception (the perceptions of temperature and pain), and interoception (awareness of sensations within the body). A person who is embodied can utilize somatic sensations to increase awareness of affect, cognitions, and impulses. They are also more able to access parts of self by utilizing somatic means. Thus, body-based therapies that increase somatic awareness can be a means of increasing cohesion among parts of self. Disembodiment occurs when people are unaware of somatic sensations and are often frightened to focus attention on their bodies. It is not uncommon for us to encounter clients who have disconnected from their internal experience, being left with an intellectual understanding of themselves but a sense of alienation from self. In people who are quite fragmented, one part may somatically "hold" certain memories or internal experiences, leaving other parts disconnected from those experiences. Engagement of the body in treatment is also essential for clients who are highly disembodied, but the pacing must be adapted to allow these clients to remain within their window of tolerance as they slowly reestablish connection with their physical selves.

The last dimension, level of resources, refers to the degree to which clients are able to access parts of themselves for healthy coping. Clients who are underresourced tend to have difficulty tolerating uncomfortable feelings and limited capacity to understand their parts of self as a system. Their parts are often more extreme and are not channeled toward effective current-day living. For instance, on one hand, a self-protective part may tend to act out in rage versus being assertive. On the other hand, a client who has more access to internal resources has at least some capacity to tolerate difficult emotions and some coping mechanisms. She has some capacity for self-reflection and is able to harness the adaptive purpose of different parts of self. She has some understanding of how her personality is constructed and can become curious about, and compassionate toward, her parts of self. This understanding allows her to harness the adaptive purpose of her different parts of self. Clients often develop or gain greater access to internal resources held by different parts of themselves as they progress in therapy.

DISSOCIATION IN CHILDHOOD

Because they live in the present moment, focused on their immediate needs, infants do not appear to have a coherent sense of self. As their experiences multiply, they have rapidly shifting self-states related to current actions, sensations, emotions, and relationships. According to Bowlby (1973, 1980, 1982), infants develop internal working models of self and others that develop through their experiences within their primary attachment relationships. Over time, with adequate parenting and early attachments, the child begins to develop a more coherent, if somewhat illusory (Bromberg, 2001), sense of a unified self. In his observations of infants, Wolff (1987) described an initial cluster of self-other states that began to come together into the experience of a unitary self. This coalescing identity allows the child to begin to develop a somewhat stable perception of "me" and allows his or her parts of self to become somewhat more coordinated. In "good-enough" families, a concept derived from the work of Winnicott (1965), babies and toddlers learn how to be nurtured and loved, and demonstrate through imaginative play with dolls, pets, or peers that they are internalizing the ability to nurture. These skills later translate into a generally continuous sense of self across time and situations, the ability to soothe and care for oneself, and the capacity for healthy relationships.

Despite this growing sense of coherence, dissociation is an inevitable part of childhood. In normative child development, some states or parts are often pushed into the background or never formulated to emerge into awareness because their narrative content and/or emotions are not acknowledged by or acceptable to the family or to the child's cultural context. Stern (1997) refers to states that are never formulated as "dissociation in the weak sense." These forbidden or neglected topics—whether aspects of sexuality, anger at loved ones, family finances, or other taboos—become increasingly cut off from conscious awareness because the child is emotionally alone in the experience and has no words with which to think about them and no dialogue or response to help give shape to inchoate sensations. If there is a good-enough attachment and a robust-enough child, having these cut-off areas is not likely to cause major difficulties in living. However, even with good-enough attachments, early relational experiences of suppression and shame often continue to influence adult life. The child part that holds the experience may continue to react when triggered, and this can affect one's emotional state and relationships throughout adulthood.

In unresponsive, neglectful, or abusive families, children often cope through disconnection from certain aspects of themselves. More recently, we and others (e.g., Chefetz, 2015; Chefetz & Bromberg, 2004) have emphasized the interpersonal aspect of dissociation and see it as tied directly to the internalization of attachment relationships. In this frame, it becomes an intersubjective or interpersonal phenomenon as well as an intrapsychic one. In his study of institutionalized children, Bowlby (1980) found that the lack of adequate early attachments resulted in splitting apart a child's internal working models. He noted that, when early caretaking interactions go badly, infants develop multiple internal representations of self and attachment figures instead of more unitary or cohesive representations. In these situations, the attachment figures subtly induce the infant to disown personal, firsthand experiences (e.g., "I am very angry at Mommy") and instead accept a false version of their experience in order to maintain the attachment relationship ("Mommy loves me, and if I am a good girl, I will not feel angry with her"). This process of disowning one's own experience results in a fragmentation of parts of self.

Parts, then, are the internalization of aspects of attachment relationships as well as toxic affect and sensory experience from early trauma. In neglectful and emotionally abusive families, children internalize aspects of the neglectful and emotionally abusive parent and, under certain circumstances, can enact hostile or withholding parts of the caregivers. The child begins to implicitly understand that the very act of seeking nurturance or support leads to further withdrawal or emotional abuse from her caregiver. Thus, these children develop internal parts whose entire role, at the beginning, is to protect themselves by silencing these young parts of themselves that hold their unmet emotional needs. One part initially may be focused on silencing or even trying to destroy the part that seeks nurturance; another may have that same relationship with a young part that holds rage. These parts also begin to play a role in relationships with others in the child's world. So, for example, the part of a child that developed to manage her own disowned longing for nurturance may be aggressive toward a younger sibling who expresses the need for nurturance. Later, without treatment, that part may also become triggered by the dependency needs of the client's own young children, leading to dissociated resentment and anger; in some cases, this pattern can contribute to intergenerational cycles of attachment-related trauma.

In contrast, some parts might develop to fill gaps in caregiving and attempt to create safety or structure. For example, if the caregivers' impairments leave them disorganized and unable to keep up with the household or get the children ready for school, a parentified part of the child may take on those functions and perform them effectively, although at great cost to the child's larger system. For instance, a divorced professional woman was a responsible mother and was well respected at work, but whenever she was home alone, she fell apart emotionally and was paralyzed with fear and helplessness. When she and her therapist explored this pattern, this woman realized that she had a parentified adolescent part that was overwhelmed and exhausted by her efforts to be successful as a mother, keep up with challenging work demands, keep emotions at bay, and manage her presentation to everyone around her.

CLASSIFICATIONS OF DISSOCIATIVE PARTS

Theorists and clinicians have conceptualized and identified parts in different ways. For instance, Sullivan's interpersonal theory identified three types of self: "the good-me," "the bad-me," and the "not-me" (Howell, 2005; Sullivan, 1953). The good-me holds the thoughts and feelings that were approved of in the infant's world, and the bad-me those disapproved of by that world. Both are accessible to consciousness. The not-me, according to Sullivan (1953), is associated with severe anxiety, horror, and dread and is dissociated and thus inaccessible to consciousness. Putnam's (1989) seminal book on the diagnosis and treatment of "multiple personality disorder" introduced a conceptualization of parts, or "personalities," that were based on their functional role. In their theory of structural dissociation, which draws in part on neuroscience and Porges's (2011) polyvagal theory, van der Hart and colleagues (2006; also Steele & van der Hart, 2009) describe the dissociated personality as being divided into two broad systems, which may or may not be broken into subsystems. What they term the "apparently normal part of the personality (ANP)" is the constricted and avoidant part, mediated by the ventral vagal system, that tries to go on with normal life while avoiding any reminders of trauma. In contrast, the "emotional part of the personality (EP)" involves the defensive systems developed during traumatization that reenact the trauma in emotional and sensorimotor ways. Although the entire system is traumatized, the ANPs and the EPs are inevitably in conflict because of their roles in the person's inner system. Schwartz (1995) has perhaps best captured the way that different parts play different roles in an internal system much like the system of a family, with different parts holding strongly to the roles they have been given in their family of origin. He labels the parts that hold the trauma and other excluded emotions, thoughts, and attitudes as "exiles." "Managers" are the parts that try to block the expression of these exiles and are strategic, proactive, protective, and motivated to try to control the environment. "Firefighters," in Schwartz's terminology, react quickly to diminish distress, such as by drinking or cutting, when the exiles are triggered. In his view, these parts are inevitably polarized.

In CBP, the language used to talk about these parts varies but should feel comfortable to both client and therapist. Our language is typically drawn from the way our clients describe their parts of self. We consider parts of self from a developmental as well as a functional lens. Accordingly, we often use developmental terminology of "child/kid parts," "adolescent parts," and "adult parts." In other situations, we may use the functional language of "vulnerable parts," "protective/defensive parts," and "wise or compassionate parts/self." For the sake of consistency and clarity, we rely primarily on developmental terminology throughout this book.

Child parts, or vulnerable parts, carry intense and unmodulated feeling states such as longing, fear, sadness, abandonment, need, hopelessness, and shame. These parts often represent either the normal feelings that were not tolerated in the family and had to be dissociated, such as the longing for nurturance, or traumatic dissociated feelings such as terror. These young parts can also hold a full range of physical sensations, such as pain, shakiness, agitation, coldness, or intense hunger. Child parts often function at the developmental level of early childhood or even infancy, with some being preverbal. These parts' cognition is often undeveloped, both because of their developmental stage and because of their trauma exposure and lack of adequate support or nurturance. Even when these parts become calm enough to think, their early narratives about the trauma are often fragmented, primitive, and/or missing. When these parts are fully present in our offices without any adult self present in the client, it can feel like we are sitting with a young child or infant. These parts may hold the client's desire for connection and support and may develop a strong connection to or reliance on the therapist. Child parts can be very fearful and dysregulated; however, they can also be highly creative, playful, and spontaneous. When they are cared for, usually by the therapist initially and then eventually by the adult self of the client, they can feel a greater sense of safety and connection, including feelings of adoration or love. With an increased sense of security, they may also be able to grieve their losses and experience sadness and empathy.

Adolescent parts, or protective parts, sometimes hold intense emotions such as anger, rage, self-hatred, or sexuality. They may be experienced by other parts as dangerous, threatening, controlling, or abusive. Functionally, the parts that may have developed to protect the child from escalation of childhood abuse are vestiges of early coping efforts. They may also protect the client by holding off more vulnerable states, denying needs that could lead to further disappointment or hurt. They often have negative reactions to authority, insist that they don't need anything or anyone, and may have more resistant or con-flicted therapeutic relationships. Like adolescents, they often think in black-and-white ways and may be quite passionate about what they think and believe. In their zeal, conviction, and rage, these parts can become destructive toward parts holding the trauma. Other adolescent parts may be numb, indifferent, or feeling too hopeless to try to engage in life. These parts may become "bur-dened" (a useful term coined by Schwartz, 1995) by early abuse and neglect in their caregiving environments. In an example of this burdening, an adolescent part develops that mimics a young woman's psychotic mother who raged over disorder in the home. This adolescent part initially developed to prevent less controlled parts of herself from ever leaving a mess in the house, in an attempt to increase safety. This part, who views herself as a long-suffering and harassed adult, is extremely punitive toward her own younger child parts, as well as to her partner and flesh-and-blood children when they "leave a mess." This attempt to experience some sense of control over her mother's dysregulated behavior leaves the child vulnerable to blaming herself for her mother's rages. However, it appears to be in some way preferable for children to see themselves as blameworthy for the abuse rather than helpless in the face of an uncontrol-lable and intolerable environment created by attachment figures (discussed in Grossman, Sorsoli, & Kia-Keating, 2006).

We see the adult self or wise self (Schwartz, 1995, refers to this as a broader "Self") as the part that carries the real wisdom, compassion, and curi-osity of the client. Some clients initially have little or no adult self or, perhaps more frequently, have fragmented aspects of adult functioning that are not integrated into an adult self; that makes the work much harder and the prog-nosis worse. In such instances, we may refer to the "most grown-up part" or the "most adult part." In other cases, the adult self is just a glimmer or emerges momentarily before being overtaken by another part. If there is an adult self, it may be the part that continues to function in the world, and often has some or many age-appropriate behaviors, knowledge, and skills (though some-times parentified adolescent parts carry those types of skills and attitudes). In people whose parts of self are more fragmented, the adult self tends to be compromised by lack of energy, which is bound up in the dissociated parts and by the effort it takes to keep these parts dissociated. The adult self may or may not know anything about the other parts.

Figure 7.2 shows a person who is highly fragmented. The circles in this illustration may represent child, adolescent, or adult parts; the number, names, location, size/strength, and interrelationships of these parts vary by individual. The commonality is that these parts tend to have firm boundaries and to be separated from each other. This illustration is based on representations of the layers of the ocean, which, in this context, represents access to awareness. The parts of self in the Sunlight and Twilight areas are those that are most commonly shown to others and that are in—or are accessible to—conscious awareness. Parts of self that are in the Midnight zone are often outside of conscious awareness of the adult self; however, sometimes certain parts of a client can communicate with or access information from parts of self residing in this zone. These parts of self can often be accessed in therapy, particularly after a strong therapeutic alliance has been established. In addition, therapy can often be utilized to increase access to parts of self in this Midnight zone. Parts of self that are in the Abyss are completely outside of awareness and are typically identified when other people point out unusual behaviors or interactions that the client does not recall. These parts of self are also sometimes observed (in treatment or elsewhere) in reaction to trauma triggers, traumatic reminders, or perceived threat; they are often seen through various expressions of acting-out behaviors (e.g., aggressiveness, self-harm, risk behaviors, hypersexuality, and so on). One goal of the parts component of CBP is to build awareness of parts of self that reside in the Midnight zone and

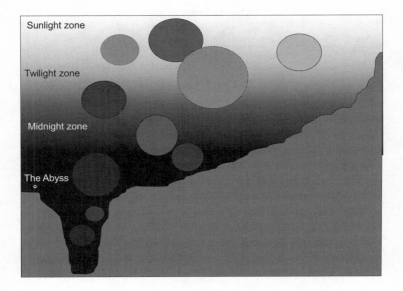

FIGURE 7.2. Fragmentation in parts of self.

in the Abyss and to build connections between parts of self residing in all of these zones.

Figure 7.3 shows a person with more cohesive parts of self, perhaps later in CBP treatment. The adult part of self is larger and encompasses many of the parts of self. Although some of these parts of self continue to be separated, have rigid boundaries, or are partially outside the person's "gestalt" sense of themselves, the parts of self tend to have generally more porous boundaries and to be more interconnected. Thus, we are not working toward "integration," or the collapse of self-states into one whole, but instead toward greater awareness, acceptance, and interconnectedness in parts of self. Although various models of dissociation can be helpful in orienting the treatment, we caution against making assumptions about a particular person's inner world and emphasize the need to listen and learn from our clients in an ongoing way.

The application of a parts framework in CBP can be helpful in "holding" and contextualizing the experience of a range of clients, from highly dissociative clients who cope by disconnecting from aspects of their emotional experience to less fragmented clients who have ambiguous and often contradictory feelings. This framework also offers the opportunity for clients to develop self-compassion for their most vulnerable, helpless, or dependent states. This framework supports trauma integration and the development of a narrative of self that encompasses multiple aspects of experience and the complexity of each person. As a result, we use the language of parts with the majority of our

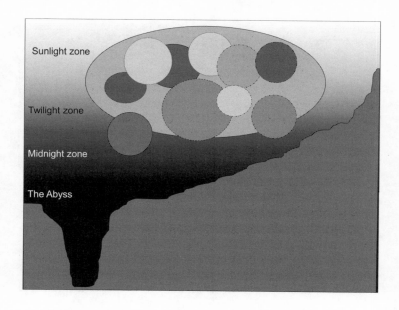

FIGURE 7.3. Cohesion among parts of self.

clients, even when dissociation does not immediately appear to be a primary presenting issue.

PARTS-BASED CASE CONCEPTUALIZATION WITH DAVID

Beginning with his first several years, David had little opportunity to make adequate attachments. He appears to have developed an avoidant attachment style, as reflected in his holding his therapist at a great emotional distance, in his description of his withdrawing from relationships in his family, and in his wife's complaints of his inability to make emotional attachments. David likely has a part that carries deep shame and self-hatred about his (normal) infant and childhood needs for nurturance that drives this avoidant style.

Child parts hold David's desperate need for connection and nurturing, which his therapist senses behind his initial emotional distance. For a man so typically closed off from his feelings, it is remarkable that David is willing and able to tell his therapist that when he fell off his bike and hurt himself at age 6, "a part of me just wanted my mom to scoop me up, tell me I was going to be okay, clean me up, and then give me a big bowl of ice cream." This hunger for connection is held by a very young part of him and is also a source of resiliency.

David has developed other protector parts. As a young boy, David learned to be independent and strong on the streets and in the orphanage; in a parts framework, a slightly older part of him came into being that was resilient in these settings, often presenting as tough or angry. This may well be the part of David that got so angry with his therapist when she gave him inadequate warning of her upcoming vacation. This part also likely plays the role of criticizing and silencing younger vulnerable parts of himself, having learned that showing these early needs led to intolerable disappointments.

David becomes increasingly clear in his therapy that his adoption by the white family was very complicated for him, bringing him significant new strengths and vulnerabilities. On the positive side, he came to have adolescent parts who knew how to live and function well in white mainstream culture, which served him well in his career. These skills included literally speaking the language of the mainstream culture, developing high-level academic skills, and functioning in a highly organized way. Although these skills have served him well, David almost certainly has adolescent parts that are deeply pained and perhaps enraged that many aspects of his identity were disparaged by his new family and that he was forced to give up his early sense of self; as David put it, "They changed me into what they wanted me to be." Echoes of this younger adolescent part who was forced to shut down and submit are seen in his relationship with his wife, who criticizes David for his "sullen resignation and inward retreat"; as was the case with his adoptive parents, David never felt accepted by his wife, nor was he ever able to stand up for himself with her. This submissive, resentful part of David also shows up in therapy from the first session when Susan conveys that her assessment will require several more visits. David is obviously not pleased but instead of clearly stating his wishes, his voice trails off "to almost a mumble and his head [turned] downward and away from Susan." It is important to note that this shift of gaze, voice, and apparent state is a common marker of a dissociative shift.

David tells his therapist that one way he silenced the parts of him that were not acceptable to his new family was to learn to lock his feelings away (i.e., he developed one or more protective parts to do this). He poignantly described spending hours alone in his room feeling terribly sad, which are likely child parts. He knew there was no place in his new family for his feelings; he had to appear perfect and grateful. David says that, as soon he could do that, his sadness went away; we understand that it was instead dissociated. The price he paid for this relief from unrelenting sadness was the loss of access to his feelings and of his ability for closeness and intimacy, which requires feelings and vulnerability. We understand David's feeling when he tells his therapist that the Beatles' song, "Nowhere Man," is him, since without access to his early history and his feelings, and without the self and relational development that comes from good-enough attachments, he is indeed "nowhere." Susan's early awareness of her lack of connection with David is a reflection of her initially intuitive awareness of the extent to which his feelings and his ability to relate are inaccessible to him and thus also to her.

With all the obstacles he faced in his development, David shows remarkable resiliency. His strengths in functioning in the world of school and now work are obvious and almost certainly due to his innate intelligence and robustness, as well as the education he was able to access through his adoptive family's financial resources. David's commitment to his wife and family suggests a strong longing to have emotional ties. His developing connection with his therapist also suggests some ability to form relationships, although this process is likely going to be very slow in his therapy, as he has to learn to trust. Furthermore, it seems clear that he does have an adult self, albeit underdeveloped, with capacities for curiosity about and compassion for himself. In his early 40s, when he came for therapy, David's dissociative adaptation seemed to be coming apart. He had become more withdrawn from family relationships and/or the demands for intimacy and engagement from his wife and now troubled teenage daughter were requiring more than he could provide. That David became openly angry with the "snotty new Ivy League recruit" at work and that he was physiologically triggered by his therapist's telling him at the last moment that she would be away, suggest that his ability to dissociate from his buried anger was decreasing. This process is not unusual, even among people who have effectively relied on dissociation for many years. Although it can make clients' lives more openly difficult and painful, this breaking-down of the effectiveness of the dissociative process is actually a first step in building awareness and connection to all parts of one's experience.

HIGH FRAGMENTATION AMONG PARTS

The stronger the dissociative barriers between parts, the greater the likelihood that parts will develop a unique sense of identity, as is seen in DID. These more fragmented parts often have a distinct view of their own history, which can be significantly different from the experienced history of other parts, and they feel their thoughts, actions, feelings, and values are their own, in contrast to the experience of other parts. In some cases, fragmented parts can gain executive control of the body, which means that part determines the thoughts, feelings, behaviors, and bodily responses of the client during that period, leading to sometimes radically differing presentations of a client with DID.

There is variability in awareness of the larger system and connection to other parts, with some degree of amnesia being common in highly fragmented clients. Some parts carry only a particular traumatic memory or a particular emotion, such as anger. Other parts that were central to a child's early coping are more complex and can be composed of substates. For instance, if a child spent a great deal of time in a compliant state in order to minimize the threat from a mentally ill parent, a complex part may develop who is generally compliant but whose behavior can vary from passive aggressiveness to robotic-like agreement. Fragmented parts get frozen in time, seeing the world through the film of their abusive and neglectful childhoods. To varying degrees, these parts may perceive themselves as still living in the world of their childhoods. In highly fragmented clients, the major dissociated parts in the system tend to be highly motivated to continue their existence because they believe in the importance of their role for survival.

For fragmented clients, it is important to remember that what you see is often not a full or accurate reflection of what is going on "behind the scenes." Kluft (2006) gives an excellent description of the often hidden nature of parts (what he refers to as "alters") in DID. Even when clinicians don't see any "switching," according to Kluft, other parts often pose as, alternate with, or greatly influence the adult self (or "host personality," as he calls it). Schwartz (1995) refers to the "blending" that occurs when the client's adult self (which he calls the "Self") is being taken over by thoughts and feelings of a part, while still being somewhat present. In an example of the obscurity of parts, a woman had a part she called "Father" who presented as an internalized version of her actual 40+-year-old father, constantly criticizing and berating her. In a visualization exercise called the "Dissociative Table" (Fraser, 1991), this client was imagining all of her parts sitting with her adult self and therapist around a conference table, talking over an issue. At one point, "Father" took off a mask he was wearing, revealing himself as a 5-year-old boy, no longer willing or needing to be encumbered by this parentified role.

Conflict between parts is an inevitable aspect of a system in which adolescent or protector parts are built to inhibit more vulnerable parts. Most extreme symptomatic behavior seen in survivors of complex trauma—self-harm, suicidality, aggression, extreme anxiety, severe somatic symptoms—represents internal conflict and can be informative about parts of self. The mental health system can inadvertently reinforce these behaviors if, for example, the client is only able to get adequate attention by exhibiting aggressive or self-destructive behaviors.

ROLE OF THE THERAPIST IN WORKING WITH DISSOCIATION

When the therapist uses empathetic attunement to notice and reflect the client's internal states, over time parts of self that have been banished can be acknowledged and shared. Because many of these dissociated feelings can seem intolerable to parts of the client, the therapeutic relationship is used as a container to help hold, modulate, and tolerate overwhelming feelings. Another aspect of our role is to hold the client's ambivalence and to validate *all* parts of her. That requires understanding the adaptive role of each part. We cannot be truly allied with a client unless we understand and build a working treatment relationship with all parts of him or her.

Chronically neglected and emotionally abused individuals need significant support from the caring and nurturing capacity of their therapist for many aspects of the work, especially when beginning to directly experience the trauma-related emotions of dissociated parts. At the same time, we understand the risks when the therapist sees him- or herself as the only person providing the nurturing and caretaking that was missing from the client's early years. In the 1980s, when therapists were learning how to treat severe dissociative disorders, they routinely worked with child parts without any "co-consciousness," or the presence of what we call the adult self. They then discovered days or years later that the rest of the self had not learned anything from these child therapy sessions, and the child parts continued to look only to the therapist for support. As Shusta-Hochberg (2004) suggests, therapists need to walk a fine line between nurturing and supporting child parts and also continuing to teach the client to nurture these parts, as well as to set limits and not let them control the entire system with their desperate needs. For this reason, we rarely do direct parts work until an adult or relatively adult part of the client is invested in doing the work and is able to stay present when a dissociative part is evoked. In CBP, therapists often take a more active role in supporting and nurturing all parts of the fragmented self early in treatment, gradually encouraging the most mature part of the client to take on that role.

Like Alice's adventures in Wonderland, exploration of dissociated experience is often unexpected, disorienting, and emotionally complex. Therapists may feel that they understand a client, have a working alliance, and have a good treatment plan, when suddenly that perception is turned on its head. Parts of the therapist often become activated in turn, with fear, self-doubt, or defensiveness emerging. CBP highlights the importance of supervision in framing, clarifying, and unifying this work. Because dissociation is not a primary topic covered in most graduate programs, the supervisor may take on the role of introducing a parts framework to therapists who are new to trauma treatment. A CBP supervisor supports their supervisee in understanding the interaction between the client's and supervisor's parts of self, including enactments (see Chapter 4). CBP supervision can guide the therapist in the use of specific techniques to engage dissociated parts, such as the imagery exercise that we describe in the next chapter. Supervisors also work to bring awareness of their own parts of self into exploration of the supervisory relationship and parallel processes between the supervision, the therapy, and the client's relationships in the world.

CONCLUSION

We have found it invaluable to incorporate a framework of dissociative parts of self into our work with adults who have experienced early relational trauma. Notably, this frame is beneficial for all clients, even those who would not traditionally be considered to have a dissociative disorder, and it can be used to better understand and work with internal conflict and contradictory reactions. We consider the dissociative process on a continuum across several dimensions, including cohesiveness, engagement, embodiment, and level of resources. CBP takes an individualized approach to considering each person's parts of self, using the client's language to understand the function of each part of self and the degree to which that part is dissociated from conscious awareness. The role of the therapist is to support the client in building awareness of, and respecting the adaptive role of, all parts of the client. In the next chapter, we describe CBP's process of intervening with dissociated parts of self. We describe three levels of intervention that may be used depending on the client's level of fragmentation, the therapist's training and skills, the client's inner and outer resources and vulnerabilities, and the particular stage of the treatment.

CHAPTER 8

Working with Dissociative Parts in the Depths of the Abyss

*I*magine that, several months into therapy with Katherine, Nicole is describing her Aunt Victoria, with her appealing wildness and sense of humor. Suddenly, Katherine notices that Nicole's voice has shifted, and she looks younger and much more energized. Nicole says, with a sly giggle and a provocative expression, "I still have the fake ID she got me, in case I ever need it." As quickly as she says this, she reverts to the somewhat constrained and adult-sounding style she has displayed since Katherine has known her and, sounding puzzled, says, "I don't know why I said that. I haven't used a fake ID since I was 17." For a moment, Katherine feels she has lost her grip on their conversation. Then she understands that a part of Nicole that Nicole is not very aware of had popped up to contribute to the conversation. "Maybe some part of you still craves that feeling of taking risks," Katherine says. Thus, they begin an exploration of this part of Nicole.

WHY WORK WITH DISSOCIATIVE PARTS OF SELF?

Although disowning internal experience can have adaptive value when a child does not have the resources to manage overwhelming situations, the fragmentation that sometimes results can create difficulties in self-awareness, consistency, ability to draw on internal resources, stability in relationships, and other areas. Working with dissociative parts in CBP has several goals.

The first goal is to help these clients understand the role of dissociated parts of self in their life's difficulties, to explore how different parts get triggered, to strengthen the adult self, and to help them manage these parts' activation in their lives. Second, CBT aims to help the adult self and the parts understand why the parts developed as they did, which involves reworking distorted narratives and building appreciation for each part's role in survival. The third goal is to create more permeability and communication among all parts, particularly between the adult self and other parts of self. Finally, parts work helps heal distorted attachment relationships of parts. As CBP therapists, we, like the relational psychoanalysts (e.g., Bromberg, 2001) and an increasing number of other trauma therapists (e.g., Chefetz & Bromberg, 2004; Courtois & Ford, 2013; Fosha et al., 2009; Pearlman & Saakvitne, 1995a; Schore, 2010), pay a great deal of attention to the relational world created by ourselves and our clients, with a particular focus on any subtle or not-so-subtle state changes in either us or them—what Lyons-Ruth (2005) and others call "implicit relational knowing."

Like many other theorists and therapists (e.g., Bromberg, 2001; Chefetz & Bromberg, 2004; Davies & Frawley, 1994; Schwartz, 1995; van der Hart et al., 2006), we see the importance of working directly with dissociative experiences. As Perry and Hambrick (2008) say, the only way to change a neural system is to activate it. However, because learning is negatively impacted in the face of intense hyper- and hypoarousal, we continue to attend to the window of tolerance as we engage in work with dissociative parts. We also emphasize engagement and at least partial, if not full, participation in this process of the adult self, or the most mature self that can be identified.

CBP'S CLINICAL PERSPECTIVE ON PARTS

In an assessment or therapy session, a clinician may first see a notable shift in a client's mood, or notice what sounds like a different point of view than the one the client had just been expressing. Strongly expressed internal conflict often reflects the activity of parts. Depending on the client's degree of dissociation, the therapist may see a notable shift in the personality of the person he or she is talking to, including change in voice, facial expression, language, attitude, body language, and access to memories. This type of variable presentation occurred with a man named John, who often dissociated into a younger rage-filled part of himself during arguments with his wife. Although he was interested and motivated to learn more about himself, he had little access to his feelings and had no memory of these apparently dissociative episodes at home. During one therapy session, John's generally reasonable and open stance gradually changed to a more argumentative tone as he questioned his therapist. After several minutes of noticing this change, the therapist asked if he had noticed some shift in himself. With assistance, John was able to notice that his body had become tense and, in particular, his abdomen had tightened. The therapist wondered if another part of him was present that did not have much confidence in her or her motives. (He was, of course, doubtful!)

More problematic, and particularly common early in treatment, the therapist may have no idea that dissociative states exist. People with dissociative disorders are often very successful at hiding these aspects of themselves, even if they are aware of these secret parts of them, having learned through early experience that it is safer to stay hidden. They may be constantly assessing, both consciously and implicitly, if the person they are talking with is likely to be able to tolerate hearing about the darker aspects of themselves. Even if the therapist is skilled at inviting and tolerating these darker aspects, some parts may still stay hidden.

ASPECTS OF PARTS WORK IN CBP

In this chapter, we describe CBP's three aspects of parts work: use of a dissociative parts framework in conceptualization and treatment planning; indirect parts work with a client; and direct engagement to increase communication with and among different parts of self. The first aspect includes the therapist's awareness of potential dissociative processes within the client, the use of supervision in consideration of the role of parts, and psychoeducation about dissociation and parts of self. The second aspect of parts work involves working indirectly by acknowledging and exploring a client's parts of self through discussion, exploring difficulties associated with dissociated parts, communication barriers between parts, and the adaptive role that each part has served in a person's life. The third aspect of parts work involves direct communication with or among a client's parts of self, whether it be between the client's adult self and a younger part, among different parts of self, and/ or between the therapist and different parts of the client. In some cases, we use an experiential engagement technique that involves the use of imagery to facilitate a therapeutic encounter between the client's adult self, a younger part of the client, and the therapist.

Conceptualization with a Parts Framework

From early in the therapy process, we are attuned to potential dissociative processes within our clients, noticing strong ambivalence, types of feelings that are rejected or not allowed, or variations in presentations. As we notice these markers, we begin to introduce the idea of dissociation and the language of parts of self. We discuss dissociation as a typical process and normalize the existence of parts of self.

When clients are uncomfortable with the terminology of "parts," we use other descriptors—*states, feelings, voices, selves, sides of themselves,* or whatever word(s) clients use to describe their parts. When talking about specific parts, we use language that is consistent with the way the client has named or described them, such as "the part that holds the terror/anger" or "the frightened part" or "the 8-year-old." In general, we stay close to the client's language about the part. We avoid using gender terms to refer to parts until the client has; the gender of the part is not necessarily the same as that of the client's adult or presenting self.

After Nicole's disclosure about her "bad side," imagine that Katherine asks Nicole if she thinks it might be useful to hear how Katherine thinks about the mind. Nicole agrees it would be. Katherine says that all of us have parts; it's normal. When things go well enough in childhood, those parts get more or less integrated so that the person can function comfortably in the world and feel that he or she has a relatively cohesive identity. When things go badly in childhood, as they have in Nicole's, these parts stay much more separate from each other, like the part of Nicole that is excited by taking risks, and the part of her that deeply disapproves of that behavior, instead coping through attempts to please others. Katherine shows Nicole a figure depicting the structure of parts, beginning with the very young parts that carry the early deprivation, rage, pain, and other traumatic memories and feelings. She explains that there may be other young parts that can't tolerate this pain and defenselessness, so they reject or shut down these vulnerable parts. Katherine wonders whether this part of Nicole who craves excitement might be protecting her by shutting down more vulnerable parts of her. Nicole responds that it could be the case, but it makes her anxious to think about it; she soon changes the topic. As Katherine does, we pay close attention to a client's reactions to early discussions about dissociation and parts of self, which provide important information about pacing parts work.

Indirect Work with Parts

The second aspect of parts work begins when the client is open to exploring his or her own parts. This stage may begin very early or much later in the work, depending on the capacities of the client. At this point, if a clear example comes up in which a client might recognize parts involvement in him- or herself, we might address what we experience as happening by saying, for example, "It seems like some parts of you are in disagreement with what I just said," "So, one part of you really wants to change, but another part wants everything to stay the same?" or "I just noticed a big shift. I'm wondering if a part of you had a reaction to that?" We then invite the client to respond and to explore these different parts of self.

This phase of work can also be initiated by a client naming a part of self; for instance, "I want to tell you, but there is a part of me that's petrified about how you'll respond" or "When I think about going back home, I feel like a little kid." It is very important from the beginning of this work to enlist the involvement of the adult self or the most mature parts of the client. Ulti-mately, the most effective model involves the adult self of the client and the (adult self of the) therapist together discussing, strategizing, and undertaking parts work.

The bulk of this second phase occurs through conversation about the cli-ent's different parts of self. Because each part has its own regulatory processes, we might support the client's awareness of behavioral, emotional, somatic, and/or cognitive patterns that repeat in certain situations. For instance, it is not uncommon for younger parts of self to become activated when a person visits with his family of origin. Enactments (discussed in Chapter 4) might also highlight certain parts of self. A woman named Farrah identified an angry, defensive part of herself that she called the "monster lady" that attacked when she felt disregarded by her therapist. Farrah was later horri-fied and ashamed by the vitriolic voice-mail messages that she left after her therapist was late for their scheduled appointment. Further exploration in the therapy uncovered a very young, scared part of Farrah, whom she called "little me." This young part's unmet needs had been activated by the caring approach of Farrah's therapist, and she became petrified at the slightest sign that this relationship would be taken away. Farrah's therapist assisted her in building empathy not only for "little me," but also for the "monster lady," as she began to understand that this angry part was trying to protect her from further abuse and abandonment.

In addition to building this type of frame around understanding the role of parts, the therapist might also indirectly share information with the client's younger parts to engage him or her but will address it to the client's adult self. For example, we might say that, although a young part of her feels like it was all her fault, a child is not responsible for her parents' behavior.

Direct Parts Work

The third phase of parts work focuses on increasing communication with and between a client's parts of self, as we cross the dissociative barrier to engage in direct parts work. As this framework becomes increasingly comfortable, a client may pause in session to "check in" with a part or parts, perhaps closing his or her eyes and having a silent internal interaction with dissociated parts. The therapist might cue the client to engage in this type of communication in session, suggesting a pause to check in with other parts that might be pres-ent. Some clients are easily able to identify internal conflicts in this way. For instance, after one young woman agreed with her therapist that she would go to an Alcoholics Anonymous meeting, she noticed a clenched feeling in her abdomen and lot of internal "noise." After bringing awareness to these activated parts, she recognized that a part of her was terrified at the idea of giving up the one thing that helped her to feel soothed, while another part of her was angry and resentful of the therapist for trying to interfere and telling her what to do.

Teresa, a woman in her mid-40s, came into session early, troubled by her recent interactions with her teenage daughter. She reflected to her therapist that, although she was generally calm around her daughter, she had recently found herself enraged in an interaction and was troubled by the rage. Her therapist suggested, "It sounds like some part of you got very set off by her insolence, even though another part of you knows that adolescents often behave that way." Teresa agreed, so her therapist wondered if she knew anything about that part, whether it came out in other situations, and how she felt about it. After some time learning about this part of her, the therapist asked if Teresa's adult self could talk directly to this "enraged" part (Teresa's terminology), explaining her desire to help and asking about this part's reactions to the conversation. These kinds of conversation have to be paced thoughtfully, with continued engagement and participation of the client's adult self, ensuring that the part does not fully emerge and eclipse the adult self.

As this dissociative barrier is crossed in therapy, we may initially see more fragmentation for a time. As the client's younger parts are acknowledged, they might be more likely to show up in the therapy. If a younger part shows up in the office, we will communicate directly with this part, with the goal of soothing the part and accessing the client's adult self or more resourced parts. We particularly want to be thoughtful about safety at the end of the session if a younger part has shown up, making sure that the client's adult self or at least a more regulated or functional part of self (such as a caretaker part or a worker part) is available as the client leaves the office, and that the younger part has received some containment and safety.

Occasionally, parts will be interested and able to befriend or support another part, as in an older part explaining something it has come to understand to a younger part or providing emotional support. This is very helpful when it happens. However, caution is recommended against overreliance on resourced parts, to ensure that we are not keeping the protective part stuck in an old role. Older parts are often convinced that it is best for them to keep protecting themselves/the adult self/the younger part by behaving as they have been for many years, for example, being angry and defensive. For this to change, there needs to be a connection with the client's adult self, and often with the therapist, that helps that adolescent part feel understood and cared for as well. Ideally, because our goal is to support the development of internal resources over time, we want the client's adult self to be present to communicate with the younger part or to witness the communication.

As would be expected, communication barriers tend to be stronger for clients whose parts are more fragmented. For instance, Gabrielle, a client with DID, had an intense fear of flying, which was required for her job. After Gabrielle had a greater understanding of her own parts and their various concerns about flying, the therapist suggested an internal "group meeting" to see what each needed before her flight. She came in after her trip and ruefully described her experience. Gabrielle said one part wanted a teddy bear to hold, another wanted her to drink herself into oblivion, and another part was berating her for these childish ways of trying to cope. She complained, with some amusement, "It's like dealing with some ridiculous bureaucratic committee trying to get everyone on board!"

Imaginal Technique to Facilitate Direct Engagement with a Part

In some cases, direct parts work may involve entering into the client's dissociated experience in the session through the use of imagery, with a technique developed by Grossman (Grossman & Zucker, 2010). Howell (2005) describes Davies and Frawley as being "among the first contemporary analysts to contemplate the desirability of entering into the patient's dissociated experience, which can be a 'royal road' to memory and experience that is otherwise unavailable" (p. 110). This aspect of parts work targets healing attachment-related wounds, recognizing the pain that is held by younger parts of self and addressing some of their unmet needs, particularly the need to be seen and cared for.

Before using this technique, we carefully assess whether the client has sufficient coping skills and capacity to tolerate difficult emotions without seriously impairing his or her ability to function in life. Working with the young parts, particularly inside the dissociated traumatized state, exposes the adult self and the rest of the system to the traumatic affect held by that part. We generally do not do this deeper parts work with clients who are currently abusing substances or behaving in other ways that may endanger life or life structure. An exception is made when it seems to be the only way to intervene to minimize dangerous activities; we are always very attentive to safety issues and to careful pacing in working with parts. This work requires a strong alliance between the therapist and the adult self of the client; some continuing presence of the client's adult self; and a clearly activated part whose reactivity has created the presenting problems for the client. The clinician should get the client's permission to explore a triggered part. If the client is able to recognize the presence of a part, the therapist might ask, "Is it okay for us to try to find out more about this part?" Although people often say yes, if they show some reluctance, the therapist should accept that, perhaps revisiting the issue at a later time. Trying to persuade clients to engage in this imaginal technique is not helpful; they sometimes have more awareness of their capacity than we do.

If we have clear permission from the adult self of the client, we briefly describe the entire process, acknowledging that it may initially feel uncomfortable or strange to talk to a part of oneself in this way. This process involves several steps: increasing access to a part of self through mindful awareness; linking current state to an earlier memory or experience; increasing vividness of the scene through sensory details; introducing the adult self and therapist into the imagery; engaging in ongoing consultation between the therapist and client's adult self; making an empathic connection with the part; identifying the main issue; responding to the main issue; creating a safe space for the part; ending the parts work imagery exercise; and processing the experience with the client's adult self. Each of these steps is described next.

Increasing Access to a Part of Self through Mindful Awareness

In order to create a connection with the dissociated part, the therapist can guide the client in identifying the somatic and affective experiences of that part. The therapist invites the client to give a detailed description of the strong emotion she has or recently had, including body sensations and emotional experience. If the client is experiencing the intense emotion or conflict in the moment, we might ask her to focus on the feeling and body sensations and try to intensify it. If she is not experiencing it in the moment, we ask her to recall the most recent time she felt it and try to reexperience it fully. We explore the associated emotions and body sensations both carefully and thoroughly, helping the client find words to describe sensations, if needed.

Linking Current State to an Earlier Memory

To develop the imagery, the therapist assists the client in linking the current emotions and/or body sensations to an earlier memory or experience. Some clinicians may want to use a technique such as the affect bridge (Watkins, 1971), in which the therapist asks the client to hold onto the emotion and the body sensations and go back as far as he can in time to when he first remembers having that feeling. Sometimes a client will have an image/memory from childhood in which he had a similar feeling. If he remembers a general scene but not a specific image, we invite him to find a visual image of himself in that scene. If a client comes up with an adult memory, the therapist can talk with him a bit about it, partly to encourage him to connect to the feeling, and then ask if there is any earlier time he can remember. Clients rarely find the earliest time the feeling actually occurred or even the youngest memory they have when we begin this work, and that is not a problem. Ultimately, the therapist can work with whatever memory or image the client offers; it is important that the client does not feel shamed and feels successful in the experience.

Increasing Vividness of Scene through Sensory Details

After identifying this early memory or image, the therapist asks the client to give the most vivid, detailed description possible of the scene she is imagining, including physical details such as what the younger part of her looks like, what that part is wearing, what the environment is like in the scene, where the part is located, and whether or not anyone else is present. We ask how the part seems to be feeling and about how old he or she seems. We generally don't ask for a name, since many parts don't have names, and we do not want to create more separateness in the system than necessary. Often clients have powerful and emotionally laden images; although this can be related to verbal facility and communication style, clearer and more vivid images often indicate greater access to the part.

Introducing the Adult Self and Therapist into the Imagery

After this description of the scene, we invite the adult self of the client to experiment by bringing himself into the image with the younger part. If the client is able to do that, the therapist talks with him about precisely where his adult self is located in the setting and whether the part is comfortable with his proximity. For clients who are able to come up with an image but cannot bring an image of their adult selves into the scene, we understand that the dissociative barrier may be too great. The therapist can normalize this for the client, remind the client that this is simply an experiment that can be tried at another time, and suggest a return to the adult world.

For many clients doing this experiential aspect of parts work, it can be beneficial to introduce an image of the therapist into the imagery in order to help them tolerate the intensity of the experience, to bolster their confidence in the new situation, and sometimes to talk directly to the part. When this approach appears likely to be useful, the therapist may ask the client how she would feel bringing an image of the therapist into the scene. If she agrees, the therapist can pause while the client adds to the imagery, and then the therapist asks her to describe in detail what has transpired, such as where the therapist is in the scene and the part's reaction, including whether the part has noticed the presence of the one or two adults who have entered the scene. Occasionally it does seem appropriate for the therapist to "go alone," as long as the client's adult self is clearly and actively participating in developing the imagery and the interventions. However, we avoid this whenever possible because we don't want to be seen by the part as the only source of comfort and healing.

Engaging in Ongoing Consultation between the Therapist and Adult Self

In this exercise, the client is moving back and forth between the imagery, directly engaging with the younger part (in words but generally not out loud) and the adult world, where he or she and the therapist are consulting about this process. Thus, at this point, a three-way conversation is occurring, with the therapist and the adult self of the client frequently consulting about what to do next, and the young part conveying his or her thoughts, feelings, or verbalizations to the adult self, who then relays them to the therapist.

Making an Empathic Connection with the Part

For clients who are quite fragmented, such as those with DID, some parts may want to know who these unknown adults are that have entered their world.

Parts who have been locked behind the dissociative barrier still experience themselves living in their childhood and often don't know either the therapist or the fact that there is an adult self in the body. If they seem curious or ask, the client's adult self may say something like, "I am the person you grew up to be" or "I'm someone who wants to help you"; the therapist can briefly explain, "I'm someone who helps kids and grownups who feel bad." This initial meeting can create intense emotions. In one case, an angry and disengaged adolescent part did not believe that the man in the scene was his adult self until the client showed the adolescent a scar he had gotten in childhood.

At this point, the therapist and client often consult to decide how the client's adult self can make an emotional alliance with the part, as one would do when meeting a child or adolescent of that age for the first time. They may decide that the client's adult self will reflect on the child's apparent emotional state, noting that she looks sad or scared or angry, for instance. We find that virtually all dissociative parts are responsive to empathy, even if they initially take a tough and defensive stance, as they often do. Kluft regularly teaches that DID "is that form of psychopathology that dissolves in empathy" (2006, p. 293). Usually, the child part will respond to the adult self of the client, verbally or nonverbally.

Identifying the Main Issue

The therapist and client work to identify the main issue that the young part is facing. In the interest of effective pacing, we strongly recommend against attempting to address multiple issues in one visit, since this work disrupts the dissociative barrier and can release traumatic affect, which can destabilize the system. When working with a young and traumatized part, an older defensive or reactive part can sometimes become activated. If this happens during work with the younger part, we recommend going to the older part first and doing this same process with her. If this occurs, it is important to provide guidance, emphasizing, for example, that all parts have an important voice, that no part can silence any other part, and that all parts will get a turn. It is very important to return to the younger part and finish that piece of work after addressing the older part. Sometimes the part will share something about her feelings, while at other times, the therapist and client's adult self may already understand the context—for example, that the young part is upset because she is being neglected by her mother—and can address it directly.

Responding to the Main Issue

In responding to the main issue facing the part, the client's adult self and therapist often provide support and sometimes clarity. They may decide that the client's adult self will say to that child part, "You're upset because your mother has left you home alone again. That's very hard." The adult self of the client, coached by the therapist, may then engage in a short conversation with the part about the primary issue, saying, for example, "It's not right that someone your age has to be alone so much" or "That must be frightening to be alone at night," depending on the circumstances. The young part may give its version of the narrative, such as, "It's my fault; my mother only leaves me alone when I've been bad." This uncovering process raises the opportunity for the therapist to talk with the client's adult self about her view that the child is not responsible for inadequacies in caretaking by the parent and to determine if the client's adult self can convey that message to the part in the imagery. If the part argues, as sometimes happens, the therapist may suggest that the client's adult self say to the child, "You don't have to believe me, but that is what I think." In some cases, the therapist may request permission to speak directly to the part to communicate similar messages.

In some instances, this type of parts work can address specific behavioral issues that are driven by a part's attempts to cope. Ruth, a psychiatrist and the daughter of a Holocaust survivor, struggled with spending a great deal of money on things she did not need, leaving her constantly on the edge of financial disaster. After identifying the emotional and somatic feeling she has just before she goes on a spending spree, Ruth was able to locate a scene in which her 9-year-old self was outside a shoe store intensely longing to buy a fancy and expensive pair of women's shoes in the window.

Ruth and her therapist both agreed that the 9-year-old needed help, but when asked about going into the scene, Ruth said she was too angry with that girl to directly interact with her; she noted, however, that it was fine with her if the therapist went. As we've mentioned, the therapist typically does not go alone into the imagery, to avoid being "the only mommy" to the younger parts. However, in this exception, the therapist felt that Ruth's adult self was involved enough to witness and participate from outside of the imagery.

Ruth imagined the therapist standing on the sidewalk, near but not too close to the girl. The 9-year-old noticed the therapist but was not enthused about her presence; the girl did not know who the therapist was but seemed not to care. The therapist acknowledged that the girl looked like she was having a hard time and conveyed her understanding that the girl desperately wanted to buy the shoes. The 9-year-old agreed and let the therapist talk with her about what it's like to want something so badly and not have the money to buy it. This young part became more relaxed as the conversation went on. Ultimately, the therapist said she knew the girl had had a lot of bad things in her life and not many good things or things she wanted, and the therapist thought they could go into the store and at least look at the shoes. At that point, Ruth's adult self was able to enter the imagery and go with the girl and the therapist into the store. In the store, the three of them had a discussion—with the girl nonverbal but actively conveying her feelings. The therapist shared her feeling that the girl should have the shoes if she wanted them so badly, but with this acknowledgment, Ruth's adult self shared that the girl did not feel she needed them anymore.

Creating a Safe Space for the Part

In some cases, the image may involve the younger part in an actively abusive situation. A client named Paul cognitively knew that his mother had been emotionally neglectful of him but recalled very little of his childhood. After he and his therapist had been engaged in parts work for some time, he came to a session quite distressed, saying he had had an image of a small boy lying on the kitchen floor, terrified as his mother screams at him. This was his first clear image or memory of early emotional abuse. Paul's adult self and the therapist agreed that both of them needed to go into the imagery, one to get the mother out of the kitchen and the other to sit with the small boy. When offered the choice of which he wanted to do, he quickly selected to be with the boy, reluctant to have to deal with his dominating and often disinterested mother. So in the first part of the imagery, the therapist talked with the mother after getting advice from Paul's adult self to try to get her out of the room. She was not interested in the therapist's thoughts, so Paul's adult self whispered in her ear that there was an attractive man in the other room, and she immediately left to investigate.

The therapist then coached Paul's adult self about responding to the boy. Some parts are too young or too frightened to speak. However, they often manage to convey their feelings to the adult self, as happened in this case, who can then report to the therapist. For therapeutic purposes, we find it's not helpful to get caught in the rational logic of these states and their precise ages and capabilities. Van der Hart and colleagues (2006) use ideomotor signaling (e.g., raising a finger if the part wants to say yes), drawing, or asking another part to come forward and help with the communication in those circumstances. Sometimes after the adult self has been empathic with a very young part, the client reports that the part seems less frightened or has allowed the adult self to move closer in the image. With support from his therapist, Paul's adult self said to the boy, "You're scared because your mother was so mad at you." Paul reported that the boy calmed down but conveyed nonverbally that it was his fault that his mother was so angry. After further discussion with the therapist, Paul's adult self was able to say to the boy, "I know you believe that, but it isn't true. Your mother is angry because of grown-up issues that have nothing to do with you." When the boy conveyed that he didn't believe this explanation, the therapist coached Paul's adult self as he told the boy, "You don't need to believe me. I just want you to know that I don't think it was your fault."

As in the case of Paul, sometimes it is clear to the adult self of the client and the therapist that we cannot leave the parts in the setting they are in because, for example, they feel that they are being actively abused or they feel desperation at the thought of being abandoned, pleading with the therapist, "Don't leave me." Responding to this plea reveals the beauty and flexibility of working with imagery. Typically, at that point the therapist and the adult self of the client consider where the part might go, in the client's mind's eye. For some clients, being helped to find a safe place in imagery can be one of the most constructive aspects of this work. If a move has been made in imagery, it is often appropriate to ask the client to check in on the part during the week before the next therapy session. It is important for the therapist to check in about this transition early in the next session to see how it is going. In this case, Paul had an emerging memory of being nurtured, held, and supported by his grandmother, who had lived upstairs when he was quite young. He created an imaginal safe space for the boy and other young parts of him—a loft in his living room, with an image of his grandmother to take care of these younger parts. Paul and his therapist were also able to find moments of humor in this work. For instance, Paul shared that, when he was checking in with everyone in the loft in between sessions, his very traditional grandmother complained that she needed a kitchen since she was always cooking and feeding her grandchildren when she took care of them. He obligingly expanded his imaginary loft to include a kitchen, and she was content.

Ending the Parts Work Imagery Exercise

In ending the parts work imagery exercise, it is important to prepare the younger part for the upcoming transition. The therapist may coach the adult self of the client to say to the client, "In a few minutes, I [or we] will be going back to the adult world. I [we] would like to visit you again. Is that alright?" Usually, the parts do want a return visit; sometimes they desperately don't want the adult self of the client to go, and they may need to be brought along with that adult self in the client's mind's eye. Finally, before ending the imagery exercise, the client's adult self can ask the part, "Before I [we] go, is there anything you would like to ask, or show, or tell?" This question opens the door for communication from the younger part and gets some amazing responses.

A young man named Anthony was struggling with a lot of anger from an adolescent part. When he had discussed with his therapist what he thought the adolescent was so angry about, he had talked about his rage at his mother, his mother's own uncontrolled rage, and the pain of being an outsider with peers. When parts work was attempted to access this adolescent boy, the boy was very unenthused about meeting with the adult self of the client or the therapist and had only grudgingly agreed that they could come back and visit. However, when asked whether he had anything he wanted to show, ask, or tell, he asked, "Do you know my father?" referring to the father who had abruptly left the family when the client was 5, after which there had been no mention of the father in his religious and upwardly mobile Irish Catholic family. The therapist knew that a 5-year-old part of Anthony thought a lot about his father and why he left, but the therapist had no idea the adolescent was preoccupied with that. With coaching, the adult Anthony responded to the adolescent part's question, saying, "It's a wonderful question. I do know your father" (meaning he had met him several times in adulthood) "and next time we meet, I will answer any questions you have about him." Both Anthony and his therapist were astonished and delighted with this question. The next session, the client immediately went back to the adolescent, who was filled with questions about why the father had left, why he hadn't written to the boy, and what he was like. Most of the session was spent with the adult self of the client trying to figure out, with the therapist's help, what to say to this boy he had been. Although Anthony and his therapist had had many of these discussions, and he cognitively understood the reasons for his father's absence, he had not previously been able to access the sadness and self-blame he had experienced over his father's sudden absence in his life.

If it's possible for the therapist or the client to make a brief response to the part's last question, it's good to do so. For the more complex questions, such as the one asked by Anthony's adolescent part ("Do you know my father?"), it's better to make a brief response and set the stage for a longer answer in the next session, in order not to open up more than can be contained at the end of a session.

Processing the Experience with the Client's Adult Self

It is also important to take time to bring closure to the experience and talk with the client about what this exercise was like for him and for the therapist. Often clients are astounded by what has transpired and are very interested and engaged. Sometimes at this point they begin to feel more compassion for the younger part of themselves, although we have found generally that this step of the work cannot begin until the client's adult self has become more curious and open about the younger parts. To that end, we generally offer some psychoeducation to help the client empathize more with the traumatic feelings held by the part, which lessens the dissociative barrier. We may say something like: "You may notice more of the feelings this part has held, and you can continue to talk with the part. We want to thank this part for letting us know more about the experience."

Whatever deeper version of parts work we have done, we recommend checking in at the beginning of the next session (and in between sessions, if needed) about whether there were any aftereffects from this exercise. Often the part will have gotten more activated, and the client feels the part's wishes as well as distress. For instance, a rather private man named Anthony had never talked about his absent father with anyone other than his therapist. However, after engaging in this imagery exercise, he stopped to help change a man's tire out of goodwill. When he realized that this man was a veteran, Anthony was astonished to find himself telling this stranger that the best things his father ever did were to join the Marines and later to leave the family.

In the case of Ruth (described above), the discussion of the imagery exercise helped her to make sense of her compulsive spending as an adult. After the closing of the imagery exercise, Ruth was able to remember the searing pain she had felt when she realized that her mother seemed not to find her appealing or lovable, and Ruth's own belief that if only she were beautiful, her mother would see her that way too. For Ruth, buying beautiful, grown-up, expensive things was a way to attract her mother's positive attention, even though another part of her knew her mother hated it when Ruth bought inappropriate things, and even though her mother was long gone, having killed herself many years before. Ruth and her therapist mourned the unmet needs of the girl she had been and recognized that this part of her needed love and affection, not more material things. As Ruth was increasingly able to accept and nurture this younger part of herself, she felt more mastery over her compulsion to buy things.

Return Visits

We have found that it is usually not indicated to go back to see the part during the next session; most clients need to take a break or spend time metabolizing what they have learned. We encourage therapists to watch and listen for what comes up in the session, and if it's unclear what the best strategy is, we consult with the adult self of the client. We particularly listen for the ways the triggered part may be more powerfully influencing the client's life. It is important to remember that the dissociative part usually has been promised a return visit, and it's not good to make the part wait too long—no more than a few weeks. Like many children, these parts often keep close track of promises and are desperate for more attention.

For many of our clients, the easiest way for them to return to the part, at least initially, is through the body states, such as tightness in the chest or a headache, that they noticed the first time they identified with the part. We then ask them to explore the physical states they're experiencing. Often during the second visit the part is in the same internal place it was found initially, such as on the floor in the mother's apartment or in the woods hiding, and there it may remain for a number of visits. Sometimes if the part has been moved to a safer, more supportive environment, the part remains there. In this second and any subsequent visits, we invite the client to imagine him- or herself (and often the therapist) in the scene and describe what is happening. We continue to approach the part as we would any traumatized child of that age and gender and continue to coach the client's adult self in interactions with the younger part. The primary goals of this parts work are increasing communication and trust between the part and the adult self, healing the part with empathy and understanding, shifting maladaptive attachment patterns, and contributing to narrative development (discussed in the next section) by ensuring that dissociated aspects of a client's experience are included in their trauma narrative and broader life narrative.

THE THERAPIST'S ENGAGEMENT IN PARTS WORK

Therapists need to know themselves and their own parts very well to ensure that they are responding to the client's needs and not their own in making therapeutic decisions (see Chapter 4). As Pearlman and Caringi (2009, pp. 217–218) put it, "To understand adequately and attune to the client, helpers must listen with respect and an open mind and heart." This implies entering the client's world and imagining his or her experience. It means feeling the pain of the victimized part and the fear and confusion of the survivor. And it means respecting boundaries.

It is vital that we, as therapists, are attuned to our own bodies and the subtle and not-so-subtle reactions we have to our clients. As Schore (2003b, p. 80) says, the clinician's body "is the primary instrument for psychobiological attunement and the reception of the transmission of nonconscious affect." Client and therapist mutually regulate each other's behaviors, enactments, and states of consciousness. Schore also points out that if the therapist is not receptive to getting emotionally "mixed up" with the client in these subtle ways, clients likely won't be able to go through the necessary regression and higher level of structural integration. As we actively engage with different parts of the client through his or her adult selves, we may learn more about different parts of ourselves. Our supervisors become essential allies in navigating this sometimes murky process.

CONCLUSION

CBP recognizes the impact of dissociative coping mechanisms on adults with early relational trauma. The less cohesive connections between a client's parts of self, the greater the importance of utilizing a dissociative parts frame in conceptualization and treatment planning. However, as described in Chapter 7, because all people have parts of self that are more or less interconnected, and because of the utility of this model in working with internal conflict, CBP incorporates a parts framework whether or not a client has an identified dissociative disorder. While conceptualizing a client's presentation through this lens, we may invite our clients into a discussion about parts of self, providing psychoeducation about dissociation and about parts work. After establishing this framework, our early engagement with clients regarding dissociated parts of self often involves indirect parts work in which we work collaboratively with our clients to identify and learn more about their different parts of self. We support our clients in exploring these different parts of self, identifying the role that each part has played, honoring those attempts to cope with traumatic experience, and learning about interrelationships between their parts of self. The final aspect of parts work involves increasing communication between the client's adult self and younger parts and within the system as a whole. For clients with a strong therapeutic alliance and an ability to regularly engage their adult self in the work, we might use a structured imagery technique to enter that part's dissociated world, with the goal of supporting healing engagement between the client's adult self and younger parts of self. Table 8.1 summarizes the therapeutic emphasis of CBP within the parts component, including conceptualization using a parts framework and therapeutic intervention with dissociated parts. In the next section, we explore the role of narrative development in CBP.

TABLE 8.1. Intervention Strategies for Parts Component of CBP

Client

- Maintaining awareness that the current presentation might be reflecting only one part of self; understanding that parts hold, embody, and/or express unresolved traumatic material
- Developing a curious, compassionate stance toward all parts of self; building empathic engagement toward fragmented self-states
- Acknowledging and supporting strengths of parts
- Reducing fragmentation: Building cohesion, linkages, and communication among parts of self
- Engaging in indirect and direct work with parts

Parts × Relationship

- Engaging relational parts of self as resources
- Identifying and learning to meet parts' relational needs
- Using the therapeutic relationship to co-regulate parts of self and to facilitate direct engagement with dissociated parts
- Exploring enactments

Parts × Regulation

- Recognizing patterns in affective, cognitive, somatic, and/or behavioral responses that may reflect parts of self
- Expanding each part's repertoire of coping skills
- Reflecting and soothing dysregulated parts; regulating the whole by regulating specific parts
- Tailoring regulatory tools and strategies to developmental stage of parts

Therapist

- Developing a curious, compassionate stance toward all parts of ourselves and toward all parts of the client, honoring the role they have served

Parts × Relationship

- Maintaining compassion for all parts of the client
- Building awareness of the ways in which parts of us are activated through interactions with parts of our clients
- Being able to acknowledge and communicate about our role in enactments

Parts × Regulation

- Noticing activation of our own parts of self and regulating them in the moment
- Identifying and drawing on parts of ourselves as resources

Supervisor

- Offering a mindful, reflective environment to build awareness of all parts of the client and therapist
- Exploring interactions between therapist's and supervisor's parts of self
- Using a supervisor's group to explore reactions of own parts of self and to consider when and how to bring these into supervision

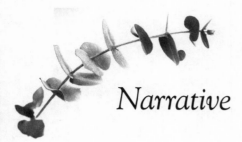

Narrative

CHAPTER 9

Constructing a Narrative, Constructing a Self

with Jodie Wigren

*P*eople seeking psychotherapy frequently introduce themselves with a story. When Nicole first contacts the trauma clinic by phone, she finds that she has a lot she wants to say. She is having trouble with her husband. She used to feel close to him, but they are mostly alienated now. She feels like she just shuts down around him, and she wonders if it has something to do with her childhood, but that thought just makes her panic. The clinic's intake coordinator interrupts her: "You are starting to tell me your story. Why don't we make an appointment for you with one of our therapists so that we can create a safe space for you to tell her more fully and for her to really listen." Nicole laughs awkwardly, then agrees to make an appointment.

In the office, Nicole launches into her story. She has been in therapy in the past; it has not been very helpful. There is something wrong with her, she thinks maybe childhood trauma—she isn't sure. She wants to feel close to other people, but something always stops her. Nicole wants to understand what is wrong. What drives this urgency to tell a story? People use the story form to

Jodie Wigren, PhD, a clinical psychologist in private practice, specializes in integration of psychoanalytic, psychodynamic, and narrative approaches to the treatment of complex posttraumatic stress and dissociation. She is an instructor in the Psychology Department at Emmanuel College and for many years served as a clinical supervisor for the Trauma Center in Brookline, Massachusetts, during its tenure within Arbour Health System. She has published articles on therapeutic alliance and narrative work in trauma treatment.

describe things that are meaningful to them. Conveying a story relays meaning, but more, conveying a story *constructs* meaning. When life makes sense, emotions can be contained, and the self can begin to feel organized and calm.

In this book, we have introduced you to a group of people who grew up without adequate parental support. Because of the difficulties and deficits they experienced as children, these people came into adulthood without an adequately developed self. Too much overstimulation, and too little protection and recognition, force the growing child to defend in the psychic spaces where they need to be developing. Experiences that under more optimal circumstances would become metabolized as psychic structure are instead held in the psyche in primitive, inchoate forms that subjectively represent threat to a desperately and prematurely autonomous self. From a narrative point of view, these are people who struggle with making meaning of the most salient aspects of their life experience, in part because their story is difficult and in part because the part of self that would tell the story does not have the psychological resources to do so.

Stories construct meaning in two ways. First, the story synthesizes or integrates strands from the multiple cognitive, emotional, and somatic systems we use to register and process experience. In this sense, the story is a form that works by creating connections. At the same time, the story creates perspective. It allows a person to disembed from experience by stepping back from it, looking at it through the measuring eye of a narrator.

Adopting the narrator's voice impels us to put our own unique experience into social or cultural contexts. Telling a story to an audience helps with this objective since the narrator must construct a story that the audience can understand. The narrator introduces us to a character and describes experiences that either have been defining or are confusing and need to be understood. The audience grasps the story and comes to care about the character, allowing itself to be informed and moved. The interplay between the attempts of the narrator to render some life episode meaningful and the effort of the audience to grasp and recognize the meanings that emerge are the form of the story and the work of constructing meaning.

When we pay attention to our clients' stories, we are paying attention to people while they are in the process of trying to make meaning. Often the meanings that people are seeking in therapy initially have to do with something that happened to them. Something happened, it was distressing, they are not sure exactly what or why, but they feel that if they could understand what happened, they could come to a better understanding of themselves. As this story emerges, other stories follow. The story about what happened "out there" yields to a story about what happened "in here": How did I feel? What did I do to adapt and cope with the difficulties I faced? How did these experiences shape my ideas about the world and my habits of psychological response? And finally, who am I? Who did I become as a result of my experiences, and is this the person I want to be?

ORIGINS AND EVOLUTION OF NARRATIVE WORK
IN TRAUMA TREATMENT

Contemporary models of trauma treatment have evolved from divergent theoretical perspectives. Ever since Freud (1896) discovered the "talking cure" while listening to his patients' memories of traumatic childhood experiences, the telling of a trauma story has been a core aspect of treatment across models. Following Freud and his contemporary Pierre Janet, psychoanalysts have listened deeply to their patients' stories and have articulated rich and clinically useful understandings of the ways that early mistreatment and neglect reappear in adulthood as transference, repetition, reenactment, and dissociation. When trauma and/or neglect deprives those afflicted of fundamental developmental needs and disrupts internal attachment systems, we see adult survivors who are propelled toward recurrent patterns of seeking and avoidance, alternatingly enacting and eschewing behaviors and relationship dynamics that are thematically or literally associated with their histories of trauma. These patterns are explained as compulsion and self-punishment, striving for mastery or desperate hope for a new and different outcome, for the reparative parenting that will yield an undamaged self (Herman, 1992b; van der Kolk, 1989). Resolving these posttraumatic responses entails helping clients to revisit their trauma in narrative form—reexamining and reframing it in the presence of an empathic witness. Such work allows people to grieve and differentiate past from present experience and to process memories in order to create new and more sustaining meanings.

Frequently, a narrative emerges not in words but in unrecognized enactments with intimate others, including the therapist (see Chapter 4). Trauma-sensitive analysts have developed relational methods for working with the trauma story embedded in interactions that might otherwise lead to impasse or treatment failure. Particularly notable in this regard is the work of Alpert (1995), Bromberg (1994), Davies and Frawley (1994), Ferenczi (1980/1933), Grand (2000), Reis (2009), and Slochower (2013).

Prevailing evidence-based trauma treatment models grew out of the intersection of three predominant theories of behavior in the second half of the 20th century: learning theory, emotional processing theory, and social-cognitive theories (for a fine review of this literature, see Cahill, Rothbaum, Resick, & Follette, 2009). In each of these theories, the crux of traumatic stress was seen as a consequence of perceptual and physiological changes that occurred when people were exposed to terrifying experiences. Traumatic exposures were observed to reshape human fear networks so that they tended toward hypervigilance and hyperarousal, to stimulate behaviors designed to avoid further exposures, and to shatter the survivor's confidence in a benevolent world and a worthy self. These theorists saw that this triad of changes tended to impede social engagement and to limit the healthy risk taking and curiosity about new experience that foster growth and development. From the vantage point of these theoretical frameworks, mechanisms of therapeutic action with those afflicted by posttraumatic stress involved some combination of (1) desensitization and extinction of conditioned fear reactions and (2) confrontation and revision of maladaptive beliefs. Telling and retelling the trauma story in the context of a safe, supportive, and reparative therapeutic relationship and environment was a vehicle for both desensitization and revision of trauma-saturated beliefs.

In another important body of work, explanatory models of the effects of trauma have been extrapolated from neuroscience. Pioneers of this framework have observed how exposure to overwhelming experience disrupts or "fragments" memory processes and evokes dissociative coping (van der Kolk & Fisler, 1995). Ensuing intervention models emphasized the necessity of integrating the processing of traumatic memories and experiences into phase-based treatment plans (van der Kolk et al., 1996b).

The host of contemporary trauma treatments that include a narrative, memory processing, or storytelling component is quite broad and ranges from widely disseminated practices that have amassed a large amount of empirical support to innovative approaches practiced only by a select few (see Foa, Keane, Friedman, & Cohen, 2008). Each model varies along a number of dimensions relevant to the narrative process. Some, like prolonged exposure (PE; Foa, Hembree, & Rothbaum, 2007) and EMDR (Shapiro, 2001), attend carefully to the "micro" details of a trauma story, linking narrative memories of "what happened" with persistent affective, physiological, and attributional correlates. Others, like cognitive processing therapy (CPT; Resick & Schnicke, 1993) and Susan Roth's approach to resolution of thematic trauma adaptations (Roth & Batson, 1997), adopt a more "macro" vista in relation to the trauma story, concerned most with elucidating and loosening the stranglehold of traumatic experiences on current thinking, beliefs, coping, and relationships.

Trauma treatment models vary considerably as well, along dimensions of length, primacy of work, and sequencing of narrative intervention elements. For example, narrative exposure therapy (NET) was developed by international complex trauma experts as a brief and focused protocol to transform fragmented traumatic memories into a coherent narrative through construction of written testimonies of autobiographical experiences. It is especially useful as a process of partnering with torture survivors and other human rights victims from cultural backgrounds or remote locales in which participation in extended psychotherapy is inaccessible or culturally incongruent (Schauer, Neuner, & Elbert, 2011).

On the other end of the spectrum, the Victims of Violence Program's long-standing phase-oriented approach to trauma treatment pioneered by Judy Herman gradually builds toward increasing immersion in the trauma story as clients establish greater capacity for emotional, relational, and behavioral safety. This work typically occurs in the context of long-term psychotherapy

(Herman, 1992b). In between lie models such as Marylene Cloitre's skills training in affective and interpersonal regulation followed by narrative story telling (STAIR/NST; Cloitre et al., 2006), which distills from Herman's approach a mid-duration session protocol that could be manualized, evaluated empirically, disseminated and trained widely, and replicated reliably by less experienced trauma therapists.

Just as the time dimensions of narrative treatment approaches vary, so do social structures. On the one hand, we see Pesso Boyden System Psychomotor (PBSP; Pesso, Boyden-Pesso, & Cooper, 2013), Albert Pesso's highly structured group intervention. Pesso undertakes to alter the trauma story by inviting individuals to create interactive theatrical "structures" within which archetypal moments of childhood attachment trauma are revisited. Participants select group members to role-play actual attachment figures, while others are selected to embody alternative, "ideal figures" coached by the client to enact verbal and physical expressions of caregiving that fulfill unaddressed or denied core needs for nurturance and security from primary attachment figures.

At the other extreme, James Pennebaker has explored that most private of narrative venues, personal journaling. Over a period of decades, his research has illuminated the healing potential of journaling and other forms of emotionally connected written reflection on experiences of trauma, stress, and loss (Pennebaker & Evans, 2014). Others have drawn on various disciplines of the expressive arts as mediums through which the trauma story can be entered and transformed, some of which are explored in Chapter 10.

Despite the variety in these approaches, all of our contemporary trauma treatment models respond to the impulse we see so clearly in Nicole's initial request: the exigent need of humans to speak the unspeakable, to tell their story, and to be heard. In point of fact, more than a century of psychoanalytic, developmental, existential, humanistic, and feminist theories have all offered explanatory perspectives on the nature and impact of trauma that culminate in recommendations that integrate some form of a "talking cure" or, more accurately, a "storytelling" one.

NARRATIVE DIMENSIONS IN CBP

We acknowledge several commonly accepted goals of narrative processing, including acknowledging and naming the injury; shifting responsibility to decrease shame and self-blame; understanding and accepting posttrauma reactions; decreasing trauma-related symptoms; and engaging in meaning-making. CBP highlights the importance of both micro and macro types of narrative processing, addressing both specific memories and larger themes, with an emphasis on matching the particular type of processing to the individual needs of each client at different points in treatment. This type of matching is influenced by all of the components of CBP, including the following dimensions of the narrative component: traumatic memory, identity impacts of trauma, engagement regarding trauma narrative, and integration of life narrative (see Figure 9.1).

In terms of traumatic memory, a person may experience frequent intrusions, including triggered reactions, flashbacks, nightmares, and reactivity to traumatic memories. Clients who have strong intrusions often have easier access to microlevel trauma processing, with the major challenges being downregulation and pacing the trauma processing. Because their trauma exposure is often diffuse, involving pervasive omissions (e.g., the absence of loving attention), many adults who experienced early emotional abuse and neglect have vague or composite memories or feel emotionally disconnected from memories of early mistreatment. Although they may have some discrete intrusive memories, their intrusions often take the form of intrusive emotional experiences such as sadness or self-hatred or somatic intrusions such as heaviness throughout the body or tightness in the chest. Clients at this end of the traumatic memory dimension often "tell their story" somatically and may benefit from alternative means of trauma processing, such as accessing somatic states or exploring in-the-moment enactments within the therapeutic relationship. Through trauma experience integration, clients can move more toward the center of this continuum, in which they have the ability to access and engage trauma material when needed.

Trauma exposure can be isolating, particularly when shame leaves a person feeling like he can't share major elements of his experience or worldview with people around him. One end of this continuum is marked by secrecy about one's trauma narrative, which can reinforce the erroneous idea that the traumatic experience reflects something bad about the person who survived it. At the other end of this continuum, some people have difficulty containing memories or feelings about their experiences and struggle with effectively filtering when and how they share the story of their trauma. For instance, after arriving late to his new job, one young man tearfully shared with his boss details about his extensive early trauma exposure as a means of explaining his tardiness. Our goal is somewhere in the middle of these two extremes, where

---

Intrusions ------------------------ (Acceptance of Memories) X --------------- Avoidance/Numbing

Secretive About Trauma ------------- (Mindful Sharing) X ------------- Spilling Trauma Narrative

Identity Disavows Trauma ----------- (Defined by Trauma) ---------- X Identity Beyond Trauma

Compartmentalized Trauma Narrative --------------------------------- X Integrated Life Narrative

---

FIGURE 9.1. Dimensions of narrative component. X denotes therapeutic goals.

a client is able to share aspects of her trauma narrative, building connection and intimacy through sharing defining experiences, while building her confidence in her own ability to decide when, what, how much, and with whom to share information.

In terms of the impact of trauma on identity, on the one hand, a person (or part of him) may disavow the trauma, which often impacts his sense of self. For instance, a client with an early history of emotional neglect described his childhood as "fine, I guess" and his parents as "just normal, busy professionals," but he had a chronic, nagging sense that something was wrong or missing in his life. On the other hand, when a person's (or part's) identity is driven by or defined by the trauma exposure, she may view herself as damaged or victimized. Her activities might revolve around healing activities, and her relational connections may be based on mutual experiences of injury. A person's identity moves beyond the trauma when he is able to accept his painful experiences and the ways these experiences have influenced him, while also developing his strengths, interests, and other sources of identity.

Regarding the life narrative dimension, phobic avoidance of or hyperfocus on one's trauma exposure can lead to the development of a compartmentalized or fragmented trauma narrative. For instance, one young woman did not identify her early childhood as difficult but had flashbulb images of her father's distorted angry face superimposed on her partner's during adulthood incidents of domestic violence. Dissociated parts of self might hold different aspects of a client's personal narrative, leading to disconnection in her identity and life story. The person who has a more integrated life narrative has a more complete understanding and acceptance of how she has been impacted by her history and context, a rich sense of her personal identity, an awareness and development of her strengths, and an imagined future self to guide her personal change.

Assessment of where a client falls on these dimensions can guide decisions about the role of trauma processing and need for narrative work and positive identity development. A rather constricted man is filled with self-loathing but avoids talking about or even thinking about his early experiences of emotional neglect. For this client, there is a strong intersection between the relationship and narrative components in CBP: he is slowly able to open up about these experiences only after he has developed a great deal of trust in his warm and accepting therapist. His chronic depression and self-hatred is a marker that his identity is built around a part of him that has internalized the emotional neglect. As he acknowledges this early maltreatment and allows himself to experience anger and grief about the love he didn't get, other aspects of his identity have more space to begin to develop. Alternatively, for a woman who is consumed with fragmented, intrusive memories of emotional abuse, beginning in childhood and continuing through several episodes of domestic violence, attempts to independently process all of her experiences of abuse would be overwhelming and destabilizing. Instead, regulation plays a central role in her early narrative work, which focuses on themes versus specific incidents, as she identifies messages she learned during childhood about her worth and how these early messages initiated a cycle of repeated abuse. While exploring the past, narrative work with this client also focuses on her present life, and she works with her therapist to notice her impulses toward fearful compliance in relationships. She also works to practice more assertive behaviors and somatic presentations in order to build a new cognitive, emotional, and somatic narrative about herself as a person who is worthwhile and has the right to express herself.

THE STORY IS AN INTEGRATIVE FORM

The story is the fundamental form for human meaning (Polkinghorne, 1988). As a form, it is integrative. In making a story, we create a storyline that embodies logic and orders events in relation to characters and other events so as to reveal intentionality and cause and effect (Bruner, 1990). We do this by synthesizing qualitatively different information from the separate but interacting learning and memory systems that form human intelligence (Stiles, Honos-Webb, & Lani, 1999). A story often appears to be simple because it so effectively captures information from a number of conceptual levels and organizes this information in a way that reveals logic (makes sense) and conveys emotion (resonates, rings true). We assess the adequacy of stories by their impact. They *move* us. They make sense in the colloquial sense of, "that makes sense," and more profoundly in the formal sense of, "that *creates* meaning."

Early on, as we recognized how often our psychotherapeutic work involved listening to trauma stories, we were struck not only by what they described but also by what was missing. Other authors were beginning to talk about gaps in posttraumatic narrative accounts. Kingsbury (1988) wrote about a lack of resolution in persistent posttraumatic nightmares and suggested hypnotic techniques for helping people follow the narrative of a nightmare all the way through to its end. In an iconic early paper, Laub and Auerhahn (1993) catalogued a range of ways in which traumatized people both "know" and "don't know" their experience of the trauma.

Understanding that the essential form of the story is integrative, we began to see how many components of a person's biological, psychological, and social experience need to come together to complete a story. We explored different ways to work therapeutically with "incomplete" stories of trauma (Wigren, 1994). We discovered that some people literally left off the end of their stories—they stopped short of the material they were unable to digest or symbolize. These people sometimes benefited from gentle encouragement to consider "what happened next." Other people could not bring strands from different memory systems together. For example, some knew in their bodies what they could not know in their minds. For them, bringing language to body sensation often led to startling and helpful insights (e.g., "If your belly could speak, what would it say?"). Some people stood too close to their experience; they could not see it as separate from themselves and found the whole business of internal scrutiny overwhelming. They needed help stepping back. Other people stood too far away, and their stories failed to move them or us. They needed help finding ways to safely engage with their own material.

Some theorists propose that a story of trauma is inherently ineffable and can virtually never be truly or satisfactorily completed (Caruth, 1996). But attending to the gaps and elisions in the stories clients struggled with kept our focus on the relationship between sufferers and their accounts of their suffering. And it turns out, this relationship is a very fruitful locus of therapeutic work. Over time, we have become very concerned not just with trauma stories, but with trauma "storying": the ongoing act of creating meaning as people attempt to offer their experience to be witnessed and recognized by an Other.

The meaning of a story is a property not only of the teller but also of the listener. If a story cannot make sense to a listener, it is not meaningful. The efforts of the audience to understand are an essential part of the act of creating meaning. When we try to tell a story to someone who cannot understand what we are saying, we quickly falter. The creation of a story requires an engaged and recognizing audience.

In sum, the story is fundamentally integrative and fundamentally connecting. It gains its power by capturing enormous complexity in a relatively simple form. It addresses the relationship component of CBP by eliciting connections between the person whose story is being told, the teller, and his or her community. It interweaves the regulation and parts components by integrating aspects of experience, and in many cases parts of self, as we develop the narrative. At the same time that the story integrates, it can also create some distance, allowing us to step outside of the story to view it—and ourselves—from a broader perspective.

THE STORY CREATES PERSPECTIVE

Every story has three voices: the voice of the actor, the voice of the teller, and the voice of the audience. The narrator speaks to the audience about the actor. The narrator steps outside of the actor's immediate experience. The narrator exercises a great deal of license in how the story elements are chosen and arranged, and this selection process gives the story its particular meaning. Without this selection process, we have only blunt action and affect: the narrator begins with these elements but adds intention, sequence, cultural resonance, and some moral or conclusion. Narrating a story can help the client step out of the immediate experience of the story to develop a broader perspective or awareness. The narrator speaks to the audience, making sense of the character for the audience and bringing the audience into connection with the character. These three voices can all be voices of the self; certainly much of our storying happens in internal dialogue. But even our internal dialogue references cultural mores and, by separating the teller from lived experience, allows a wider perspective. And while we do frequently "talk to ourselves," the actual perspective of an outside listener is extremely useful. The audience's distinctive "hearing" of a story plays an important role in making meaning. This is why we often find that talking to a friend or a therapist moves our inner experience in ways that our internal dialogue cannot.

Consider the following example of an early story. A toddler, just beginning to use language, hears her mother's car pull into the driveway. "Mommy's home!" she calls out, running toward the front door (Wrye & Welles, 1994). This is a complete story, with the logic and meaning carried by her ebullient tone and gleeful movement. We can imagine the affective response of the nanny who is standing nearby. What does she feel as she watches the little girl? She is probably tickled, pleased, and amused, and it shows on her face and in her posture. Now imagine some other possible responses. What happens to the story if the nanny says, "Wait, watch out, you might fall!" or "Shh! Quiet!" Or what if she stands by with no response at all? The child's rising joy and ebullience will be replaced by hesitation, shame, confusion, and deflation. The audience response to a story is part of the meaning and is part of the creation of meaning. Every telling of a story is a performative act in which actor, narrator, and audience come to some agreement about some aspect of lived experience that has some importance. We live within these meanings created by our stories, but stories can be retold.

TELLING STORIES THAT CAN'T BE TOLD

Dan McAdams (2008), an academic researcher who has read and thought deeply about narrative, comments that "some stories are so bad that they simply can't be told" (p. 253). As trauma therapists, we know a great deal about these stories. Judy Herman (1992b) wisely brought our attention to the difficulties that both individuals and cultures have "knowing" about trauma. Individuals struggle to grasp the meaning of traumatic events, often knowing and not knowing (Laub & Auerhahn, 1993) or knowing and defending against knowing (see van der Kolk, 1989, for a history of clinical thought).

Children in particular struggle to grasp the meaning of experiences that are distressing and troubling enough to be disorganizing. When trauma happens within the context of the family, the child's experience is often actively disqualified and denied (Summit, 1983). This leaves children vulnerable to a terrible confusion (Gelinas, 1983). They have to decide whether to trust their own senses and constructed meanings at the cost of alienation from the people to whom they belong. Most children faced with such a choice choose to belong at the expense of trusting their own knowing. This decision has survival value, but its great cost emerges as people struggle with the tasks of adulthood: creating a coherent and consistent identity, engaging the challenges of meaningful work, and forming loving romantic relationships. Then the traumas of childhood express themselves in self-doubt, triggered responses that are disorienting and don't seem to make sense, and aversive responses to the very things that are most desired. Storying experience allows people to make use of it (Stiles et al., 1999), and many young adults seek therapy when they can't make sense of themselves. As they try to tell the stories of their lives, the difficulty of storying these lives quickly becomes apparent.

Some people can't tell a story because they "don't know": they don't have enough factual information, or they don't have access to the information they do have because of encoding and memory problems. Some people can't tell a story because the dissociated experience is too threatening to personal constructs, feels overwhelming to the point of psychic disintegration, or feels disloyal to the point of rupturing crucial relationships. Some people know things they can't tell because they have been threatened into silence or have not been given the kind of recognition that helps them trust their knowledge. It can be difficult to discern the differences among "I don't know," "I can't say," and "I don't want to tell" in the disrupted attempts survivors bring to telling the stories of difficult experiences in childhood (Sorsoli, 2010).

LISTENING INTO SPEECH: NARRATIVE AND RELATIONSHIP

Posttraumatic anxiety and dissociative attempts to escape from that anxiety form and deform personality. A trauma narrative—a story that says trauma causes negative feelings and behaviors, that says, "I'm not crazy, something really bad happened to me and my reaction to this bad thing is normal"—has been liberating for people suffering the aftereffects of a broad range of traumas. People found that being able to talk about what happened and to have their account accepted and understood was enormously relieving. Once there is some connection within the therapeutic relationship and basic self-regulatory capacities are in place, therapy can begin to focus more centrally on creating this narrative. What story does the client need to tell? The therapist moves into the role of an audience. By audience we do not mean passive listener. An audience has a critical role in the development of a narrative. The quality of an audience's receptivity affects a narrator's interest in her own story, her capacity to bring energy and attention to what she is expressing. Furthermore, each audience listens in a unique way, helping to shape both what is talked about and how it is understood. And finally, an audience receives the story and in doing so brings the personal into the communal. But the ability of others to hear and understand what traumatized clients are trying to say cannot be taken for granted. As Judy Herman observed, psychiatry and the culture at large have repeatedly grasped the fact of trauma and its impact, and then subsequently discredited or forgotten it.

Therapists tend to be good listeners by both temperament and training. However, they need to learn to listen to trauma stories. People are naturally fascinated by painful or horrifying experiences, but they also turn away from them. Many of the stories we hear from our clients have to do with the isolation and alienation they feel; people don't want to listen to them and don't hear what they are saying. In the face of such responses, they stop trying to speak. When we really do listen, what we hear affects us; it changes our views about the world as a safe, benign, and predictable place. Like our clients' friends and families, like our clients themselves, we often want to turn away. *Bearing* witness is an apt phrase and takes considerable intention.

So our first job as an audience is to bring our presence to the encounter. Our presence matters. Psychologist Judith Jordan (1987) shares a moment in a therapy session when her mind wandered. Her client had been telling a story, and as Judith turned back, she realized that the client had faltered. "I feel lost, like I'm in a fog today. I don't know what I want to talk about," the client said. In sorting out what was happening, both Jordan and her client realized that the client had become lost because Judith hadn't been paying attention. Stories that have not been told by people who have not been able to tell them can and will be told to a receptive, attentive, and recognizing audience.

What are we listening to when we as therapists take on the role of audience? This is an important question because our attention is guided by our clinical theory, and clinical theory often treats the story as a source of information about various things aside from the story itself. CBP therapists work to develop their ability to hear both the text and subtext of their clients' stories, and through this role, participate in the unfolding meaning of the storytelling. From a narrative perspective, we need to listen to stories in a way that self-psychologists call "experience near." That is, we listen, first, in order to understand what the story means to the person who is telling it. CBP teaches a narrative stance that is simultaneously active and nondirective. We want to be quiet enough to make space for the client's specific story to emerge on its own terms, and at the same time we are often quite active as we check to be sure that they are safe in the telling and feel heard accurately.

In order for the story to develop, we need to be quiet in our listening. We are not silently analyzing, or mentally finishing their story, or searching for words to phrase our understanding, or taking mental notes for a cognitive intervention or exposure protocol—all useful activities at some times, but here distractions from the emerging story. When we are quiet in this way, we often experience confusion as our client makes his or her way toward something that is not yet understood. We have learned to appreciate this confusion. It signifies a place of not-knowing and makes a space for truly new thought. This is what the 1980s feminists were talking about when they coined the term "listening into speech" (Morton, 1985). The joint project of speaking and listening invites new stories—stories that are not yet in the realm of culturally shared experience, stories that give meaning to inchoate experience. Our attentive listening as an audience helps a client invest in her effort to tell her story. It signals that her story is important. It creates a space for the client to open up to emergent thoughts and feelings. It supports her efforts to metabolize her experience in new ways.

Finally, sharing a story brings the personal story into the communal body of knowledge. An audience that receives a story welcomes the teller into relationship with the community. This relationship shapes the story: if an audience hears something that is too alien they will mishear or forget (Bartlett, 1932). The selectivity of the audience's response helps guide the teller. It conveys cultural norms, ensuring that the personal story will not be too idiosyncratic to support social connections. At the same time, the understanding of the audience revises collective awareness to include experiences that have so often been elided from our collective his or her story.

Many clients want to start by understanding what happened out there. Nicole, for example, needed to start by speaking about external conflicts— her deteriorating relationship with her husband. But the subsequent work of psychotherapy is grasping the reality of what happened here: How did I feel? What did I do? Who am I? How did I get this way? Who would I have been if life had been different? Am I okay? What about me needs to change?

After listening to stories about neglect and mistreatment, we find ourselves listening to stories about anxiety, depression, and dissociation; about the child's loss of hope and the adult's struggles to tolerate criticism on the job or closeness in the marriage. The narratives that emerge as therapy deepens end up being about the impact of adversity on our clients' abilities to live up to their full potential, their shame over enduring vulnerabilities, their anger and sadness when they recognize that some opportunities are forever lost. And finally, as a more fully recognized self begins to recover vitality and resilience, we begin to hear stories of hope.

Narrative therapists have in common a belief that the story is a primary meaning structure. Throughout their lives people story and re-story their life experiences to create a narrative that supports a continuous, coherent, and congruent sense of self. When the life story is disrupted, people develop symptoms of anxiety and dissociation. Processing a difficult experience by telling the story of it contains anxiety and diminishes dissociation, allowing difficult material to take its place in the ongoing history. This is what clients typically come to therapy to do. Our job is to identify and help them overcome obstacles to storying, and then to listen.

Recognizing (Re-cognizing) Enactments and Developing the Relational Narrative

The storying experience is a synthetic action that brings together information from multiple processing systems within the human brain and psyche. So much of what goes into a story is unconscious—processed and stored without awareness, and also processed and stored in somatic systems that don't lend themselves to words. Not surprisingly, the life experiences that have been the most difficult to comprehend remain encoded viscerally and somatically, in the memory systems that tell us how to do without telling us what to think. As we've discussed, this material inevitably comes into the room through enactments, moments when we engage with our clients in interactions that resemble their most hurtful experiences. As we recognize and repair these ruptures in CBP, a new relational story is developed, unfolding the possibility for different types of connections.

BUILDING RESOURCES SO STORIES CAN BE TOLD: NARRATIVE AND REGULATION

When we meet new clients for the first time, we invite them to tell their story. We encourage them to start in the present: What is it that makes them seek help now? If the help is helpful, how will things be different? Since we think that the psyche is organized narratively, we want their story to direct our conversation from the outset. But people often can't tell a story. And as therapists, we need to be prepared to help them develop the psychic resources that creating a story requires. An adequate story recognizes and contains their experience. Such stories, cumulatively, form an autobiography, and the autobiography brings coherence and continuity to one's sense of self (McAdams, 2008). Typically, as people attempt to speak of experience that has not yet been storied, their difficulties with self-regulation emerge. Some people quickly become hyperaroused and have a hard time continuing. Other people become flat, affectless, disengaged from the emotional meanings of the material as they talk about it. Victims who have protected development through the use of dissociation may lack access to relevant information that is stored in affective states associated with a personality fragment, or part. Finally, some people present for therapy with secrets—stories that are well known to themselves but embedded in shame and shared with no others. At the level of brain and memory, all of these stories reflect problems with arousal. Self-regulation and the capacity to create a full and adequate story are deeply interconnected.

As we discussed in the relationship and regulation sections, the securely attached child is both well regulated and able to use thoughts and feelings to construct knowledge about his world; he is well positioned to begin to make stories as soon as he is developmentally capable of putting ideas together. Children who have not had such fortunate experiences with attachment are less well regulated and less capable of efficient and accurate use of cognitive and emotional information. Their lack of confidence that events are predictable, their lack of trust in the authenticity or usefulness of emotional expression, and their sense of being on their own to manage, all interfere with the kind of free exploration that leads to rich life experiences *and* to the capacity for self-regulation that allow people to explore their own experience within the context of their story.

Some stories are hard to tell because they are so stimulating that the person telling them fears being overwhelmed to the point of coming undone. And some stories are hard to listen to because the person telling them is too disconnected from the telling, which makes it hard for the audience to engage with the story. Some stories are fragmented because the experiencing "I" is separated into different parts of self. A primary job of the therapist is to teach and assist in regulation as the story is being told, so that the client/narrator can become more skilled at recognizing dysregulation and making appropriate moves to become more grounded and centered, to upregulate (become more energized) or to downregulate (calm down) as needed.

Telling a Story That Is "Too Hot to Handle"

Sometimes, the obstacle to thinking and speaking about difficult material is that it can feel dangerously arousing. At a certain threshold, anxiety kicks in, and our client feels that to continue will lead to "too much." We begin to hear statements like, "If I start crying I won't ever stop," or "I think I am going to throw up," or we see the sideways glance that conveys, "If I move a single muscle right now, I am going to break into pieces." The therapist needs to be attuned to changes in the client's arousal and to the threshold, after which increased arousal is overwhelming.

Nicole makes this easy. Consider this scenario. Nicole shares a memory of a verbal attack by her mother, and when she does, her shift to hyperarousal is sudden and marked. Her breathing becomes quick and sharp; her face reddens. She leans forward, her head in her hands. Katherine feels compassion for Nicole here, but she is not polite, doesn't offer sympathy, and doesn't inquire about the thoughts and feelings behind the tears. Both begin to feel hopeless, and treatment reaches an impasse in that moment. In moments such as these, the potential for enactment is high, with risk for client and therapist alike to slip back into the abyss. Now imagine instead that Katherine leans forward to join closer to her in this moment, and says, "I have some things I want to teach you about arousal and emotional regulation. Are you present enough that you can listen? Would that be okay?" In response to a direct but gentle invitation of this nature, one that simultaneously empowers the client with personal choice while also conveying her therapist's confidence about proceeding in this vein, Nicole would likely be receptive to undertaking this piece of work and allowing Katherine to teach her about the window of tolerance and some simple downregulation tools.

Working with a Story That Is Too Cool

Nicole's story was too hot. Some stories evidence the opposite kind of dysregulation: Instead of triggering hyperarousal, it seems as though they are not stimulating enough. This is usually a sign that the narrator of the story has defensively disconnected from the protagonist, from the self or part of the self who experienced the story she is telling.

Stories create perspective by creating a separation between the part of the self that tells and the part of the self that experiences. The narrator informs us of the actor's intentions, actions, feelings, and how things work out, without necessarily endorsing these. The narrator can see meanings in the story that are different from those of the protagonist. This perspective-taking is one of the things that makes storying so powerful as a vehicle for making meaning.

But sometimes people move too far away from their experience. As they tell their stories, they move beyond decentering into disconnection. The stories that result are emotionless and flat, and they leave the audience cold. When we find ourselves bored while we are listening to a story, it is likely a sign that the person telling the story is defending against his own story, against himself. This disconnection is common among people who have grown up in overstimulating and underrecognizing environments. When children find that expressing their feelings causes trouble at home, they begin to keep those feelings to themselves. The more a child withholds her felt experience, the less the world shapes itself to what is happening inside her. Over time, a split develops, and the child begins to believe that in order to fit in, she needs to be not-me.

David provides a good example of this adaptation. He has concluded that he cannot both be himself and belong. As a child he suppressed his livelier and his grief-filled sides in order to make himself a "good" candidate for adoption and to fit in with his white adoptive family. As an adult, David feels pressure to be more expressive of his black heritage, something that would require him, he says, to "undergo an entire personality lobotomy."

David's therapist Susan registers his disengagement in their first meeting. She finds *herself* detached and wonders if the affectively flat way David brings his story to her is similar to what his wife is complaining about. She explores his willingness and capacity to move closer to his story by asking what he is feeling as he talks, but he is not responsive to these questions. Sometimes the simple overture of asking after feelings helps people reconnect with their own emotions, but David isn't ready for this step; in response to Susan's queries, he changes the subject or he launches into complaint.

Sometimes we can help people become more engaged with repeated and persistent inquiry. It is often helpful to ask after body experience: Where do you have feeling or sensation in your body right now? What can you notice about that sensation? Does anything come to mind as you feel it? What do you think that feeling might be about? Do you think it has anything to do with what you are talking about? Put your attention on that burning feeling in your abdomen and just free associate; let your mind go wherever it wants and just notice what comes to mind.

Susan has identified a problem in David's regulation as he tells his story: he is too disconnected from himself as well as from his audience. She focuses on looking for ways to increase his engagement. After a few sessions, David complains that he doesn't feel he is getting anywhere—or rather that his wife feels he isn't working hard enough in therapy! Susan asks him to tell her about his wife and notices that the story he shares, judging by her own response, is much more engaging. From this she moves to a discussion of the therapy, and for the first time David engages more directly with her in a way that is thoughtful and emotionally connected. This is good technique on her part: often people who cannot engage with themselves about their feelings can make an affective connection to feelings that are happening in the here and now in the relationship with the therapist. David and Susan talk about his frustration with himself. He talks about his difficulty expressing feelings, his efforts to entertain Susan by keeping things light, and his sense of not knowing how to go deeper. He is able to be self-observant during this conversation, aware of feelings as they come up, and he ends the session with a comment that they have made progress.

When David's affect begins to be better regulated in session, he is increasingly free to act in emotionally regulated and affectively connected ways outside of session. His more open curiosity about his early life coincides with a serendipitous discovery of a letter from his aunt to his adoptive mother. The aunt's letter reveals her deep distress at having to place David in care and her wish for further contact. David's adopted mother had not informed him of this letter, but finding it revived long-lost memories of time spent with his aunt and cousins. David brings this information into the session with considerable excitement, feels understood by Susan's response, and begins to share his adoption narrative more fully and with much more feeling.

THE UNDERDOG VOICE: NARRATIVE AND PARTS

When we listen with fully open minds and open hearts and with deep resonance for the person whose story is being told and the person who is telling the story, we will begin to hear things that have not been said before. Sometimes what we hear are secrets. Take the case of Amos, a middle-age black man who has sought an opportunity to talk about his early experiences of sexual exploitation. He begins by letting his therapist know that he wants to say something that he has never before revealed. "I think I'm ready to talk about the sexual abuse," he says. "I think I'm ready to talk about it."

Frequently, it isn't just a secret, but a secret *self* that needs to come into the story (see Chapters 7–8). In fact, Amos's memories of sexual abuse may have been largely compartmentalized and held by a part of him. It is pretty hard to come into adulthood with a sense that all parts of ourselves are lovable and welcome. What most of us do with those parts that have been unwelcome in the past is to try to leave them behind as we come in the door. Faced with a choice of being fully ourselves or belonging to our family, most children, most people, choose to suppress aspects of the self in order to belong.

It is now widely recognized that the "self" is not a singular structure and is impacted by dissociative adaptations to trauma (Bromberg, 2009; van der Hart et al., 2006). In the context of the story, this perspective is important in two ways. First, the emergence of a submerged voice often represents a disclosure and a "coming out." This part or these parts are private, they have been kept secret, and the aspects of life that they contain and express are separate from the overt structures of our clients' lives. Second, these parts are often shameful, or repudiated. Pamela Tanner Boll's (2011) movie, *Who Does She Think She Is?* follows a number of women struggling to sustain primary commitments to both art and family. Most of the women portrayed in this film have sacrificed some aspect of family in order to pursue their art. Sculptor Janis Wunderlich is one artist who is successful at integrating the two. We meet her in her home studio, surrounded by busy children and bizarre, beautiful clay figures of mothers rent and devoured by their children. All of the maternal figures have two heads. Wunderlich says, in an almost off-hand way, "Yes, they all have two heads. I guess that is a second part of me, a part I don't like." A part I don't like!

When clients bring the not-liked, exiled, dissociated, or secret part of themselves into the therapy room and therapy relationship, they are risking disdain in order to create intimacy. As one client commented, "You probably know that when I let you see this part of me I am always watching you for signs of disgust." This client's wish, like that of Nicole, David, and others, is to be able to bring the parts of themselves that have been exiled into their primary relationships: to integrate the parts of themselves that know how to relate to others with the suppressed parts that carry the spark of desire, excitement, intensity, shame, loneliness, and/or aggression.

When Nicole's therapist Katherine asks, "What gives you the spark now?", Nicole realizes the time has come to tell Katherine about her "bad" side. Nicole's bad side has affairs, brief relationships, or sexual encounters that bring her an excitement she can't find at home. These encounters are striking for what they both are and are not. They are not emotionally compelling. In fact, Nicole's impressively precise recounting of the sequence of her affairs, and the various shifts in her emotional and energy states preceding, during, and following each encounter, reveal that she is almost certainly functioning in a dissociative state while carrying them out. Still, there are aspects of the affairs that Nicole experiences as intensely arousing, and she spends days planning and anticipating them, and further days regretting and atoning for the betrayal they express. These days of private contention with herself are thrilling and enlivening. That they feel dangerous is part of the appeal, but they are beginning to get out of hand. Nicole fears the disruption of her marriage and family if this part of her gets exposed, and she also fears her escalating involvement in its affairs.

When they tell stories *about* what this exiled self is doing, clients are, more importantly, giving a voice *to* the exiled self. Sometimes this is enough to initiate a greater cohesion among the parts of self. Bringing exiled parts of self into therapy is the first step and a step that all by itself changes the relationships among the voices as well as the relationship with the therapist. Nicole shares that she is both enlivened by and afraid and disgusted by her "bad" side. She is afraid that if she lets her guard down, other people will discover this part of her and will reject her. At the same time, she also recognizes that this side of her might be trying to protect her by preventing her from getting close to people who could reject or abandon her.

Many of us adapt to the relationships we belong to by locking up some less desirable aspects of ourselves into a second self, a forbidden self, a shadow self. But the cost of this adaptation over time is a gradual depletion and dissatisfaction, and/or, perhaps, a growing sense of danger when the life of the secret self threatens to come forward. The work of therapy is to integrate the exiled voice into the main story. Perhaps Janis Wunderlich's graphic representation of her two-headed selves supported her successful integration of artist and homemaker. Wunderlich said, "I *guess* it's a part of myself." Coming to recognize the dissociated selves as a part of the self and bringing those selves into an integrated awareness that is owned as "self" are essential steps of a major project to develop a more cohesive identity and narrative.

CONCLUSION

Trauma in childhood—the active trauma of abuse or exploitation or the passive trauma of neglect with its failure to provide protection, recognition, and containment—leaves a child ill equipped to make meaning of life's experience, with many experiences hidden or disowned. Narrative work in CBP includes processing microlevel elements of the trauma, such as specific memories of maltreatment; macrolevel processing of themes, such as the impact of these early experiences on one's ability to trust, hope, or believe; and life narrative and identity construction. As we co-create the type and pacing of narrative work with each individual client, we consider each of the CBP components, including four dimensions of the narrative component: traumatic memory, identity impacts of trauma, engagement regarding trauma narrative, and integration of life narrative.

Storytelling serves an integrative function, bringing together aspects of memory, emotions, somatic states, cognitions, and behaviors; it also creates perspective and supports meaning-making. As CBP therapists, we should support the client as she builds awareness and tolerance for the increasingly *embodied experience* she holds as the protagonist of the story, develops the more *measured perspective* of the narrator as she makes sense of her story, and receives *comprehension* of the audience as we actively engage with her storytelling. The roles of protagonist, narrator, and audience shift as we reflect back portions of her narrative, while she processes her emotions and makes sense of her experience in increasing layers over time. The act of storytelling enhances the relationship component of CBP, as intimacy develops through sharing aspects of experience; the idea of "listening into speech" guides us in the active, receptive stance that is required as we convey the importance of the client's experience, open a space for her emerging thoughts and feelings, and invite her to metabolize her experience in new ways. As we actively engage with our clients in this storytelling process, we also become part of the story. We hold the essential role of supporting our client's regulation through this storytelling, helping him manage stimulation in stories that are "too hot" and increasing engagement when he is disconnected from stories that are "too cold." In narrative work in CBP, we should also listen for and invite "secret selves," or parts of self that have been suppressed or split off, into the story, building a narrative that integrates all aspects of our client's experience. In the next chapter we explore how CBP seeks to transform work with adult survivors of complex child trauma around their trauma stories into life narrative construction and identity development, impacting both client and therapist.

CHAPTER 10

Transcending the Abyss
Life Narrative and Identity Development

Nicole and David come into therapy with a focus and, beneath and surrounding it, a story. David's focus is marital strife. His story is one of not fitting in, of being alienated and misunderstood. This story unfolds into a trauma narrative of profound childhood loss, emotional neglect, and self-loathing engendered by impossible caregiver expectations. Nicole's focus is interpersonal recklessness and promiscuity. Underlying this story is a narrative of pernicious childhood emotional abuse and rejection and the ensuing lifelong search for identity and self-love.

Katherine and Susan also come into treatment of these clients with their own focus, stories, and identities. Katherine enters treatment with Nicole as a young but relatively experienced therapist who is skillful and conscientious but has not done quite enough work on herself. Susan is older and more seasoned, and she is quite able to talk about her own anxieties with her supervisor. Like those of Nicole and David, Katherine and Susan's narratives and identities evolve over time. More importantly, they intersect with those of Nicole and David, impacting the course of treatment by influencing what each therapist notices, what they fail to see, and what needs of their own they endeavor, consciously or otherwise, to meet in the context of this work.

In Chapter 9, we talked about the essential role of story in complex trauma treatment and about how this story changes over time. Far too often, adult survivors of childhood emotional abuse or neglect spend years "chasing ghosts," desperately searching for memories of "real trauma." Typically, this manifests as the search for evidence of some experience of physical or sexual violence horrible enough to justify how miserable and stuck they have become in their lives, to account for how short of their aspirations they have fallen. Many of these individuals endured and have access to memories of profound emotional abuse or neglect more than sufficient to account for their suffering, but they have internalized societal, cultural, or contextual beliefs or assumptions that discount, minimize, or overlook these experiences. In these instances, narrative work in CBP begins with helping clients come to a different appreciation of these insidious experiences and their qualification as legitimate forms of trauma. From there, CBP seeks to advance clients' understanding, organization, and communication of how the sum of their adverse experiences intersected and combined to profoundly shape their functioning, identities, and life course.

In intervention with adult survivors of chronic and complex childhood trauma, this storying routinely goes far beyond our clients' often presumptive, initial focus on the processing of their trauma narratives and into construction of a life narrative. Even when treatment is heavily focused on maintaining the safety and stability of highly vulnerable, dysregulated, or reactive complex trauma survivors, we observe the driving influence of the implicit narratives clients have internalized about their lives and their place in the world. The CBP therapist holds this narrative frame in his or her meta-awareness during these early stages of treatment until clients are ready to engage in narrative processing as an explicit element of treatment. This is especially important given how readily the narrative component of trauma treatment gets put on indefinite hold in the general psychotherapy of many childhood trauma survivors. In that context, problematic attachment dynamics from unresolved childhood trauma narratives frequently get triggered in the treatment relationship and play out in enactments between client and therapist. CBP emphasizes the need to heed the emergence of our clients' (and our own) explicit and implicit trauma and life narratives beginning with our first moment of contact. As we see in Nicole's vignette, there is far more to be gleaned about her story and sense of self in the nuance of her initial verbal and nonverbal communications in her first session (and even more so in her pretreatment assumptions and expectations about therapy) than in any detailed, objective rendering of her demographics and history. Likewise, each cultural or contextual assumption made by the therapists in these vignettes about David and Nicole based on their own implicit biases and stereotypes adds another layer of obfuscation, clouding their understanding of their clients and distancing them from authentic connection.

In Chapter 4, we described Martha Stark's (2000) characterization of two-person therapy, one that is relational and authentic. CBP takes this a step further. We do not merely recognize the inevitability of enactments; to some extent we invite them. We view the personhood of the therapist not only as an essential ingredient in the treatment alliance, but also as one of the greatest potential detriments to, and catalysts for, therapeutic change. CBP uses the supervisory process to attend carefully to the ways in which the professional *and* personal narratives and identities of the therapist permeate the work, and at times impede it, intersecting with and influencing those of our clients. We are also mindful of how the relationship between the therapist and supervisor can get caught up in these enactments and distortions. It is for these reasons that we describe CBP as aspiring to go "beyond two-person therapy" in its effort to glean the "macrolevel" influence of the extratherapeutic life narrative and experiences of the therapist on the "microlevel," moment-by-moment treatment process.

Most trauma-focused treatment models share a belief that the "core work" of trauma-focused psychotherapy involves helping clients build the capacity to manage and in some form or another contain, process, or resolve their traumatic material. Most trauma-focused interventions hold as a stated or implicit assumption that the narratives they are helping their clients to construct derive from material belonging primarily, if not exclusively, to their clients. In contrast, in CBP, we view the story of the therapeutic relationship as belonging to, and invariably integrating, language, understanding, and experiences from both client and therapist. In turn, the unfolding trauma and life narratives in CBP are ultimately understood as co-creations of client and therapist, and occasionally the supervisor. Over the course of CBP treatment, our client's stories take form and are inevitably altered and transformed through not only the therapeutic act of listening into speech, but also by residue from the intentional and unintended contact with the personhood of the therapist

Figure 10.1 graphically visualizes the process of narrative development over time in CBP. The therapist and client both play a role in the unfolding "story" of the therapeutic process. Each is changed by this process. There are shifts in the relational narrative, as the therapeutic relationship develops, has ruptures and repairs, and often strengthens over time. As the adult self or most adult self of the client is cultivated, there is a greater capacity for integrating dissociated aspects of the trauma narrative. Parts of self that were holding fragmented elements of the trauma narrative become less isolated and more able to share the burden of these memories and the related distress. The experience and meaning of the trauma often shift; instead of being denied or all-defining, these experiences are increasingly accepted as a part of and assimilated within the person's larger life experience. As the client develops a more sophisticated current identity, he is able to hold and tolerate ambivalence, acknowledge positive and negative experiences, and incorporate discrepant characteristics. Acknowledging and accepting one's past, while not being defined by it, allow adult complex trauma survivors the freedom to explore hopes and desires and develop increasingly resourced future selves.

Mirroring this process, CBP therapists will ideally engage in continual self-reflection throughout treatment. They will work to increase their awareness of how the work is being influenced by their own personal needs,

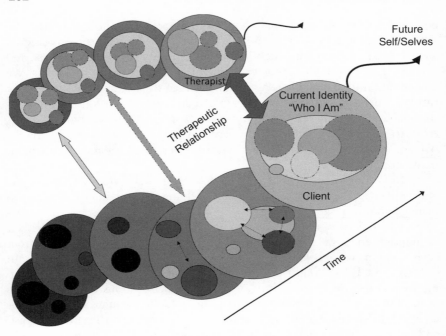

FIGURE 10.1. Narrative and identity/self-development.

reactions, and views of self, endeavoring not solely to temper their personhood in the therapeutic relationship but to utilize it in the service of therapeutic growth. They will strive to continually cultivate their sense of self as both professionals and persons.

TELLING STORIES ABOUT "NOTHING": NARRATIVE WORK WITHIN THE ABYSS

For many adult survivors of chronic emotional abuse and in particular emotional neglect in childhood, their traumatic "experience" was as much, if not exponentially more, about what did not happen than what did. Their childhoods were characterized by ①pervasive experiences of isolation, ②caregiver rejection, ③or emotional deprivation. Narrative work in trauma therapy is almost always most challenging with individuals whose formative years were defined by the *absence* of experience. For one, identifying focal or "index" memories to target and process with these clients as part of trauma-focused therapy can be akin to searching for a particularly important grain of sand in a desert. On a more profound level, for clients raised in a family environment shaped by pervasive emotional abuse or neglect, once they adopt a complex trauma frame and come to recognize their histories as having indeed been characterized by chronic and profound trauma, the number and immensity of the emerging stories can seem as overwhelming and endless as the desert itself.

Of necessity, narrative work in CBP more often centers on deeply entrenched, archetypal experiences of identity and relationships. By the time she enters treatment, Nicole's internalization of self as a "disgusting creature" can no longer be tied to the one specific event that led her father to make this comment. It has come to reflect the essence of her overarching experience of self in the eyes of both of her parents. It typifies Nicole's personality, her behavior, her body, her sexuality. It will not simply be "cleared" out and resolved with a trauma-processing protocol targeting a particular memory. More than that, it has become integral to her sense of self. Despite and within its negativity, it has become the locus of Nicole's power and passion, her most alive, agentic, and embodied experience of self. Perhaps even more challenging, David's sense of self as a "Nowhere Man" has evolved into far more than the sum of his experiences of abandonment by his family of origin and the chronic alienation, perceived incompatibility, and inferiority he experienced within his adoptive family. Even if one could help him to achieve a sense of acceptance or resolution of the specific traumatic memories, this would not in itself be enough to fill his void of self-love, nor would it equip him with the capacity to give and receive love from others. Rather, attempting to engage David in traumatic memory processing may serve to accentuate his awareness of these deficits and voids, deepening his sense of hopelessness and despair.

This is not to say that traumatic memory processing should not be undertaken with adult survivors of complex attachment trauma. Doing so is in most cases an essential element of ultimate growth and recovery. However, narrative work in CBP rarely begins or ends here. In addition to processing as necessary specific urgent, intrusive, or pivotal traumatic memories and telling and reconstructing the trauma story (see Chapter 9), the narrative component of CBP is directed toward a number of clinical objectives related to broader life narrative and identity development.

Echoing Roth's important model (Roth & Batson, 1997), one function of narrative work in CBP is the examination of maladaptive schemas or attributions of self and relationships formed as a consequence of emotional abuse and neglect dynamics experienced within formative early attachment relationships. Here we seek, for example, to help clients recognize when the negative attributions of self they have internalized and the unfavorable identities they have constructed were formed in the context of efforts to protect parents, siblings, or other important attachment figures from responsibility for harm inflicted on them or nurturance withheld. Reconciling these distortions in clients' stories often involves reworking their narrative to see that their parents were not equipped to adequately parent, whether because of their own histories or other limitations. It also involves helping clients see that the abuse or neglect they endured was not committed because they themselves were not good enough or attractive enough or some other deficit they believe they must have had (and often were told they had).

Expanding on the work of Korn and Leeds (2002), a second objective of narrative work in CBP is the internalization of reparative experiences and establishment of adaptive reframing of life narrative and identity. Here we work with clients to identify, increase access to, and augment the narrative salience of important past experiences of personal mastery, relational connection, or protection; as well as to cultivate and integrate new positive experiences and facets of identity into a forward-looking life narrative. This latter element of CBP becomes a bridge to the vital therapeutic "work" that needs to happen outside of psychotherapy. As glimmers of personal interests, talents, and goals begin to emerge within treatment, it is essential for the CBP therapist to encourage, reinforce, and support client efforts to return to or take interest in new self-care regimens, hobbies, community activities, or friendships that serve to increase their sense of connectedness to life, other people, and the world.

A third facet of narrative work in CBP bridges elements of our Center's child complex trauma treatment model approach to working with fragmented self-states (Kinniburgh et al., 2005) with relational psychoanalytic approaches (e.g., Bromberg, 2001) to working with dissociative parts. Here we work with clients to integrate fragmented, disparate, and seemingly incompatible parts of self into a cohesive sense of identity and life narrative. Often this involves helping clients to acknowledge and disentangle (or "unpack") the trauma-based origins—and ultimately accept, if not embrace, the survival-based functions—of behaviors and personality characteristics that have been hidden, disavowed, or suppressed out of fear or shame. Each of these elements shares the goal of interlacing meaning-making into the life narratives of adult survivors of complex childhood trauma. Finally, harkening back to the phased approach delineated by van der Kolk and colleagues (1996a), a fourth element of narrative work in CBP is meaning-making.

Casting Light into the Void: Meaning-Making and Resiliency in Narrative Work

It is fundamental to humans to make sense of their experiences and to bring that understanding into the rest of their lives (e.g., Cohler, 1991; Grossman et al., 2006). Because childhood is the "cradle for the construction of meaning" (Garbarino & Bedard, 1996, p. 467), children who are subjected to chronic trauma beginning at the youngest ages may be most susceptible to lifelong struggles with meaning-making. The complications inherent in doing so are only magnified when significant aspects of early traumatic experiences are partially or fully inaccessible to narrative memory. Being repeatedly emotionally abused throughout childhood and enduring prolonged emotional neglect are such extreme experiences that they are very difficult for survivors to make sense of, to create meaning for these experiences, that is not further damaging to the self. And when these traumatic experiences of emotional neglect or abuse occur in the context of primary caregiving relationships, the taproots to self-love and relational intimacy can be severed.

For most of our clients, at some point in their recovery process, it becomes essential to find some way of making meaning out of experiences of childhood trauma and the ensuing years or decades of suffering they have engendered. *"Why did it happen to me?" "Why did she do that to me?" "Why did he give up on me?"* Such laments are endemic to adult survivors of attachment trauma. Frequently uttered early in the therapy process, they can evoke dismay in compassionate clinicians who often struggle to provide what will almost invariably be received as unsatisfactory responses to these crucial identity-defining questions. As Silver, Boon, and Stone (1983) articulated, an important component of the meaning-making process for most trauma survivors is the attempt to answer these questions—and in turn for therapists to support them in grappling with this undertaking.

It has long been noted that many survivors adopt a cognitive frame to help them try to understand their abuse (e.g., see Harvey, Orbuch, & Weber, 1990, who call it "account making," and Pipher, 2002, who writes of "healing stories"). Early research on this topic revealed that children often construct narratives of self-blame to make sense of as well as gain some semblance of control over what is happening to them (Silver et al., 1983). This tactic also allows the children to stay connected to pivotal attachment figures if they are the ones carrying out the abuse (e.g., Feinauer & Stuart, 1996). We have encountered such self-blame repeatedly in our clients regarding the neglect and emotional abuse they experienced. This aspect of narrative work in CBP is much less about helping our adult clients to understand rationally that they are not to blame (they generally already know this on a cognitive level), but to integrate this knowledge into their life narrative and identity on embodied, emotional levels.

In a common example of narrative work on meaning-making, Samantha, a client who suffered incredible emotional abuse and neglect throughout her childhood, continued through several years of therapy to feel and believe that if she had only been nicer and not so angry and difficult when she was a child her parents would not have treated her as they did. As she and her therapist periodically revisited this topic and worked with some of her parts who totally blamed herself, the client reluctantly began to see how young and completely vulnerable, trusting, and defenseless she was when it all started—an infant, in fact—and to accept that she could not have been to blame. As is often the case, Samantha's resistance to exonerating herself was entangled with fierce efforts of some of her child parts to preserve an idealized view of her parents.

For many clients, one important but challenging facet of this work involves shifting the blame from themselves to their perpetrators (Grossman, Cook, Kepkep, & Koenen, 1999). For other clients, or the same ones at different junctures in treatment, contemplation and decision making about cutting ties with, forgiveness of, or reconciliation with emotionally abusive and neglectful parents, family members, or significant others become important foci of the work. Our aim in CBP is to support each client in whatever position they need to take on this complex issue and, moreover, to emphasize that decisions to forgive, reconcile, or sever attachment bonds are by no means contingent on whether one's perpetrator is still alive.

In a seminal series of qualitative studies, Frances Grossman and her colleagues examined factors supporting resiliency and processes of adaptive meaning-making in resilient adult survivors of childhood abuse (Gartner, 2005; Grossman et al., 1999, 2006; Kia-Keating, Grossman, Sorsoli, & Epstein, 2006; Lew, 2004; Sorsoli, Kia-Keating, & Grossman, 2008). This research highlighted the importance for resilient survivors of not only making sense of the suffering they endured, but also of "constructing an alternative view of the world in which this suffering is not the dominant feature" (Grossman et al., 1999, p. 190). A second factor involved challenging and reframing negative and self-blaming attributions about their traumatic experiences based on memory fragments or stories passed down by family members. Third, many resilient clients constructed or adopted broader, contextually based, and less binary frames of understanding of how many positive as well as problematic aspects of their identity were shaped by their early histories. Frequently, this entailed recognition and exploration of how these histories themselves were created by much larger forces than simply their parents' inadequacies. Attention to the intersection of individual trauma histories with culture and context (e.g., generational influences; historical and intergenerational trauma; poverty and racism; religious oppression; restrictive familial views about gender and sexuality) is of particular importance here. Fourth, almost all survivors studied emphasized the importance of helping others as an integral part of their healing journey.

Finally, for some complex trauma survivors, embracing one's unique spirituality was observed to enhance self-acceptance and sense of agency, while illuminating new means of engaging in life with increased purpose and meaning. For those whose traumatic experience has been justified, reinforced, or intensified by intolerant religious beliefs or hypocritical practices, processing past harmful religious experiences may be essential to reclaiming, redefining, or finding an adaptive system of belief. Interestingly, research has found that a history of chronic childhood abuse, in contrast with exposure to acute or impersonal forms of trauma exposure, leads to a more ambivalent relationship with religion and often disrupts the spiritual well-being of individuals (for a comprehensive review of this topic, see Walker, Reid, O'Neill, & Brown, 2009). Not uncommonly, one element of narrative and identity work in CBP involves examining, challenging, and revising harmful self-beliefs and meaning-making forged in the context of shame and guilt inflicted by clergy, parents, or other important adult caregivers in the name of religion. (For a more detailed treatment of the intersection of spirituality, religiosity, and complex trauma, see Pressley & Spinazzola, 2015, 2017).

THE IDENTITY CONTINUUM IN TRAUMA RECOVERY

Our narrative work with adult survivors of complex childhood trauma involves a substantive exploration of and quest for identity. Historically, psychotherapy and advocacy with individuals impacted by interpersonal forms of trauma have proffered a victim–survivor paradigm of identity development. In CBP, we regard this as a problematic binary in its limitation of the human potential. CBP adopts a five-"stage" or "-state" metaphor of identity: No Self, Damaged Self, Victim, Survivor, and Person. We view this paradigm as not only more helpful and empowering to clients, but also as more accurate in its characterization of the aftermath of complex trauma and the trajectory of recovery.

The first stage in this representation of identity, No Self, most closely corresponds to the state of the abyss. It reflects an identity characterized by a sense of profound emptiness and disconnection. Through David's poignant recounting of being the "Nowhere Man" and Nicole's description of being trapped in a "black hole," we know that both are intimately acquainted with this desolate, hopeless stage of identity. While this is unlikely the primary identity stage of either David or Nicole at the time of their entry into treatment, it is clear that part of each of their identities resides primarily in this stage of development, and likewise that other parts of self primarily inhabiting higher stages of identity development can sink down into this more primitive state of being when triggered. Both David and Nicole are susceptible to being swallowed back into the depths of an identity abyss at a moment's notice in response to relational conflict and perceived or actual rejection, abandonment, or betrayal.

The second stage, Damaged Self, represents a meaningful progression on the continuum of trauma identity development. Here the individual does possess a tangible, substantive sense of self and a frame of reference for self in relation to others and the world, albeit a highly negative one. Affective valence is typically heightened when clients inhabit this stage or state of identity; above all, shame is its master. In the initial phase of treatment described in the vignette, this is the stage Nicole most frequently occupies.

The third stage or state in this continuum, Victim, reflects equal parts progression in empowerment and complication. Here individuals impacted by trauma have attained some belief in the wrongness or injustice of what they experienced or were denied, and with it some measure of relief from inward-directed blame and loathing. And yet here the risk of getting sucked into a binary black hole is greatest, as the external locus of hatred and blame, however justifiable, exerts a consuming magnetic pull that can draw individuals away from the self-reflection, awareness of limitations, and acceptance of personal responsibility for change that are necessary for true recovery. We see David's susceptibility to getting locked into this state of identity when he feels put upon or forgotten by his intimate attachments, including his therapist.

The fourth state or stage, Survivor, is the prototypical end point for the vast majority of trauma-focused interventions. Here individuals have overcome their trauma, learned from and often grown in meaningful ways as a result of working through their adversity and suffering, and are commonly focused on giving back to others who have endured or are at risk of exposure to similar experiences. As empowering as this stage of identity development is for the traumatized individual, in CBP we regard this as a false summit. Like the Victim identity, this state still clings to an identity that is centered around and defined by traumatic experiences.

Accordingly, the end goal for identity development in CBP is that of Person. This stage of identity development entails transcending trauma and forging a life whose whole is greater than the sum of one's experiences of adversity and loss. Some adult survivors of complex childhood trauma inhabit this stage of identity much of the time, getting pulled backward periodically by triggers and relational upsets in their current life. For clients with more fragmented parts of self, efforts for their adult self to remain in this state of being for extended periods of time can be more challenging. For other adults with histories of chronic and complex childhood trauma in general, and profound emotional abuse and neglect in particular, accessing this state of identity can be more elusive and for periods of time can often be perceived as impossible. Nevertheless, even in these situations, it is more often glimpsed than perhaps realized by client and therapist alike. This can happen when the adult or most adult part of a client has the experience of being truly seen and accepted by, or being in rhythmic connection with, another adult with whom they are in a meaningful relationship. We encounter this at the end of the Nicole vignette, when Katherine achieves a repair of their chronic underlying therapeutic rupture and we witness nonverbal synchrony in affect and breathing of client and therapist. In CBP, we work to help our clients increasingly access this state and direct their attention to an awareness of it. In doing so, irrespective of how fleetingly sustained or how rapidly extinguished, we generate a flicker of belief in its future possibility, some small but real proof of its existence.

Advancing the client's progression through these stages of identity is an important element of narrative work in CBP. We undertake this work directly with the adult or most adult part of the clients, beginning by educating them about our understanding of the stages or states of the trauma identity continuum. Over the course of treatment, we listen carefully for opportunities to draw their attention to and name the state or states that their adult self or other parts of self appear to be primarily inhabiting or shifting into in response to internal or relational triggers. We normalize parts of self being stuck in stages of identity that are perceived as more hopeless and forsaken, in the context of lived experiences and survival adaptations, and we promote movement, within and between parts of self, to states of identity that clients experience as more empowering, connected, and life-embracing.

For parts of self lost in the abyss (No Self), we might use disclosure of our own emotional response as we visualize the abuse or neglect clients endured during childhood in an effort to evoke in them an authentic affective or somatic response—be it sadness, longing, or self-pity—that might shift them into a higher state of identity (Damaged Self or Victim). For parts of self adhering to a sense of permanent damage and hopelessness, we might first provide validation by expressing anger at the social injustice of what they experienced in an effort to evoke in the client a shared sense of outrage that might shift them into a Victim state. Often this effort is more safely and effectively undertaken, at least initially, through displacement: focusing our emotional expression on a safer target—for example, drawing on contemporary events portrayed in the media or imagining how the clients would respond to mistreatment similar to their own inflicted on a beloved niece or nephew. Then, we may work to assist them in accessing other, more agentic or resourced parts of self to comfort, accompany, and help them through these dark places and periods of their lives.

For clients or parts of self embroiled in a Victim identity, we work to reframe the adaptive nature of their current state of being: the degree of power, control, and predictability they have afforded themselves in cultivating and remaining entrenched within this stage of identity. Eventually, and gently, we challenge our clients' dependency on this identity, helping them to recognize its limitations and supporting them in mustering the immense courage and sustained effort necessary to work toward a higher state of identity development. For clients whose adult self has attained the identity of Survivor, we mix validation and reinforcement of their progress with persistent encouragement to engage with us, in session and in their outside life, in mindful, embodied attention to present-focused experiences of joyful connection and engagement to self, others, nature, and the world.

It is our experience that movement across these stages of identity development is quite fluid and episodic; in turn, upward progress tends to be episodic and rarely linear. Many of our clients inhabit one primary stage of identity, but particular dissociative parts embody other stages of identity. Others fluctuate between two or more stages of identity; these are not uncommonly two or more steps removed from each other. Likewise, some people will experience transient states of distress or moments of present-focused engagement during which they temporarily leap forward or revert to an "earlier" or "later" stage of identity. Finally, some of our clients had sufficient resources in early childhood during their formative periods of self and identity development to have never experienced the most impoverished stages or states on this continuum, whereas others could not yet envision the possibility of ever attaining a state of personhood unfettered by their trauma history.

FORSAKEN IDENTITIES: NARRATIVE AND SOCIOCULTURAL CONTEXT IN CBP

For adult survivors of childhood trauma, especially chronic familial emotional abuse and neglect, there is inevitably yet another layer of complexity. For the preponderance of these clients, one or more (sometimes all) fundamental aspects of personal identification have been altered by virtue of their traumatic experiences. For many of our clients, experiences of being victimized, betrayed, or physically or emotionally abandoned by one's family result in an inextricable sense of being severed from or cast out of the family's associated cultural identification. For David, this process involved a disconnection from his racial identity and complicated his adoption of a confident and secure masculine identification; for Nicole, it despoiled her religious upbringing and contaminated her view of self as a sexual being. For other clients, trauma histories may intersect in problematic ways with community-based, cultural, or geographical ties. These struggles steep many of our clients in a profound sense of cultural alienation through which they feel they belong to nothing and to no one.

In CBP, our work with clients to integrate cultural experience into treatment is engaged on many levels. For some, it unfolds as a component of their specific trauma narrative. For others, it becomes an essential component of their identity development and life narrative. For many, it operates most often on a larger implicit level, running under the surface of much of the work. And for most, it inevitably involves some combination of working with clients to grant themselves permission to alternately retain, reject, transform, reclaim, or forge new cultural identities for self.

In CBP, we strive to address the complicated intersections of these cultural and contextual dimensions with our client's histories of complex trauma exposure. For example, in treatment with Nicole, we would explore how her sexuality and femininity became directly tied to the seat of her emotional abuse and primarily held in fragmented, shame-ridden parts. We would also explore how the implicit hypocrisy of her mother's religious righteousness in the context of her pervasive emotional cruelty and verbal debasement drove Nicole away from what otherwise might have served as a protective resource in her life, resulting in her becoming an adult alienated from the solace a spiritual connection might offer. We might then undertake the even more complex work of unpacking Nicole's internalized racism and its dual protective and distancing effect in her relationship with her husband. Finally, we might contemplate how her middle- to lower-middle-class upbringing has afforded her an affinity for "underdog" characters and role models but also contributed to a chronic sense of inferiority to those perceived to be of higher educational, professional, or economic status. Here we might wonder if Nicole's husband's career progression, marked by his steady movement over time from lower-middle-class supermarket clerk to upper-middle-class franchise owner, has led to a sense of inferiority, further contributing to her sense of emotional distance from her husband and her defensive coping in the form of affairs and ethnic devaluation. Through careful and gradual disentangling of cultural, contextual, and traumatic experiences, CBP endeavors to increase the client's capacity to retrieve, discover, and create facets of identity that are not predicated upon or defined by traumatic experiences and that envision and work toward positive connections to affirming cultures, contexts, and systems of meaning.

TRANSFORMING THE ABYSS: INTEGRATING EXPRESSIVE ARTS AND PROJECTIVE TECHNIQUES IN NARRATIVE DEVELOPMENT

The need to integrate alternative approaches to healing, addressed in the regulation section of this book, is also highly relevant to narrative work and has become increasingly relevant in light of the compelling research of Raio, Orederu, Palazzolo, Shurick, and Phelps (2013). Their fascinating study empirically demonstrated on a physiological level that cognitive approaches to emotion regulation established to be efficacious in controlled experiments with individuals in a state of calm break down and cease working when attempted with individuals who are in states of acute stress. Our colleague, Bessel van der Kolk, has asserted that effective treatment of complex traumatic stress requires bypassing the dorsolateral prefrontal cortex, the part of the brain that is most associated with working memory, planning, and rational analysis of situations. This portion of the brain, most directly targeted in cognitive approaches to trauma therapy, has been demonstrated in neuroscientific research to lack a pathway to the limbic system, the emotional center of the brain (LeDoux, 2000). Drawing on LeDoux's (2000) research, van der Kolk has theorized that true and lasting resolution of traumatic stress may entail activation of the center of the brain responsible for *interoception*, or self-awareness: the medial prefrontal cortex.

In CBP, we regard the medial prefrontal cortex as a critical "side door" of the brain, access through which can facilitate the processing of traumatic experiences by building synaptic bridges to the limbic system. Accordingly, and as exemplified throughout this book, CBP draws heavily on nontraditional approaches to trauma treatment to engage this critical area of the brain, including activation and working within dissociative states of consciousness; therapist use of self as an energy barometer and pressure gauge; use of metaphor; and storytelling. In the same vein, we frequently incorporate expressive arts approaches and projective techniques within the narrative component of CBP as other potent mediums providing passage through this side door. Specifically, we have found that engaging our clients in the use of metaphor, creative writing, expressive arts, drama, and projective techniques can help them to tell "stories" about their trauma and life experiences that is more integrative and linked to limbic experience than can often be achieved through traditional talk therapy. Here we provide select examples illustrating the role of these approaches within the narrative and identity development component of CBP.

River Maps

Confronted with the unspeakable in many of her clients, particularly in the treatment of adolescents and young adults, our colleague Annie Rogers (2007) created a metaphor-rich, visual arts–based narrative timeline exercise that elaborates on a preexisting theater arts technique. Using a long scroll of paper, which they revisit periodically across multiple and often many sessions, clients chart the course of their lives. They can begin and pick up this exercise at any point of their life history—present, past, or future. Symbolic imagery is used to represent salient adversarial and protective people, epochs, and events in their lives. For example, clients may draw a lightning storm to represent a terrifying traumatic event; a section of shallow rapids filled with treacherous jagged rocks reflecting a tumultuous period in their lives; a deer on the river bank indicating the unexpected befriending of a safe and gentle person; a log jam representing a stuck time in their life; a fierce beaver representing a complicated caregiver who simultaneously serves to protect them and stifle their growth; and so on. This fluid and evolving client drawing can become an inroad to clinical dialogue, often providing language for clients to talk about trauma and its influence on life's journey that was previously unavailable We have frequently used this exercise and other visual arts–based exercises within the overall context of CBP narrative work to provide clients a simultaneously containing and freeing artistic structure that integrates difficult and painful traumatic experiences into a forward-moving life narrative.

Complex Trauma Imprints

Developed by Spinazzola, this individual or group visual arts exercise is predicated on the notion that every person's traumatic and protective experiences create a tangible, "visible" imprint that is simultaneously unique and resonant of the collective human experience. In this exercise, an inexpensive spin art kit, commonly available at most craft stores, is used to create artistic patterns formed by drops of paint on cards or sheets of paper. Clients begin by selecting an initial color representing a traumatic experience they have endured, allowing a single drop of paint to fall on the sheet of paper that is spinning on the art wheel. Even if the therapist (or another client in a group intervention) selects precisely the same color to represent his or her experience of trauma, the two patterns formed will be similar and distinct, much like two fingerprints. Additional colors may be added to represent other types of adverse and protective life experiences, and multiple drops of the same color may be administered to reflect repeated or prolonged exposure to particular forms of traumatic experience. The final product expresses, contains, and ultimately transforms traumatic experience into a work of art. In group intervention, clients may each elect to create their own imprint as well as a communal representative of trauma and resilience. As with River Maps, the creation that emerges in this exercise often provides a vivid and moving path of access to affectively charged material within the context of a creative structure. It also provides sufficient containment, displacement, and distance to enable clients to tolerate inhabiting these dark places and to begin to process and integrate formerly overwhelming traumatic memories and sequelae.

One-Sentence Stories

Not uncommonly, and often very early on in treatment or even during the screening or intake process, our clients poignantly convey a comprehensive story of their lives in a single sentence. Almost as frequently, we overlook this sentence, only later realizing its critical importance.

> "I've gone through life as a two-legged stool."
> "I'm like a small animal: there's just one of me."
> "It doesn't matter; no one listens or cares anyway."
> "If you knew me, you'd leave me too."
> "They can't make me!"

These visceral statements reflect more than complaints or cries of despair; often, they epitomize and encapsulate a life. We encounter such statements multiple times in Nicole and David's clinical vignettes:

> "I've spent the majority of my life trying to please everyone in it for as long as I can until I simply can't hold out anymore and have to escape."
> "[I'm the] Nowhere Man."

At times, we even uncover the clinician's one-sentence story of his or her work with a given client: *"I feel like I am everything and nothing [to this client] all at the same time."*

These stories are often held by a part; in other instances, they are tied to an encompassing sense of identity. In many cases, they are internally conflicting and contradictory, as in Nicole and Katherine's dualistic and shared struggle between conversely expressed views of self as a "good person" versus a "disgusting creature." Listening for these stories is an important facet of narrative work in CBP. They inform case conceptualization and provide a language or foothold from which to approach and anchor emotionally laden identity development and narrative work. Moreover, they often reveal the nexus of defensive coping and with it, more often than not, a portal to wounded, forsaken, terrified, or exhausted child parts shouldering the immense burdens of unresolved trauma.

Superhero Narratives

Adult survivors of complex childhood trauma are often most seen and defined by society and the people in their lives for their defects, problems, and maladaptive consequences. Challenging this stigmatizing vantage point, CBP reframes the immense and often miraculous acts of courage, ingenuity, hardiness, and strength necessary to survive complex trauma. In CBP, we view adaptation to complex trauma as an act of power and resilience, and we recognize the potent energy fueling even the most destructive and self-defeating patterns of coping. Accordingly, we find the superhero metaphor to be quite apt for adult survivors of complex trauma. As with most superhero characters in fiction, our clients share poignant histories of relational loss, victimization, or betrayal that have become both defining cornerstones of identity and life narrative and the source of incredible adaptation. Table 10.1 examines a number of common problematic clinical presentations observed in our clients, recasting each presentation from the vista of the superhuman survival adaptation it represents. With some of our CBP clients for whom this metaphor resonates, we engage in expressive arts exercises, generating a storyboard in which they retell their origin story or reframe their chronic maladaptive coping from this vantage point. With others we might imagine, draw, or even construct their superhero costume or emblem or compose their theme song. Finally, we work with clients to visualize and chart the course toward a future in which they gain the ability to master and channel these powerful energies and instincts to achieve a different way of being in their lives.

CBP AND CLINICIAN NARRATIVES AND IDENTITIES

Whereas a handful of psychotherapists have written about the relationship between their personal and professional identities and associated role confusion, conflicts, and emotional challenges (e.g., see Allen, 2007; Bowen, 2013; Espín, 1993), consideration of these issues within the challenging context of trauma-focused psychotherapy has been more limited. Several scholars and expert practitioners have explored the vicarious traumatization that can occur for therapists engaged in trauma-focused psychotherapy (Cerney,

TABLE 10.1. Latent Superhero Narratives: Adaptive Reframes of Client Psychopathology and Maladaptive Coping Behaviors

Problematic behavior/pathology	Superpower	Adaptive reframe
Hypervigilance/hypersensitivity	Superhuman senses	Threat/danger detection and avoidance
Deadly rage/destructive behavior	Super strength	Personal agency and power
Poor hygiene	Toxic blast	Interpersonal distancing strategy
Unnoticed, ignored, overlooked	Invisibility	Preserve safety in midst of danger
Recurrent quitting of opportunities/giving up on self prematurely	Clairvoyance	Predictability; buffer against disappointment; agency in the face of failure; reinforces lack of effort
Recurrent sabotage and undermining relationships; turns others against oneself	Telepathy/mind control	Agency and power in relationships; deny others the power to hurt, reject, or betray oneself
Out-of-body experiences	Astral projection	Escape pain/sensation of abuse; transcend physical limitations
Dissociative identity disorder	Multiplication of self	Generate and deploy specialized "field agents" to meet needs
Resistance to change or growth	Time manipulation (freezes time)	Predictability, familiarity, control, safety
Manipulation, deception, exploitation	Master of disguise	Make people like you; get needs met; prevent people from seeing who one truly is; conceal personal defects
Impenetrable emotional defenses/emotional analgesia	Protective force field	Self-protection against interpersonal emotional harm
Alexythymia; emotional numbing; inability to experience certain emotions (e.g., love, fear, pain)	Invulnerability	Self-protection against intrapersonal emotional harm and unbearable self-awareness

1995; McCann & Pearlman, 1990a; Pearlman & Mac Ian, 1995; Pearlman & Saakvitne, 1995b; Perlman, 1998). However, few have examined the complex intersections between their clients' developing narratives and identities and their own.

One notable exception is an important but largely overlooked manuscript by Lonergan, O'Halloran, and Crane (2004) in which these authors propose three primary stages in the developmental process of the trauma therapist. Drawing on an earlier model of a developmental approach to therapist supervision (Stoltenberg & Delworth, 1987), the authors referred to the stages identified in this qualitative research study as (1) the beginning of the journey, (2) trial and tribulation, and (3) challenge and growth. Each stage in the developmental progression of the trauma therapist is characterized by the clinician's evolving views of therapy, self, and attention to self-care. In the initial stage of their framework, treatment is dependent on more rigid beliefs and practices imposed by the therapist's formal academic training, lack of awareness of and/or underdeveloped self-care habits, and inflated view of self as holding primary control of the session and greatest responsibility for client change and healing. In the trial and tribulation stage, therapists are beset with self-doubt and uncertainty about the effectiveness of book-learned approaches to trauma intervention, and they struggle to formulate their own understanding of the therapeutic process. It is during this stage that therapists become increasingly aware of their personal vulnerability, recognizing the impact of the work on their personal well-being and the need to cultivate personal strategies and approaches to self-care. This stage is characterized by the therapist's personal experience of distress and the dual potential for burnout and meaning-making. In the final stage of this framework, the trauma therapist becomes less rigid and more integrated in his application of theory to practice. Here, more cognizant of the limits of his power in the therapeutic process, the trauma therapist paradoxically becomes more agentic and effective in his work. This final stage involves maintenance of an active self-care practice and acceptance of the therapist's role as a vulnerable human in the therapeutic relationship.

The CBP approach continuously attempts to bring to awareness the professional identities and driving narratives that evolve, often implicitly and sometimes unconsciously, by clinicians undertaking complex trauma therapy. CBP seeks to illuminate and gain understanding of the personal etiologies and unresolved needs that are being met by the primary and at times more consciously accessible identities and organizing narratives adopted by the adult self of the therapist. Each of these is typically associated with the strengths as well as the limitations of the trauma therapist; predicts greater ease or difficulty in effectively engaging clients with different clinical profiles in treatment; and influences both affective synchrony and propensity for therapeutic blind spots. In the Nicole vignette, examples of these are Katherine's implicit identity as a good person and her explicit narrative as an experienced and savvy trauma therapist, despite her relatively young age and less than a decade of practice. This implicit personal and professional identity engenders Katherine's misattunement to Nicole at several junctures, contributing to ruptures in the therapeutic alliance and triggering enactments. In turn, Katherine's more consciously accessible professional narrative as an "expert" operates as a defense against critical self-examination and serves to conceal underlying self-doubts about her competency, contributing to her avoidance of bringing uncomfortable and potentially unflattering material into supervision.

Concurrently, in CBP we pay special attention to divergent or therapist identities and narratives that manifest in response to specific clients or clinical situations. Often, these are held by younger, less fully integrated parts of self that emerge during therapeutic enactments or become activated when the therapist feels otherwise threatened, impassioned, or overwhelmed by this challenging work. Returning again to the Nicole vignette, we see manifestations of a latent identity held by Katherine's less integrated parts of self in her strong physiological and moral aversion to Nicole's expression of herself as a "disgusting creature." A judgmental part of Katherine emerges here that exists in conflict with her self-identification as a "good person" and unconsciously competes with this primary identity. Likewise, in response to her need to regard herself as a good person, an identity the stability of which both her supervisor and her fiancé threaten, a narrative as "unappreciated victim" of the trauma therapy process emerges to compete with her explicit/implicit sense of self as a trauma expert/fraud. Interestingly and importantly, while the emergence of this alternative narrative evokes a powerful protective impulse in Nicole to retreat from the work, it is only in the context of the raw emotional vulnerability engendered by this experience that Katherine finally recognizes how misattuned to Nicole she has become and musters the authentic compassion and firm determination to set things right.

Therapists' Entry into Trauma Treatment

The vast majority of practicing psychotherapists treat individuals who have experienced and been impacted by trauma, irrespective of whether this is an overt focus of the work or whether the clinician is even aware of this reality. Examination of the intersecting personal and professional identities and driving narratives of the clinician in CBP begins with an appraisal of how each therapist entered this work. For some practitioners, it very much involved an intentional decision, built on years of formal training and specialized study. Others find themselves saddled rather unintentionally with a caseload of clients whose lives have been profoundly shaped by traumatic experiences despite this not being part of their clients' language or organizing frame of reference, nor in response to any representation of expertise in this area on the part of the therapist. It is not uncommon for generalist psychotherapists to recognize the presence and effects of trauma in their clients but not be able "to not go there" for a variety of personal reasons. Others have become exhausted and emotionally depleted from being steeped in their clients' misery and hopelessness and long to escape from the mire of this work but feel trapped within it. Still other therapists overlook trauma altogether in their work with complex, treatment-resistant clients, and only come to it reluctantly in response to the client's efforts, through personal research or outside consultation, to better understand what is holding them back in therapy and, more importantly, in their lives.

In CBP supervision, we are almost exclusively working with therapists who have knowingly entered into the practice of trauma treatment and who typically are engaging in this arena of therapeutic practice willingly, if not outright enthusiastically. Nevertheless, coming to understand the motivations and identifications that brought each clinician to this work is invariably important to effective CBP treatment. In our decision to become trauma therapists, some of us are driven consciously or otherwise by a highly personal mission to help others make their way through dark and forsaken places similar to those we have endured; others are motivated by a more general calling to end suffering and promote healing; and still others by a fascination with the scientific workings of body and mind in response to extreme life experiences and ambition to figure out "what works." Finally, more than a few therapists are drawn to trauma-focused therapy by an underlying motivation held by parts of self in the abyss or Midnight zone of consciousness, to address vicariously their own unresolved trauma sequelae and thereby facilitate their own recovery.

Prominent Identities and Driving Narratives of Trauma Therapists

The CBP framework identifies several prominent identities or organizing narratives of the trauma therapist. Table 10.2 provides a detailed description of these narratives, including considerations of their functions. Each is associated with the potential advantages and risks to the effectiveness of intervention with particular complex trauma clients. The 12 narratives described represent an illustrative, nonexhaustive list and may be readily regarded as therapeutic styles or ways of approaching trauma treatment.

The vast majority of practitioners we have encountered in our training and supervision evidence facets of more than one identity or style in the work and commonly as many as five or six. In practice, we experience these identities as more dimensional than categorical. Clinicians typically exhibit varying hues or intensities of these organizing approaches to the work versus their absolute presence or absence. Rarely is the presence of one identity mutually exclusive of another within the same clinician, or even as manifested in work with the same client. Most commonly, one or more of these identities or organizing narratives characterizes a therapist's general approach to trauma treatment, whereas others manifest reactively in response to particular clients

TABLE 10.2. Trauma Therapist Identities and Organizing Narratives

Description/function	Strengths/advantages	Limitations/risks
The Rescuer		
Approach to treatment characterized by a sense of urgency to move clients through the stages of their trauma recovery and/or protect them from further harm.	Empathic. Likely to be perceived by some clients, at least initially, as a true champion or the long-awaited solution to their problems.	Heavy setup for failure and propensity to activate unhealthy reenactment patterns (e.g., initial idealization of the work can become a setup for disillusionment, resentment, or hopelessness). High risk of vicarious trauma/burnout on part of clinician, with ensuing risk of reaffirming clients' long-standing sense of futility if clinician is perceived to disengage, give up, or express disgust.
The Activist		
Approaches trauma treatment as a societal problem versus a psychological problem. Intervention adopts a peer-to-peer or consumer-driven approach.	Affirming in tangible sharing of clients' outrage over the injustices of trauma. Empowering.	Risk of overstimulating client and activating dysregulation or decompensation. May promote clients' externalization of responsibility for change. Potential to be light on technique or strategies to navigate the prolonged "middle phase" of complex trauma intervention.
The Healer		
Draws heavily and "banks" on a spiritual, mindfulness, or other energy or abstract concept-based approach to trauma recovery.	Emphatic. High propensity of success around regulation and relationship components of intervention. Instills hope.	May inadvertently affirm/collude with clients' avoidance of trauma processing/narrative/parts work, even when indicating/necessary to foster growth/recovery. Potential setup for clients whose expectations have been set too high when treatment stalls or gets stuck and the healing "aura" begins to fade.
The Coach		
Therapist as "helping hand." Active, skills-based approach to intervention.	Client-centered. Often embraces more embodied approaches to trauma recovery, with the therapists' use of self as a purveyor of tools. Strength-based.	Propensity for clinician impatience/intolerance for long-term work. Less tolerance for extensive pathology and persistent vulnerability of clients. Difficulty remaining present with clients immersed in, or needing to repeatedly revisit, dark places.

(continued)

TABLE 10.2. (*continued*)

Description/function	Strengths/advantages	Limitations/risks
The Scientist		
Adopts a planful, often assessment-driven and evidence-based approach to intervention.	Tendency to be thorough, intentional, and energetic. Systematic approach to treatment, typically with willingness to explore new interventions. Often thoughtful about pacing, combination, and sequencing of intervention.	Risk of overreliance or rigid adherence to treatment protocols at the expense of attunement to clients' needs. May be perceived as detached or less emotionally invested in the client versus "the work." May be less aware of or adept in use of self as a core component of treatment. Likely to adopt a less relational/intersubjective approach to treatment than optimal for complex trauma clients.
The Parent, Partner, or Spouse-in-Training		
Drawn to trauma treatment less by a conceptual interest in the work than by an innate caretaking or protective instinct. Often observed in young adult child trauma therapists who have recently completed their graduate training.	Often experienced by clients as authentically warm and caring early on in treatment, contributing to development of strong early treatment alliance.	Risk of motivation waning over time as the work proves to be difficult and as evolving personal relationships (e.g., marriages, birth of own children) engender redirection of emotional connection. Risk of early vicarious traumatization and burnout. Difficulty managing clients' reactivity to personal leave and extended absences. Risk of gradual reduction of caseload or clinician resignation or modification of career focus.
The Self-Healer		
Drawn to trauma treatment, consciously or otherwise, as an element or means of personal recovery from unresolved trauma.	Able to draw on personal experiences. Capacity to genuinely relate to some clients.	High vulnerability to vicarious traumatization. Potential for misattunement resulting from false equation of own/clients' experiences/needs. Risk of personal decompensation as a result of vicarious trauma. Potential for withdrawal from the work if overly triggered and/or loss of interest once own issues become addressed.
The Cat		
More traditionally reflective, interpretive stance in relation to the work. View of self primarily as a "mirror," judicious advisor, or "object" for the client.	Low risk of enmeshment. High tolerance for clients with low tolerance for emotional connection. Comfortable with long-term and slow-paced intervention. Able to recognize and appreciate modest, incremental treatment gains.	May be perceived as aloof or detached. May struggle to provide depth of intimacy, connection, active confrontation, or embodied experience necessary to advance treatment with many complex trauma clients. May collude with client's avoidance of taking risks or processing trauma. Susceptible to overreliance on an overly cognitive, overly sedentary approach to treatment.

The Dog		
More active, embodied, experiential approach to intervention.	Hard working and earnest, often perceived by clients as a champion "in their corner." Openness to try innovative therapy skills and techniques, particularly those that are interactive or energy based.	Dogged approach bears risk of clumsiness and of inadvertently triggering clients, setting off clients' defenses or otherwise contributing to misattunement to clients' needs. May rush treatment or push client too hard.
The Witness		
Approach predicated on a belief in the power and importance of bearing witness to the clients' communication/disclosure of lived experiences of trauma and adversity.	Validating, empathic approach.	Can be light on technique/strategy unless an empirically developed narrative/exposure protocol is being followed. Propensity to devolve into protracted supportive therapy that is "circular" in nature: "hanging-in-there therapy." Risk of functionally "sitting shiva" indefinitely with a life that's not over yet.
The Empath		
Therapy driven by an intuitive, instinctual, organic approach versus developed model or protocol.	Typically experienced as genuinely caring and engaged. Tendency to be thoughtful, observant, reflective. Good barometer and pressure gauge for client in promotion of regulation. Potential for wide window of engagement and likely facility with remaining present and grounded with challenging and vulnerable clients in dark/quiet as well as bright/loud places.	Propensity to reject out-of-hand, evidence-based treatments, systematic protocols, or other approaches that may be beneficial to clients. Tendency to uphold empathy and intuition as an excuse against needing to be systematic, to evaluate treatment outcome, and to question and examine personal effectiveness.
The Mountain/River Expedition Guide		
Expert-based approach to trauma treatment. Component and/or phase oriented. Evidence-based or informed, systematic approach, with heavy emphasis on development and evolution of the trauma narrative.	Tends to promote grounding of therapist and effective approach to use of power and recognition of limits of power; therapist is less prone to fall into the abyss; less likely to rush the pace of treatment, work harder than the client, or feel the need to rescue the client.	Risk of observing only what the therapist already expects to see: assuming, based on his expertise in leading expeditions and familiarity with the contours and features of terrains pervasive to complex trauma, that he knows in advance all the facets of each client's mountain/river landscape. Risk in doing so of falling into a sinkhole, sliding down a gorge, or activating a fault line that sends both clinician and climb tumbling into the depths of the abyss.

or clinical consultations. Moreover, we routinely observe, both in ourselves and in those we train and supervise, the evolution and substitution of these identities and organizing narratives over time as providers mature in their relationship to this work.

The ongoing examination and elucidation of these overt and latent clinician identities and organizing narratives is one of the primary foci of supervision in CBP. The overarching supervisory goal here is to increase the clinician's self-awareness of prevalent identities he or she adopts in general, as well as less common ones that are activated by specific clients and that may reflect enactment of younger parts of self in interaction with younger parts of clients, in the service of better attuning to clients and improving clinical outcomes. This includes working with clinicians to gain a mutual understanding over time about which identities represent their strengths and effectiveness as trauma therapists and to aid them in developing these further. Likewise, CBP supervision endeavors to increase awareness of which therapeutic styles represent a given clinician's greatest vulnerability areas in this work, and then to assist the clinician in better managing, modifying, or substituting these over time. Above all, the goal of this element of supervision in CBP is to bring these identities out of the less conscious, more dissociated zones of awareness (Abyss, Midnight, and Twilight zones) into the Sunlight zone so that they can become better integrated and most consciously accessible to the adult part of the trauma therapist, enabling the therapist to marshal and hone them to best meet the needs of specific clients.

Specifically, as clinician identities and narratives are identified, the CBP supervisor works with clinicians to determine when, and in what form, additional clinician supports are needed and to refine treatment strategies to better align with the needs of clients. This aspect of supervision most often begins with helping clinicians to bring latent identities and implicit narratives to awareness. Often, it involves helping clinicians to become aware when younger or less integrated parts of themselves have been activated by the work and require comforting, reassurance, or better consolidation with the adult self. And in some cases, it entails recognizing, in as collaborative and gentle a manner as feasible when unresolved issues related to personal trauma history, mental health, or other life adversity have (re)surfaced and require more intensive support, including potentially through the clinician's initiation, resumption, or modification of personal counseling.

CBP supervisors may help their supervisees to temper their primary or reactive therapeutic narratives to better match the unique needs of different clients. For example, through supervision Janet realized that she needed to tone down her "Empath" identity with Phyllis, a client who was too threatened by the degree of emotional intimacy it conveyed. Instead, it proved to be important for Janet, an experienced trauma therapist, to bring to the forefront her "Activist" identity, given the chronic entanglement of Phyllis's experiences of trauma within the context of enduring severe poverty and racism.

For Phyllis, these realities had chronically been misunderstood and even discounted by past providers set on adhering too rigidly to traditional medical models of case conceptualization.

In other instances, the CBP supervisor may help a clinician recognize when a particular client or clinical situation has activated a latent identity or alternate narrative held by one of the clinician's own child parts, resulting in an enactment. For example, Thomas, a normally empathic and well-boundaried clinician, needed support in supervision to redress the therapeutic process when a terrified child part of his client Kimberly had in turn activated in Thomas an urgent "Rescuer" identity held by one of his child parts. This was clouding his judgment and leading to emotional overinvolvement. Conversely, in another instance, Thomas became emotionally withdrawn in treatment when faced with boundary-threatening behaviors from a dysregulated child part of his client Simon. Here Thomas required assistance from his supervisor to recognize how this experience had led to an enactment in which one of his own protective child parts had emerged that manifested a more emotionally removed response (a "Cat" identity). Simon perceived Thomas's consequent shift in emotional engagement in treatment as an abrupt rejection and emotional abandonment that affirmed and magnified Simon's chronic sense that he was unlovable.

Finally, at times, the CBP supervisor will encourage clinicians to attempt to "try on" or cultivate identities that are more foreign to them in an effort to meet the needs of a particular client. For example, Tracy, a clinician who normally practiced trauma therapy in an intuitively driven manner, came into supervision asking for a new case to be reassigned. A psychodynamically trained therapist, she explained that her new client, Nik, came in adamantly insisting upon "11-session dialectical behavior therapy." Tracy emphasized that this case was not a good match for her as she was not a cognitive-behavioral therapist, and besides, she was pretty certain that there was no such thing as "11-session DBT." Invited by her supervisor to pause in this decision making in an effort to adopt a broader vantage point, Tracy ultimately came to recognize in Nik's request a healthy assertion from someone who from the cultural context of his gendered experiences held wary presuppositions about therapy as an experience that "goes on forever and leaves you raw and exposed." In the context of these fears and concerns, Nik's request for a more time-limited approach that involved tangible evidence of outputs and outcomes in the form of homework sheets and pre- and postassessment measures made complete sense. In this request, he was seeking a sense of agency, predictability, and control in the treatment process, the very things that had been denied him as a child in the context of his maltreatment.

Tracy's supervisor encouraged her to "try on" a "scientist" identification in order to partner with Nik around this work. Returning to this client, Tracy brought workbooks into treatment from which to choose homework assignments in a collaborative manner, incorporating weekly regulation skill introduction, practice, and review into her overall approach. Tracy agreed to the 11-session course of treatment and worked with Nik to set realistic goals to target for that interim. In turn, Nik agreed to come in for a 12th session in order to review progress, assess the presence of any continued needs, and decide at that time to either conclude treatment or to renew the contract for an additional batch of sessions. Thus began what ultimately resulted in over a year of productive CBP treatment, parceled out in a consecutive series of "11-session intervals."

CONCLUSION

CBP goes beyond traditional trauma-focused therapy in its emphasis on helping clients to generate a life narrative that integrates but is greater than the sum of even the most insidious and prolonged traumatic experiences. Pursuit of this clinical objective is met with additional obstacles and challenges for adult survivors of childhood complex trauma with histories of impaired caregiving, attachment disruption, emotional abuse, and especially emotional neglect. In these instances, the lives of clients being treated with CBP have often been as much or more defined by the stark absences and chronic deprivation of all the good, normal experiences that should have transpired in their development than by the specific acts of violence they endured. Further complicating this work for many of our clients is the intersection of their traumatic experiences with broader cultures and contexts of oppression and exploitation that must be taken into account in treatment. Toward this end, meaning-making and promotion of resilience are important facets of the narrative component of CBP, as is helping clients to foster a sense of identity that transcends their traumatic experiences. Treatment elements employed in the service of these clinical objectives in CBP include the trauma identity continuum and the incorporation of new and borrowed creative arts approaches into the treatment process.

CBP utilizes the supervisory process to attend heavily to the practicing clinician's parallel process of identity and narrative development. Here the CBP supervisor seeks to elucidate and reconcile overt and latent, integrated and fragmented, mature and vulnerable expressions of the clinician's intersecting personal and professional identities and narratives. Increasing the clinician's self-awareness of these internal processes, the CBP supervisor aids the clinician in attaining the personal resources and support needed to temper, modify, substitute, or redirect these personal features in the service of improved attunement and response to the clinical needs of each complex trauma client in their caseload. Table 10.3 summarizes the elements of identity and narrative development work for client and therapist within this component of the model.

TABLE 10.3. Intervention Strategies for Narrative Component of CBP

Client
- Linking triggers to past traumas
- Reframing behaviors as survival adaptations
- Developing a trauma narrative; integrating (verbal, affective, sensory/somatic, cognitive-behavioral) aspects of trauma-related experience and decreasing related distress
- Integrating traumatic experience and evolving the trauma narrative into a life narrative
- Redefining narrative work: instead of focusing solely on trauma memory processing, moving beyond to meaning-making and identity development

Narrative × Relationship
- Developing a narrative about relational patterns, using a trauma-informed lens
- Building new relational patterns and a new story about self-in-relationship
- Bearing witness and "holding" the developing narrative
- Building the story of the therapy and the therapeutic relationship over time

Narrative × Regulation
- Providing psychoeducation about trauma reactions and regulatory processes
- Paying careful attention to the window of tolerance and window of engagement during trauma processing
- Achieving regulation through narrative work or memory processing, including relief of alienation and shame that can emerge from being seen or witnessed

Narrative × Parts
- Listening for one-sentence stories that may hold the defensive stance and defining narrative of a part of self
- Providing psychoeducation about dissociation and parts work
- Helping client recognize implicit trauma narratives that are organizing identity and driving behavior
- Exploring different narratives held by different parts
- Supporting development of an integrated narrative across parts of self

Therapist
- Recognizing own stance or orientation to trauma work
- Acknowledging that narrative is always there, even when it is implicit or unspeakable; understanding that there is no singular narrative
- Listening/"listening into speech"
- Actively working on own trauma or life narrative (building self-awareness), with our professional narrative integrated into a larger self-narrative
- Recognizing the presence, operations, advantages, and limitations of the professional identities and organizing narratives that influence and at times drive our work as trauma therapists; working to shift and temper these as needed to increase our effectiveness in general and with particular clients

Narrative × Relationship
- Using self-disclosure appropriately
- Codeveloping the therapeutic narrative
- Acknowledging the intersections of traumatic experiencing and broader cultures and context of oppression and integrating recognition of these into the treatment process

(continued)

TABLE 10.3. (continued)

Narrative × Regulation
- Understanding our own regulatory patterns and challenges
- Maintaining effective pacing regarding trauma processing: not colluding in avoidance or overfocusing on traumatic experiences

Narrative × Parts
- Recognizing our implicit narratives of our identities as trauma therapists
- Cultivating the ability to be flexible around these—drawing on different identities/roles in response to the unique needs of different clients

Supervisor
- Bringing attention to pacing of narrative work
- Fostering increased therapist awareness of latent identities and implicit narratives driving their general approach to trauma treatment, or held by less integrated parts of self and emerging in enactment in reaction to specific clients or clinical situations; assisting clinicians in cultivating and obtaining the personal supports and resources to manage these internal experiences and cultivate them in the service of increased attunement of the needs of their clients and effective response
- Maintaining a grounded stance in the meaning of supervisory work; building mindful awareness of the impact personal and professional experiences and worldviews have on supervisory style

PART III

THE COMPONENT-BASED PSYCHOTHERAPY MODEL INTEGRATION

OUT OF THE ABYSS

CHAPTER 11

Tailoring Treatment with CBP
Individualized Adaptations and Effective Pacing

Component-based psychotherapy supports the development of a more connected, balanced, and coherent way of living. The primary goals of CBP are (1) to build awareness of, and tolerance for, internal experience; (2) to increase connection and integration, which involves connecting thoughts, emotions, somatic states, and behaviors; building pathways between parts of self; linking past and present; and developing connection to others and to community; and (3) to develop identity and create opportunities for resilience, growth, and positive experience. CBP is a framework for intervention with survivors of complex trauma, including, as we have focused on in this book, early emotional abuse and neglect.

Throughout this text, we have explored each of the four components—relationship, regulation, parts, and narrative—in depth. As we have discussed, the relationship component refers to all the interactive elements of the therapeutic relationship, as well as to other relationships in one's life. The regulation component addresses balance in affective, somatic, cognitive, and behavioral states. The parts component is essential in exploring a person's internal experience when there is disconnection from, or fragmentation in, self-states. The narrative component is the basis for integrating traumatic experiences into a larger life narrative and developing a positive future self and sense of meaning. These components often intersect, and the emphasis on various components fluctuates throughout the course of treatment with

CBP. CBP emphasizes the roles of both client and therapist in the therapy and the interactive nature of the therapeutic process over time.

But a number of questions remain. How does the therapeutic process with CBP change over time? How is CBP adapted to the unique needs of different clients and different therapists? How does a CBP therapist consider which component might be the initial focus with a particular client? How can we influence the pacing of therapy to ensure that we don't delve too deeply too quickly, or that we don't stay in a comfortable place for too long? In this chapter, we address several phases of treatment in CBP. We consider how client characteristics influence our choices about the primacy of the four components. We describe timing and pacing in treatment with adults who have experienced childhood emotional abuse and neglect, and we explore how shifting the focus of treatment can help maintain effective pacing in the work.

STAGE OF TREATMENT

Typically, all four components of CBP are at work in the therapy to greater or lesser degrees. However, certain components tend to be primary at certain stages of therapy, with different types of presentations and at different moments within the therapy. Consideration of which component and component goals are primary can serve as a useful guide regarding the process of therapy over time. The simplest example of the role of various components over time is to look at stage of treatment, similar to conceptualizations within many phase-oriented models (see Table 11.1).

Early Stages of Treatment

Because CBP is a relational therapy, early treatment typically focuses on development of the therapeutic relationship. We acknowledge each client as an expert in him- or herself and emphasize the development of a working partnership. At this point, narrative may appear to be primary because early therapy often focuses on an exploration of the client's personal history and current experiences. Narrative does have an important role here, as the therapist begins to learn about his client through "listening into" their stories (see Chapter 9) and the therapeutic relationship is built through sharing these personal experiences. Psychoeducation is another narrative approach that can help to acknowledge the impact of early developmental trauma, normalize reactions, and provide a framework for treatment. As they get to know one another early in the therapeutic process, the client and therapist frequently develop a joint narrative about the purpose and framework of the therapy.

Despite the important early role of storytelling in establishing the therapeutic relationship and treatment planning, narrative work does not tend to

TABLE 11.1. Primary Components by Treatment Stage

Early treatment	Mid-treatment	Late treatment
Primary		
Relationship (development), Regulation	Parts, Narrative (trauma integration), Relationship (working with enactments)	Narrative (identity development)
Secondary		
Narrative (sharing history and current experiences, psychoeducation)	Relationship, Regulation	Relationship
Tertiary		
Parts		Regulation, Parts

be primary in early CBP. Instead, narrative provides the context for the core of early treatment—exploration of inner experience, which is an aspect of the regulation component. The CBP therapist is more interested in the client as a person and focuses on her internal experience rather than on the details of what has happened to the client. This consideration is particularly important in trauma treatment because it establishes the perspective that a person is not defined by his experiences. The therapeutic relationship is fostered by the therapist's ability to be consistent, authentic, regulated, and attuned. In early treatment, the CBP therapist focuses on actively engaged listening, promoting mindful awareness of internal experiences (for both their clients and themselves), and providing support for their clients to tolerate and manage distress. Regulatory tools are used primarily for containment and relief at this point. Many people who experienced early emotional abuse and neglect have had limited modeling, practice, and internalization of regulatory tools. Therefore, co-regulation often plays an important role in early CBP treatment, as the therapist supports the client in building her capacity for awareness, tolerance, and modulation of internal experience by practicing these skills together in session. Awareness of parts of self may begin to emerge for either the therapist or the client at this stage, but parts work does not tend to be the focal point at this stage unless more significant fragmentation is preventing progress on relationship development and regulation.

Middle Stages of Treatment

The middle phase of treatment tends to rely much more on the individual presentation of each client; however, we can offer some generalities about mid-stage CBP treatment. When dissociated aspects of self are present, parts work tends to become the primary focus. In terms of narrative, a deeper acknowledgment of the impact of early emotional abuse and neglect often occurs during this stage. Clients often move beyond a cognitive understanding of the impact of trauma to experiencing shame, resentment, rage, loss, grief, or other reactions about their early abuse and emotional deprivation. Portions of this narrative work are interwoven with the relational component, such as telling "stories that can't be told"; unburdening secrets, acknowledging self-blame, and being witnessed and validated can chip away at the shame and alienation that haunts many survivors of childhood abuse and neglect. In this stage and often continuing into later treatment, many clients work to make meaning of their experiences and begin to integrate their trauma narrative into a larger life narrative. The therapeutic relationship and basic regulatory skills established in early treatment may form the backdrop to parts work and trauma integration during the middle phase of treatment. Work on regulation focuses increasingly on the refinement of regulatory tools in the middle stage of treatment. Clients often begin to personalize and internalize these tools and increasingly generalize their self-regulation skills for use in a variety of situations outside of sessions. The therapeutic relationship often deepens during this time, through ruptures and repairs. During this middle stage, exploration of enactments can be a fruitful means of addressing the relational impact of this early trauma in the here and now, incorporating aspects of all four components.

Late Stages of Treatment

Later in CBP treatment, narrative work often shifts to identity development, including developing a future sense of self and strengthening positive aspects of self-identity. Many clients continue to explore meaning-making and development of a life narrative that incorporates but moves beyond traumatic experiences. At this point, a sense of rhythm has likely been established in the therapeutic relationship, but the relationship often continues to deepen, and enactments may continue. Work on regulation and parts will also likely continue, with later work being more likely to focus on a more in-depth understanding of the complexity of all the parts of self and use of a greater range of regulatory tools. This stage may also incorporate more advanced work, such as the use of specific regulatory tools by different parts of self or the ability to acknowledge and draw on strengths of all of one's parts of self. In late stages of CBP treatment, these processes may begin to occur more intuitively and independently, with the therapist playing a less active role and the client requiring less conscious effort. For therapies that have planned endings, the process of internalizing the Other and saying goodbye becomes an important late aspect of relationship work. Later narrative work in CBP includes the story of the therapeutic journey, acknowledgment of change, and hopes and plans for the future.

CLIENT PRESENTATION

Beyond the stage of therapy, the client's current state will influence which component(s) are primary. As we have discussed, traditional models of trauma treatment were developed in response to acute adult-onset traumatic incidents, including combat and sexual assault. With classic PTSD, a person might come into treatment complaining of intrusive memories or triggered reactions. In this type of situation, if the client is highly resourced, we could move quickly to narrative work, providing psychoeducation and then engaging in trauma processing, in the context of a supportive therapeutic relationship. With a client who does not have as highly developed resources, the therapist might teach regulatory skills prior to engaging in narrative work.

Therapeutic work with survivors of early emotional abuse and neglect is often more complicated. There may be an absence of discrete traumatic "incidents," meaning that the clinical picture is often not marked by intrusive memories. Instead, we see a variety of complex trauma responses, with significant variability in individual responses. Some people notice feelings of emptiness, have difficulty noticing or tolerating internal experience, or have coped by disconnecting from parts of themselves. Some survivors of emotional abuse and neglect feel they are on an emotional rollercoaster or find themselves repeatedly in crisis. Still others unwittingly replay their early betrayals and injuries through relational enactments. Because of the variability in types of responses that individuals experience in response to early interpersonal trauma and also because of the unique elements of any therapeutic relationship, CBP should be adapted for each client–therapist dyad at different points in time. Consideration of a client's current presentation can guide decision making about which component is primary at any point in time in CBP. Table 11.2 depicts which CBP components are primary, secondary, and tertiary for clients with different presentations, including clients who are in crisis, are highly dysregulated, have fragmented self-states, experience repeated relational enactments, struggle with a sense of emptiness or lack of a sense of self, have strong avoidance of internal experience or trauma memories, or are marked by shame. This is not an exhaustive list of primary client presentations, nor are these responses typically discrete; each of these presentations could emerge in the same person at different points in time, or a person might fit within multiple categories at one point in time. Despite this fluidity, these descriptions are intended to illustrate the necessity of modifying the therapeutic approach based on each individual person's needs, which vary over time.

In Crisis

Current crises and high clinical acuity obviously have a significant impact on the focus of treatment. Some clients lack stability in their lives because

TABLE 11.2. Primary Component(s) by Current Client Presentation

In crisis/high risk	Dysregulated	Fragmented self-states	High relational enactments	"Empty" (lacking sense of self)	Avoidance of internal experience and memory	Shame
Primary						
Safety planning, Regulation/co-regulation	Regulation, Relationship	Parts	Relationship, Parts	Parts, Regulation, Narrative	Regulation, Relationship	Narrative
Secondary						
Relationship (ongoing crisis)	Parts	Regulation, Relationship	Regulation	Relationship	Parts	Parts, Relationship
Tertiary						
Parts	Narrative	Narrative	Narrative		Narrative	Regulation

of issues such as involvement in conflictual or unpredictable relationships or recent loss of a relationship, unstable living conditions, financial stress, lack of supports, lack of involvement in meaningful activities, significant health problems, and other destabilizing events. Others face potentially imminent safety risks such as suicidal ideation, involvement in unsafe relationships, substance abuse, and other health-related issues such as eating disorders, self-injury, and refusal of needed medical care. In cases of high risk, safety must be addressed in a concrete way by identifying needed resources, establishing additional supports, and building safety. Case management may be essential, as well as a consideration of level of care. In addition to this external focus, regulation is a central component in intervention with CBP clients who are in crisis. Co-regulation will be particularly important for clients who do not have well-developed regulatory capacity.

In situations of chronic stress or ongoing crises, the therapist should work to focus *both* on safety and on the development of the therapeutic relationship. Some beginning therapists may be reactive to indications of risk and respond solely by attempting to manage the high-risk behavior. Take the case of Kai, a young Japanese woman who lives with chronic suicidal ideation. Each day, she considers elaborate schemes to kill herself so that she can escape the pain of her life. Although she has had these fantasies for years, she has never attempted suicide. Kai often feels better after she considers what she could do and then goes on with her day, with the sense that she always has a "way out." Although the idea of therapy is foreign to her, she eventually works up the nerve to make an appointment with a therapist. She starts out talking about the relentless physical and emotional pain that she suffers and eventually shares some of her detailed fantasies of suicide. The therapist, a relatively new clinician, is fearful of what Kai may do when she leaves the office. She immediately shifts away from a focus on Kai's emotional experience to a safety assessment, bringing out paperwork and asking her a series of structured questions about her plans and whether she has the means to carry out these plans. Because Kai lives near a train track and has repeated fantasies of throwing herself in front of a train, the therapist calls an ambulance to take Kai to the emergency room. She is screened at the emergency room and released. The entire experience is frightening and alienating to Kai, who never returns to therapy. In this instance, the therapist's anxiety interferes with her ability to accurately assess the situation and to begin to develop a therapeutic relationship with Kai. When a therapist jumps too quickly to try to ensure safety (e.g., bringing up hospitalization at the first hint of suicidal thoughts), contain potentially risky behaviors (e.g., taking a behavioral focus in treatment without trying to understand the underlying function of the behavior), or "fix" the emotions (e.g., repeatedly attempting to teach new regulation skills despite their apparent lack of effectiveness), the relational element of the dysregulation is missed, and the attempts to ensure safety are often unsuccessful. Bearing witness to distress and providing support as the client builds tolerance for uncomfortable feelings can contribute to the development of connection in the therapeutic relationship. Parts work may become important in addressing early safety issues when a client is not benefiting from simple work on regulation tools. This may be an indication that a part of the client is engaging in therapy and expressing an interest in building regulation skills, while another part of her is reacting against the regulation approach. The reactivity may occur for many different reasons, including that this part of her mistrusts her therapist or therapy in general, is triggered by receiving instructions, is uncomfortable with the particular regulatory approaches that are presented, feels unseen when her therapist focuses on regulation, is not ready for change, only feels safe when in a high alert state, is holding the feelings of despair and hopelessness within her system, or other reasons. Getting to know a client's different parts of self can elucidate barriers to therapeutic change and supports treatment that is responsive to all parts of the client.

In general, CBP therapists do not engage in formal narrative work while a client is in crisis because of the focus on stabilization. One exception is an exploration of patterns of crisis for clients who tend to experience ongoing or repeated crisis situations. In this case, increasing awareness of these patterns and psychoeducation about the role of ongoing crises can be helpful. Identifying patterns can also highlight early warning signs that a crisis is imminent, activating regulatory tools, support-seeking, and problem-solving skills to avert the crisis. Trauma processing or development of a larger narrative development would likely not be undertaken until some basic level of safety is established.

Dysregulated

For clients whose main presenting problem is dysregulation, the primary component is obviously regulation. However, because complex developmental trauma negatively impacts regulatory capacity, this component is not addressed in isolation. That is, it is not enough to teach basic regulatory strategies in a skills-training format. Instead, the regulatory work takes place in the context of the therapeutic relationship. A client who is emotionally dysregulated and uncontained may benefit more from an initial containing response than from an exploratory response. The therapeutic relationship is central, as the therapist creates a "holding environment" by witnessing and reflecting the client's internal experience without becoming dysregulated herself. This process is the window of engagement that we have discussed. The therapist can also use herself as a co-regulator: As she notices her client beginning to become overwhelmed, she may slow down and lower her voice. She may help bring attention to the client's dysregulation ("I notice that your hands are in fists and that you're beginning to breathe very shallowly") and then guide the client in coming into a more regulated state ("Would you be willing to try an experiment? I wonder what might happen to the tension in your hands if we took a few deep breaths together"). This regulatory approach uses a relational frame to downregulate the client into a calmer state. While the short-term goal of this co-regulation is present-moment emotional safety, the longer-term aim is the client's internalization of regulatory skills and strengthening of regulatory capacity.

For some clients, fragmentation in self-states underlies their dysregulated presentation. In these cases, parts work becomes a central element of understanding and addressing the dysregulation. As we have discussed, different parts might have different regulatory processes, with unique expressions of dysregulation (affective, somatic, cognitive, or behavioral). For instance, a client might repeat a pattern in which a period of high anxiety and achievement orientation is interrupted by an inward retreat into isolation and despair. Although both reflect dysregulation, these varying states might be driven by different parts of self, and attempting to manage these emotional states without exploring the root causes of these responses will likely not lead to lasting change. (For further discussion, see the next section on clients with highly fragmented parts of self.)

Narrative tends to be a less central aspect early in treatment with highly dysregulated clients. The therapist focuses attention as much on *how* a client's story is shared as on the content of the narrative. The early role of narrative involves providing a framework that makes sense of the dysregulated emotions, thoughts, somatic states, and behaviors, which can help the client feel "seen" and understood. Early psychoeducation may also suggest a path for intervention, which can instill hope. Another role of narrative at this point would be to understand and identify triggers that lead to dysregulated behavior in order to notice early "warning signs" that signal the need for regulatory tools. As the therapy progresses with a dysregulated client, narrative work often forms a backdrop to more focal work on other components. For instance, relational and regulatory patterns may be identified; current dysregulated states may be linked to historical experiences; and the narratives of different parts of self can be identified. As regulatory and relational capacities develop over time, later work may include a stronger focus on narrative work and relational enactments.

Highly Fragmented Parts of Self

For clients with severe dissociation, fragmentation of self-states may be the primary presenting issue. Treating these clients without a parts perspective leads the work to be confused and ineffective. In one moment, a regulatory tool could be presented and apparently be internalized and effectively used. However, moments later, the client's presentation might be dramatically different, with the same regulatory tool being completely ineffectual. In order to treat the whole person, the therapist must maintain a larger perspective, "holding" all of the client's parts of self, whether or not they are present at the moment. Meta-awareness of the therapeutic process becomes particularly essential in this situation, both to maintain a centered stance in the face of sometimes dramatically varying states and to sustain awareness of parts of self that may be rarely shown. Through parts work, the client develops greater awareness of their different parts of self, and communication between parts of self often increases.

Because dissociated parts of self are often dysregulated, holding a polarity of experience, regulation is also a central component. Thus, parts work has a regulatory focus, as each of the client's parts of self learns to identify, tolerate, regulate, and express their inner experience. It is helpful to keep in mind that different parts of a client might respond to different regulatory tools. On one hand, for instance, a very young part of self might be soothed by coloring or by manipulating play dough or clay. On the other hand, an older part that needs to feel in control might respond more readily to resources that elicit feelings of strength, such as identifying certain forms in trauma-sensitive yoga that activate a sense of empowerment (Emerson & Hopper, 2011). Thus, the process of experimenting to identify effective regulatory tools becomes much more complex when a person has more fragmented parts of self.

Parts work always occurs within the context of the therapeutic relationship. As mentioned earlier, the therapist plays the essential role of being a container of the client's experience as a whole. The therapist may operate as a guide in negotiating communication and relationship development between the client's parts of self. For highly fragmented clients, the therapeutic relationship also often provides fodder for exploration of internal experience through enactments. The therapist holds the responsibility for working to be aware of his or her own parts of self that are activated during interactions with the client.

Over time, the client's parts of self may develop their own trauma narratives and/or life narratives. Later in the work, the client's parts may also begin to develop a shared narrative. This shared narrative reflects a developing cohesion among a client's parts of self, ideally with shared goals and visions for the future.

Insecure Attachment and High Relational Enactments

Attachment style influences the use that a client is able to make of the therapeutic relationship, including whether the therapy is experienced as a "holding environment" or whether intimacy in the therapeutic relationship is avoided or is triggering. In some cases, the client's ability to relationally connect and trust can be an additional resource that allows them to take greater risks and to engage in more in-depth work, exploring previously unaddressed experience or aspects of self. Alternatively, therapy with those who feel disconnected from other people, including their therapist, may need to focus first on establishment of safety. In these cases, the therapeutic relationship often develops over the course of months or even years. Consistency, reliability, attunement, and regulated responses can contribute to the slow development of trust, as can the repair of even small ruptures in the relationship. Further complicating treatment, clients' different parts of self often have different attachment styles. Therapists must be aware and expect that different parts may respond to the therapeutic relationship differently, working to develop safety and connection with each part.

For people who tend to feel triggered by intimacy and who experience relational enactments in therapy, the therapeutic relationship may become the central focus of the work. Parts work also tends to be a central component in work with clients with high relational enactments. People who were emotionally abused or neglected in childhood may have difficulty "internalizing" an Other and holding on to the connection when there is physical separation. Some clients are able to feel connected and utilize therapy in the moment, but they have difficulty translating that into their lives outside of the therapy office. The relational connection is fragile, and when an appointment is canceled or the therapist is out of town, the client experiences a rupture in the relationship. In this case, one part of self is able to feel closeness; however, this vulnerable part of self may only be able to be accessed in the safety of the physical presence of the therapist. Physical separation creates a sense of threat, activating a more protective part of self who is not able to acknowledge the need for connection. Some clients may seek intimacy but have difficulty experiencing a close connection, so they continually seek increased amounts of contact. The problem, however, is not the *amount* of contact but the *depth and resiliency* of the felt connection, which typically cannot be improved solely through increased contact. In other cases, clients may feel threatened when they do feel a sense of connection, causing them to become dysregulated and/or to withdraw from the relationship. This pattern typically signals the presence of a protective part of self, suggesting the need for parts work. In all of these situations, the therapeutic relationship becomes the primary working ground for practicing a slow awareness of increasing boundaried connection with an Other, often through work with parts of self. Regulation is an important backdrop to relational parts work, as the pacing is guided by the regulatory capacity of all parts.

In parallel, the therapist's own self-awareness and regulatory capacity is central in working through complex enactments with their client. Supervision can be helpful as the therapist works to become aware of dissociated aspects of his or her own reactions and to regulate themselves in the face of often intense emotional reactions to enactments.

Because this work tends to be long term, often a new relational narrative develops as enactments are processed in the therapy. New relational experiences within the therapeutic relationship can be the basis for developing other intimate relationships in a client's life. Ideally, the new relational narrative incorporates messages such as "relationships can be challenging, and people don't always agree, but it is okay to have different thoughts, feelings, and needs"; "people have misunderstandings or conflict, but they can resolve these issues and still care about each other and maintain the relationship"; and "people can internalize aspects of a relationship and feel connected to another person even if there is not ongoing contact." ⟶⟋

"Empty" Presentation (Lack of a Sense of Self)

In situations of extreme emotional neglect, the child does not experience him- or herself through a caring adult's positive reflection. Emotionally neglectful homes often lack mirroring, curiosity, labeling of experience, or acknowledgment of the child as a valuable and richly nuanced individual. Because these types of reflections provide the groundwork for the child's sense of self, emotionally neglected children may grow up with a sense of internal emptiness, the feeling that something is missing, or the lack of a strong positive sense of self. In some cases, they may withdraw in self-protection, leading isolated and lonely lives. In others, they draw a sense of identity from other people in their lives; however, this sense of identity or purpose is fragile because of its over-reliance on external affirmation.

With this "empty" type of presentation, the first piece of active work with the client typically involves regulation, through an exploration of inner experience. Because it is not uncommon for these clients to have difficulty identifying stable internal traits and amorphous emotional states, it is often useful to anchor early work through developing awareness of somatic states. Although the apparent focus here is on regulation, parts work and narrative provide an ongoing context for the regulatory work. That is, the emphasis is on connecting with and further developing a strong sense of personal identity. We often find that the sense of emptiness or blankness is held by a part of self that had to shut down or comply to survive, leading to a lack of awareness of the client's feelings, thoughts, and sensations. Therefore, although we typically do not actively engage in parts work in the early stages with clients who have a strong sense of emptiness, a parts framework offers an important context for understanding the emptiness as a survival response and for holding awareness of potential other dissociated parts of self that may have much stronger access to internal experience.

Because of the lack of connection to self, the therapeutic relationship is often impacted. It can be more difficult for these clients to develop or sustain a felt connection. The therapeutic relationship will likely continue to develop with time, consistency, and slow progress in self-connection. However, although the therapeutic relationship is important, active use of the therapeutic relationship to deepen the work often does not occur until further into therapy.

High Avoidance of Internal Experience or Trauma Memories

Many clients are aware of and able to manage their cognitive experiences but lack awareness of, or regulatory capacity over, their affective or somatic experiences. It is not unusual for survivors of early developmental trauma to cope in an intellectualized way, particularly when they are very bright. They are able to "rationalize" with themselves and to know how they "should" be reacting, but they are not connected with much of their "felt" experience. David is a good example of a client who appears somewhat fearful of internal experience. Although he is able to share stories of his early life experiences, he finds it more difficult to be aware of, or to experience, his own more vulnerable reactions. When Susan's eyes tear up after hearing David's early history, he recognizes that his story is "objectively sad," but he "feels frustrated and defective, almost alien, that he can't join her in these feelings."

Some survivors of emotional abuse and neglect disconnect from early memories. Consider Daria, a middle-age woman who suffers from chronic anxiety and an underlying sense of panic. She reports having repeated failed relationships because she can't tolerate intimacy. She noted that, as soon as a relationship starts to become serious, she unwittingly sabotages it. She has a general sense that her childhood was bad; however, she isn't able to access clear memories of childhood. Daria notes that she rarely talks to her parents and notices that her life often takes a "nosedive" after family visits. She wonders if it is normal that she only has one or two memories before the age of about 12. Obviously, an initial narrative trauma-processing approach would not work with this type of presentation because there is no content to process. Instead, a useful starting point might be the fear and panic that emerges for Daria when intimacy begins to develop in a relationship. As she brings these situations to mind, Daria becomes aware of tightness in her chest. This present-moment sensation provides an entryway into an exploration of the affect, somatic states, and cognitions that arise when she is faced with intimacy. Because her level of anxiety is dysregulating, regulation is an important aspect of the treatment. As Daria builds confidence in her ability to tolerate and contain her overwhelming emotions, she begins to have increased access to the root causes of her present-day relational struggles, with increasing memories of emotional abuse during childhood.

A client's level of disconnection from traumatic memories and internal experiences associated with those memories influences the timing and pacing of intervention. Generally, with a more phobic reaction, a slower pace of therapy is required. Instead of focusing on the early narrative, intervention generally focuses first on building awareness of internal states, as the client gradually develops a sense of confidence in managing difficult emotions and sensations. For clients who are particularly phobic of internal emotions and sensations or who have a very anxious response to therapy, a more cognitive approach that incorporates regulation and narrative components might be helpful, in which the therapist provides psychoeducation about trauma and the window of tolerance and provides reassurance that they will work together to carefully pace the therapy. As the client becomes more comfortable with the idea of therapy and as the therapeutic relationship develops, regulatory work is used to increase access to disconnected thoughts, feelings, or sensations. Somatic approaches can also be effective for some clients in providing a link to unaccessed emotional states and memories. Experimentation is key to identifying strategies that are most effective for each person in slowly decreasing their avoidance of internal experience and/or traumatic memories.

Shame

Shame is a central emotion for many people who were emotionally belittled, manipulated, and abused throughout childhood. It is a central part of identity for some who have an underlying self-narrative such as, "There's something wrong with me" or "I'll never be good enough." Work with these clients generally emphasizes the narrative component, with a goal of impacting this trauma-related identity. Some people cope with their feelings of shame and self-blame by pushing those memories and associated emotions away, either consciously or unconsciously, resulting in a dissociative process. A trusting therapeutic relationship needs to develop before a client is able to acknowledge what seems intolerable and to share what seems unspeakable. In some cases, disclosures of specific shame-laden memories emerge after years of therapy. A specific memory, emotion, or somatic experience may also not be experienced because it is held by a part of self that does not trust the therapist. Thus, relationship and parts components provide an important context for the narrative work.

Even when early trauma is acknowledged, shame can be a barrier to progress in therapy, leaving some aspects of self hidden. Consider Charlie, a blue-collar worker and the divorced father of a preadolescent son. Charlie comes into therapy complaining of problems managing his son during visits. After some time discussing his son's problem behaviors, the therapy turns to Charlie's own childhood, with a narrative focus. He describes how, when he was a child, his father constantly belittled him. His father was a "rageaholic" and purposefully did things to his sons to shame them. While the primary issues in his childhood were the constant emotional abuse and neglect, there was also physical abuse that contributed to the shaming. Charlie shares many memories of his father's abuse with his therapist John, including a time when he was 14 and his father brought in his younger brothers to watch while he made Charlie take his pants down and spanked him. He recalls his father saying, "If you're going to act like a little baby, I'll treat you like one. You need to grow up. Act like a man!" He tells John about his responses of fear—running to hide in the basement when his father came home, cowering silently in the corner of the room, hoping his father wouldn't notice him. Although Charlie was initially standoffish with John, he lets his guard down over time and begins to trust him more and more.

After a year and a half, John notices episodes in which Charlie becomes irritated with him. Charlie comes in one day, upset because his son called him a "bully." He denies doing anything to his son and seems agitated and defensive. John says, "You seem to be feeling something right now. . . . I could be wrong, but you seem a little irritated or something?" Charlie replies, "No, I would never want to feel like that." Picking up on the discrepancy between his words and his presentation, John tests out a parts framework. "So it seems like a part of you feels like it's not okay to feel angry or irritated?" Charlie quickly responds, "Yeah, well, my dad was always angry, and I'm not like him!" John says, "That makes a lot of sense. But I wonder if there's another part of you that sometimes feels a little angry or irritated, even if you don't want to feel that way?" Charlie grits his teeth and averts his eyes, muttering, "I hate it!" As John helps him to explore these two "parts" of himself, Charlie gets upset and expresses hatred for himself. The next week, as soon as Charlie walks in the door, he says, "There's something I need to get off my chest. That angry part of me? It's always been there. When I was a kid, I used to corner my little brothers and scare the crap out of them. I'd call them names and do exactly the same stuff my dad did to me. He told me to be a man, and I was just so fricking angry! I hate myself so much for doing that."

At this point, the therapy moves from processing the abuse by his father to a deeper level, in which Charlie acknowledges the shame and self-hatred that has been driving his depression and maintaining the underlying rage that created conflicts in his relationships. As he acknowledges and shares these parts of himself, the shame that had been maintained through secrecy and dissociation begins to decrease. Relational work with his dissociated parts allows Charlie to rework his narrative about himself, as he builds empathy for his younger self and begins to work on his dissociated anger.

TIMING AND PACING IN CBP

The therapeutic process is constantly shifting in depth and intensity. The treatment focus weaves back and forth, with emphasis on varied areas such as building relationship, noticing internal states, experimenting and developing internal resources and coping tools, exploring parts of self, finding lightness or joy through humor and play, addressing enactments in the therapeutic relationship, developing positive aspects of self or future plans, and integrating trauma narratives into a larger life narrative. Because these elements do not proceed in linear order, the process of therapy vacillates in terms of intensity of depth of work. Connection within the therapeutic relationship also tends to vary over time, with moments of more intense bonding and expression, instances of therapeutic rupture, and periods of more comfortable attachment. This vacillation in engagement and content contributes to the pace of therapy.

Timing and pacing is an essential part of trauma treatment. Changes in relational intensity and focus of treatment from moment to moment are important aspects of effective pacing, with the client and therapist staying within—and ideally expanding—the window of tolerance and the window of engagement. Moving too deeply, too quickly, without adequate preparation can be counterproductive, leading to a sense of failure and a fear of change, while avoiding challenges can contribute to therapy that is more pleasant but is ultimately not as effective. From moment to moment, we make choices about how to respond to what the client is telling or showing. Should we ask for more details about the story? Engage in co-regulation? Ask about what the client notices emotionally or somatically? Offer psychoeducation? Reflect postures or movements we are noticing in the client? Create space through the use of silence? Make a connection between the current story and the client's history? Explore the relational elements of the storytelling? Suggest an experiment? At these therapeutic choice points, the CBP therapist is ideally considering a host of information, such as the client's regulatory state, relational engagement with the therapist, degree to which the client is in his or her head or body, what parts of self are activated, how quickly the process is moving, and what resources the client is able to call on. To add to the complexity, we are also working to build in-the-moment awareness of ourselves in all of these areas. Ultimately, the pacing of treatment relies on an intuitive, nuanced sense of the client and therapist's present-moment interpersonal connectedness and regulatory status and capacity.

Pacing in CBP can be influenced through shifting the focus of therapy, for example, by adjusting the aperture or shutter speed of a camera. Any of the four components can be used to influence pacing by either offering containment or by deepening the work. The therapeutic relationship can be a source of support and co-regulation, or it can be fodder for exploring enactments. Regulation can be used to explore untapped aspects of inner experience, or the focus may shift to grounding and containment, assisting clients in remaining within their window of tolerance. When parts of self that contain or avoid internal experience are accessed, they often slow the pacing. Alternatively, when vulnerable or dysregulated parts of self are accessed, the pace may speed up as traumatic memories are accessed or enactments occur. Similarly, narrative work can be used to build resources or to process traumatic experiences that have been held at bay.

As we have discussed, one role of the therapist is to be able to be both fully in the moment with the client and maintain a meta-awareness of the larger therapeutic process. In the therapy itself, there is a fluid shifting between a focus on micromoments—being reflective while staying "in the moment"—and attention to the macroprocess—learning how elements fit together in a larger picture over time. Shifting back and forth between an emphasis on "big-picture" themes and patterns to a present-moment, experiential focus is another tool that can influence the pace of CBP.

The introduction to therapy often begins with a thematic focus, as the therapist invites the client to provide context for the work: "Can you tell me a little about what brings you here?" This macrofocus can be applied to each of the four CBP components. Some clients may begin with a narrative, sharing stories about difficult aspects of their lives. Others may start with a description of themes of dysregulation, a "symptom" focus. As patterns of relational, behavioral, cognitive, somatic, or affective dysregulation emerge, psychoeducation can help to link past and present within a conceptual trauma-informed framework. These patterns might also highlight dissociated parts of self. Use of metaphor is another thematic element that can contribute to meaning-making. As a trauma narrative is developed and evolves into a larger life narrative, identity development often becomes an important theme. Focusing on the future, setting goals, and developing a potential future self are other elements of treatment with a more global focus.

While addressing larger themes and narratives, the work is often deepened by exploring the current-moment experience—what is happening in the room, right here, right now. The moment-to-moment experience in the therapy may reflect any of the CBP components: a shared moment of silence may signal the relationship component; a tight feeling in the throat can reflect awareness and tolerance of somatic experience within the regulation component; a surprising and scary connection to an unfamiliar feeling of hope might suggest a dissociated child part; and a feeling of pride over a successful venture can reflect a narrative shift from failure and damage to resiliency and efficacy. Focus on the current-moment experience lends itself to the development of regulatory capacity. Exploration of internal experience can bring increased awareness of cognitive, affective, and somatic states; build tolerance for these states; and provide a springboard for change. When current experience is explored within therapy, the therapist is inherently an aspect of the experience, making relationship an important component to spotlight. For instance, the therapist might raise the issue, "What is it like to notice that choking sensation and feeling of panic while you're sitting here with me in the office?" The focus might also move more solidly into the relationship component, exploring relational interactions: "I noticed something shift right there. What just happened for you when I laughed?"

If the therapeutic process seems to be slowed down or stuck, or if it is progressing too quickly, a shift in focus can work as a regulatory tool and impact the pace of CBP. For a client who intellectualizes as a coping strategy and is stuck in her head, shifting to a more somatic approach can open up new avenues of intervention. Some clients utilize a narrative approach, focused on storytelling. In some cases, the stories serve a protective function, preventing exploration of inner experience. The use of silence can be an effective regulatory tool in these cases, creating a space for self-reflection and awareness of inner experience. The relationship can be brought into this work by the therapist noticing his or her own internal reactions as the stories are shared. Alternatively, the therapy may transition from a narrative focus to an exploration of the internal experience of the part of self that is sharing a particular story.

Some clients have the experience of bravely attempting to combat their typical avoidance by confronting difficult emotions or memories. Unfortunately, because this prospect is so daunting, there is often an urge to "get it over with" quickly and to "put it behind me." This push to confront too much, too soon, generally results in overwhelming the client—"I was right; I can't handle this"—and a retreat back into even more rigid avoidance. To shift this pattern of unsuccessful vacillation, empathetic engagement with all parts of the client is necessary when adjusting the pace of treatment.

When a client becomes flooded or is overwhelmed with intrusive imagery, the goal of shifting the focus is typically containment. There is an interaction between the relationship and regulation components, as the therapist provides support and offers guidance and teaching on regulatory strategies. Narrative work that focuses on psychoeducation and understanding trauma-related reactions can provide cognitive scaffolding to help hold the affective overwhelm. For highly fragmented clients, more resourced parts of self might be called on to help with regulation.

Misguided urges around pacing sometimes emerge from the therapist's internal processes. When feelings of emptiness, disorientation, or numbness arise, therapists frequently struggle with discomfort and an urge to rescue the client, and themselves, from these feelings. There is a tendency to shift the content too quickly because there is "nothing" to process in terms of internal experience. A seasoned CBP therapist might instead choose to focus on tracking these experiences. Doing so can build tolerance for the uncomfortable feelings (or apparent absence of feelings) and sometimes highlights the dissociative quality of these reactions, which can mask other vulnerable emotions. Other choices may be to explore the narrative component by linking this feeling with earlier experiences of developmental trauma; to explore this feeling as a part of self; or, if the experience becomes overwhelming or does not shift, to regulate through grounding techniques.

In CBP, pacing is a transactional process in which the client and therapist work together to ensure that the therapy is meaningful, while understanding that lasting change often occurs over a longer period of time. The client's and therapist's tolerance to stay with the process through the ebbs and flows of both intensity and "nothingness" allows each to get to know, accept, and strengthen themselves and each other, in all of their complexity and wonder.

CONCLUSION

CBP takes an individualized and flexible approach to treatment for complex trauma (see Table 11.3). In the treatment planning phase, we consider the four components of CBP, as well as their interactions, to determine our primary focus with each client. This decision will be based on each person's unique presentation and needs and will shift as the treatment evolves. Timing and pacing are essential elements of this decision making, as we determine when and to what degree to address various components. Shifting between various components, and between a more macrolevel and present-moment experience, can assist in maintaining effective pacing.

CBP is a complex treatment that challenges not only our clients but also us as therapists. The therapeutic process in CBP is developed collaboratively and necessarily involves reflection, awareness, and openness to new experience for our clients and ourselves. In the Appendix (also available to download at *www.guilford.com/hopper-forms*), you can find a Clinician Self-Assessment for CBP. This measure is designed for use as a self-assessment for clinicians' proficiency with CBP and for support of the CBP supervision process. It also serves as a fidelity guide for implementation of the CBP framework. With open engagement, CBP therapy can be transformative for both client and therapist, as we connect with each other across the abyss. In the last chapter, we apply these lessons to our two clinical case vignettes, David and Nicole.

TABLE 11.3. CBP: An Integrated Framework

Client

- Incorporating assessment of four components into conceptualization and treatment planning
- Individually tailoring treatment by prioritizing among components for different client presentations
- Developing an in-depth understanding of client's parts of self, regulatory processes, relational patterns, and life narrative
- Attending to timing and pacing; shifting between CBP components to contribute to effective pacing
- Engaging in complex work that incorporates multiple components, such as using the therapeutic relationship to co-regulate while engaging in parts work, trauma processing, and identity development; using enactments to explore dissociated parts of self that impact relational patterns; or accessing parts of self through dysregulated somatic states and incorporating these parts of self into a larger life narrative
- Developing greater sense of connection to self and others, improving general functioning, and increasing sense of meaning and engagement with life
- Reflecting on the therapeutic process and progress

Therapist

- Cultivating our ability to be actively engaged in moment-to-moment therapeutic interactions, while simultaneously maintaining meta-awareness of all parts of the client and ourselves, contextual factors that influence us, and how these impact the therapeutic process over time
- Parallel to our clients' experience, developing our own capacity to "show up" in our professional and personal lives, continually developing our self-awareness, regulatory and relational capacity, and cohesive identity that includes all parts of ourselves

Supervisor

- Raising awareness about relational enactments, regulatory challenges, dissociative processes, and narrative development, involving the client and/or therapist
- Supporting the therapist's present-moment attunement (to client and to self) and meta-awareness of the larger therapeutic process and the ability to effectively toggle between the two
- Attending to parallel processes in the supervisory relationship that informs CBP work

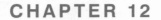

CHAPTER 12

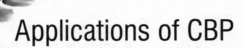

Applications of CBP

Revisiting David and Nicole

Because of the complexity of the CBP framework, we close with an application of the integrated model to David and Nicole, the two clinical vignettes that we have woven throughout this book. The two cases share some common elements, including the subjective co-construction of the therapeutic process over time by the client and therapist; therapeutic rupture and repair in enactments; the importance of the four treatment components, to varying degrees over time; and emphasis on balance between immersion in the present moment and meta-awareness of the larger process. However, because of the differences in the particular histories and current presentations of David and Nicole, the different styles of their therapists, and the uniqueness of the two therapeutic relationships, there is considerable variability in the relative roles of the components over time and the types of interventions used in each of the therapies. The comparison of treatment used with these two clients illustrates both the hallmark themes and the variability in CBP.

From the beginning of their treatment, Susan approaches David from a curious and empathic stance. As she listens, she begins to learn about David's approach to himself and to the world. Her process of learning about him is intuitive and often nonverbal, but we will try to put language to this experience.

We can consider how David might fall on the component continuums as a basis for Susan's decision-making process about the primary entryways into therapy with David (see Figure 12.1). It is important to note that this visual is necessarily an oversimplification. There is variability in where any one person would fall along these continuums based on parts of self. In this image, two points marked along the continuum reflect a dichotomy between two parts of self on that continuum. In addition, a person's placement on the continuums will likely change over time, based on current state and life circumstances, as well as on therapeutic change over time. Despite this complexity, developing a working-case conceptualization based on these dimensions can be helpful in initial treatment planning and guiding intervention over time. Susan considers each of the four CBP components as the initial focus for treatment with David. Their work together moves through a series of phases, including a general narrative approach and deepening of the therapeutic relationship, resource identification and development, regulatory and parts work through an exploration of somatic and affective experience, identification of a vulnerable part of self and trauma processing, addressing enactments, parts work, and then a relational process around ending the therapy and saying goodbye. Throughout this process, a shifting emphasis on various components is used to maintain effective pacing.

Case Conceptualization and Initial Approach

When David chooses the farthest chair and then launches into a seemingly mentally rehearsed story in their first session, Susan recognizes that, although he shares information easily, David appears controlled and is emotionally guarded. He describes a lack of connection with therapists in the past and says that he feels alienated from colleagues and even his closest family members. Susan notices David's physical posture, an "almost droopy meekness," and is struck that he has entered therapy at his wife's insistence, speculating that he tends toward compliance. Susan understands fairly quickly that the therapeutic relationship will take some time to develop and, although it will clearly be important in their work together, does not consider this as her primary entryway with David. She recognizes that she will need to respect his self-protective stance by approaching development of the therapeutic relationship slowly.

David shows a rather distinct split in his emotions, thoughts, somatic states, and behavior and seems to have parts of self that are rejected or held at bay. Susan notices that David's primary presentation is a passive, compliant, and emotionally shutdown part. She also, however, notices indications that he has another part of self that is more aggressive and emotionally dysregulated. He describes his marriage as a "constant argument" and mentions conflicts at work. This latter part of him is apparent in a rather subtle way very early in the treatment process, when David sets a time limit of 2 to 3 months for his treatment.

Relationship

Overly Open/Vulnerable --------------------- (Open) -------------------X--- Guarded/Self-protective

Uncontained ------------------------------- (Expressive) ------------------------X------ Unexpressive

Enmeshed ------------------------------------- (Connected) ------------------------------X----- Alienated

Aggressive/Self-focused -----X-------------- (Assertive) -----------------X- Compliant/Other-focused

Regulation

Hypoaroused ---------X---------------------- (Alert/Calm) ------------------------------- Hyperaroused

Volatile --- (Flexible) ----------------------X-------------------- Fixed

Internalizing ------X---------- (Adaptable Expressions of Distress) ------------------- Externalizing

Controlled ---------X------------------- (Active Acceptance) ------------------------------ Uncontrolled

Parts

Cohesive --X---------- Fragmented

Embodied --X--- Disembodied

Engaged --X----------------------- Disengaged

Underresourced --X------------------------------------ Resourced

Narrative

Intrusions -------------------------- (Acceptance of Memories) --------------X- Avoidance/Numbing

Secretive About Trauma--X------------ (Mindful Sharing) ------------- Spilling Trauma Narrative

Identity Disavows Trauma X----------- (Defined by Trauma) ----------- Identity Beyond Trauma

Compartmentalized Trauma Narrative-X--------------------------------- Integrated Life Narrative

FIGURE 12.1. David's early presentation on component continuums.

Susan understands that, over time, she will learn more about these parts of David and that she may discover other parts of him that he has not yet shared. For instance, she fairly quickly comes across another part of David that is hurt, sad, and lonely, elicited by his childhood memories of feeling abandoned and unaccepted. Understanding the complexity of David's presentation is helpful as Susan holds awareness of the different parts of him that he might not be showing in the moment. At the same time, Susan is aware that parts work is likely to be threatening to David and that she will need to broach this topic slowly over time to assess his comfort with the concepts and language. Therefore, a parts framework is very helpful in conceptualizing David's struggles, but parts work is not the focus for early intervention with him.

Susan can see that she will need to be active in the therapy and attentive to the parts of David that are shut down and at risk of withdrawing from treatment. However, she is also aware that she will need to stay out of power battles with the angrier, defended part of David that protects him from vulnerability by trying to assert control. Instead, she looks for ways to connect with this protective part by empathizing with his desire to feel more in control of his world and considering ways that he might build his own efficacy. Susan also provides David with some information on her background and a framework for understanding her therapeutic approach in an effort to decrease his uncertainty and anxiety about this new therapy.

Susan observes that David is facing a number of external situations that are stressful to him and that are causing emotional upheaval. His conflicts with his wife and the threat of losing his marriage, the threat of negative consequences at work from his recent behavior, and issues with his daughter seem to be stirring up emotions that he is having more difficulty containing than usual. Susan considers that regulation might be a promising in-road for David. However, when Susan attempts to explore David's emotional reactions, he quickly sidesteps her efforts. She notices that "every time she tried to test the limits by encouraging David to explore his feelings, he launched into another angry but flat diatribe." She recognizes his reflexive retreat from emotional content as a regulatory strategy and understands that he quickly moves out of his window of tolerance when noticing his emotions. As a result, Susan needs to focus first on helping David to identify and build up his resources, creating safety through careful pacing.

Because his cognitive realm gives David his strength and comfort, Susan uses a more "top-down" approach initially, providing psychoeducation and normalizing his reactions. Focusing initially on "making sense" of what he is experiencing might help David develop some sense of safety within the therapy. After some exploration of the different components, the therapy settles on an initial narrative approach, with regulation and parts influencing the pacing. Because David seems to feel comfortable telling stories about his history, as long as the focus is not explicitly on emotion, Susan invites him to share stories about his life, listening for somatic or emotional content. She continues to gently test his tolerance for emotion. For instance, he is able to recall being scared when his mother left him alone in the house during childhood. Susan "stops David mid-story to ask about his fear. His memories are vague, and he cannot really say anything else." This suggests that her intervention was perhaps too abrupt and emotionally difficult for David, so that he disconnected from that experience. The wonderful thing that Susan notices is that David is the one controlling the timing and pacing of the therapy. He challenges himself by engaging more and more in therapy, while a protective part of himself quickly steps in when he senses treacherous emotional territory emerging. Susan's job here is to start by respecting and encouraging this part of David, without doing extensive or exploratory parts work. She is serving the role of a witness and holder of the narratives that are emerging from David's different parts of self. She reflects what she hears in his narrative and honors his ability to cope with difficult experiences. David and Susan work together to establish a rhythm to the therapy. Over time, as the therapeutic relationship begins to grow based on shared experience, Susan has increasing latitude to notice David's somatic states or emotions, help him tolerate these states, experiment with regulatory strategies, and explore the different parts of himself.

"Nowhere Man"

Fairly early in the therapy process, Susan notes that she "feels little, and at times no, emotional connection" to David. When she does respond emotionally to one of his stories, he actually experiences it as alienating because he cannot feel the same empathy for himself. The risk is that Susan will unwittingly withdraw from the therapeutic relationship in response to David's apparent relational absence. Susan is challenged to notice her feelings without judgment and to accept them as information about David's experience in the world. Luckily, Susan is able to make good use of supervision to notice her discomfort at her emotional distance from David and to explore whether any of her distancing comes from her own parts, both of which allow her to continue to be engaged in the therapy.

Susan's continued engagement is rewarded after a couple of months of a generally narrative approach, when David is talking about his wife and describes himself as "Nowhere Man." Susan tests the limits of David's window of tolerance by encouraging him to consider his feelings about the list of therapy goals his wife made for him. Unexpectedly, David opens up about his experience of the therapeutic relationship, states that he wants to "entertain Susan and keep things 'light,'" and acknowledges that he doesn't "know how to go there." He reflects that whenever he is in situations with conflict or intense emotion, he feels cut off from himself. Wisely, Susan does not press David to explore the more vulnerable emotions (as he just indicated, he doesn't know how to go there!), but instead she helps him to stay with his fears about what might happen if he did experience or express these more vulnerable emotions. David clearly responds to this session by looking pleased, smiling, making eye contact with Susan, and reaching his hand out to shake hers. These somatic, emotional, and behavioral changes suggest a shift in the therapeutic relationship. Exploration of this moment-to-moment interaction transitions them into a deeper stage of the therapeutic process.

Identifying Internal Resources

In discussing David's history, two early memories emerge that seem to be potential resources, so Susan explores them in more depth with him. In one memory, David is completely embodied in a wrestling match with his cousin. When he recalls this memory, he is able to feel strong, confident, and connected to his body and emotions. The somatic state that is elicited by this memory provides a confidence that David needs as he faces his fears of being more vulnerable in the therapy. In another similar memory, he recalls his father representing the qualities that he wants to have, including strength and confidence. This memory, which involves a birthday celebration, also represents connection with others. David is able to fully experience the sensory aspects of this memory, down to the sounds of singing and the heat on his face from the candles. He is also able to connect with his internal experiences, feeling a sense of belonging, pride, and joy. Susan can use each of these memories to help David experience emotion in a way that is less threatening because the emotions are positive and represent strength instead of vulnerability. These resources can help David later in the more difficult work of experiencing vulnerable and painful emotions.

A Somatic Intervention Including Relationship, Regulation, and Parts Components

Imagine that, with increasing safety and trust in the therapeutic relationship, Susan begins to gently explore David's somatic experience when he becomes rigid or defensive, as a way to help him tap into his inner experience and to eventual parts work. She is aware that he manages difficult emotions by disconnecting from his internal experience, so pacing is particularly important in this work. In one instance, David is discussing a fight with his wife and reflects that he is feeling cut off from his feelings. When Susan invites him to bring his awareness to his body, David describes a busy feeling in his head and the sense of a line across his throat, with "nothing" below. They spend a number of sessions focusing on the busy activity and sense of frenetic energy in his head, as compared to the absence of feeling or the "deadness" in his body. They focus on increasing David's tolerance for "staying with" his awareness of these conflicting feelings. Because intimacy is both important and triggering to David, Susan provides implicit references to their developing relationship, without directly addressing the relationship component. For instance, she suggests that they "pay attention together" to certain aspects of his experience, uses language of "we" and "us," and asks him to reflect on the difference between his internal experience in the therapy office versus in other settings. David notices that it is easier to tolerate noticing these sensations when he is "in the office" (his terminology acknowledges the importance of the therapy, without directly naming Susan as an important attachment figure for him).

The distinction in somatic states between David's head and his body also provides an entry to some early parts work with him. Susan introduces language referencing his dissociated self-states, asking David about these two "parts" of himself and their relationship to each other. He says that the "perfect" part of him is driven by his head but that he doesn't know if he wants to know what's going on in his body. With support from Susan, he is able to pay more attention to the line at his throat. He says, "It's like my throat is trying to hold something down. It's a choking feeling." In the interest of pacing, Susan chooses not to move directly to this dissociated "something." Instead, she helps David to explore what his throat is afraid might happen if it doesn't hold this "something" down. He says, "Blackness. The blackness would just explode and take over everything. I would get lost in it. I would die." David notices that he is feeling more anxiety. Susan uses the relationship to provide some containment to David's increasing dysregulation. First, she attunes to his affective and somatic distress, while paying attention to her own regulatory state. She is able to calm her own small burst of trepidation about his increasing distress and to center herself. She says, "Let's notice that feeling together" and asks further about his experience. Bringing attention back to his somatic state, Susan reflects that his leg is shaking, and David acknowledges tension in his legs that he has not noticed before. He reflects that his legs want to move and notices that he feels like running out of the office. By "staying with" and exploring his discomfort, Susan is helping him expand his window for tolerating this type of distress.

After a few moments, David's breathing becomes rapid and shallow, and he describes feeling panicky and nauseous. At this point, Susan is aware of two things: (1) David had taken a big step by identifying two previously unexplored "parts" of himself (a desire to protect himself by actively escaping, which is different from his characteristic compliance, and an awareness of a powerful dissociated "blackness") that are experienced somatically (through the sense of nothingness in his body, a choking sensation in his throat, and tension in his legs) and emotionally (through anxiety and fear); and (2) David is moving outside of his window of tolerance. In response, Susan redirects the focus by asking, "And as you notice that, what is happening in your head?" The point of this shift is to help David regulate by staying with a somatic focus but shifting from an exploration of more vulnerable parts of him back into his "safe zone"—his head. David responds by noticing that the activity in his head is more frenetic than ever. He expresses feeling dizzy and experiencing a choking sensation in his throat.

Susan asks David to pay attention to these feelings and to notice what happens to them. She is focusing on whether David is able slowly to regulate with decreased attention to the more dissociated parts of himself or whether she needs to intervene further. She considers a few options if David moves too far outside of his window of tolerance. One would be to help him step outside of his immediate experience. For instance, she might ask, "Is this a feeling that you've had before?" (noticing patterns of experience) or "What types of things usually cause your thoughts to be spinning around like this?" (analysis of these patterns). These questions would likely encourage David to consider his experience from a more cognitive and removed perspective, and to perhaps reply, "My thoughts always spin around more when I'm anxious." Another option would be to rally David's strong defensive system: "When your head starts to swim like this, what do you usually do to help it to settle?" In this case, he may reply that he splashes cold water on his face, focuses on something else such as work, or just waits until it settles (a sign that he is able to tolerate the distress). A third option would be to use co-regulation, guiding him through an "experiment" in affect regulation such as a grounding or deep-breathing exercise.

For the moment, however, Susan does not intervene. Instead, she just encourages David to notice what is happening in his head. He says that his head feels dizzy, as if it is teetering on top of his spine. He notes that this is a strange feeling for him, to notice his head even being connected to his body. Sensing a potential somatic resource, Susan asks David to pay attention to the support that his spine is giving to his head. He notices some energy flowing through his spine, up to his head. She encourages him to focus on this energy and reflects that she sees him sitting up straighter in his chair. As they notice his posture, he says that he is feeling calmer and stronger. When David, with apparent relief, abruptly shifts to talking about his work life, Susan asks if they can take a moment to acknowledge this new feeling that he had in his body. David agrees, and they pause to notice and celebrate this new feeling of strength through his spine, before moving on to talk about David's work issue.

These few moments in the therapy session integrate all four components and provide important groundwork for David's continuing therapy. Susan was using the therapeutic relationship as a container for co-regulation, helping him to notice parts of himself and then to explore a somatic resource. Connecting with this somatic-based part of self provides David with a positive experience of connecting with his inner experience and creates the groundwork for a new narrative: "I have an inner strength that can help me feel calm and grounded."

Accessing Vulnerable Parts and Trauma Processing

As David builds more tolerance for his internal experience, a more vulnerable part of him emerges. He tells Susan about the part of himself that "had to appear perfect. Act perfect. Be perfect. And soon he *was* perfect, and the sadness went away." This "perfect" part of David protects him by meeting the demands of the external world, but it also creates a disconnection from his more vulnerable emotions like sadness. This part of him has become so strong that he is often not aware of his more vulnerable parts. As Susan recognizes David's "amazing strength" and "incredible resilience," he is "surprised to feel a wave of emotion start to rise up. 'Yeah, but I was invisible,' he finds himself continuing, the tears starting to come." Then David provides Susan with an excellent opening into parts work: "Yeah, I could take care of myself, but I also really wanted to be taken care of. It's hard to admit, but after that bike accident, a part of me wanted my mom to scoop me up in her arms, tell me I was going to be okay, clean me up, and give me a big bowl of ice cream." Susan holds the value of both of these parts of David: "What does it mean now for us to see beneath that extremely capable part of you, to see both the resilience and amazing competence, and all of the pain of feeling invisible?"

This statement really gets to the heart of the work that David and Susan will embark on together. They have moved beyond the basics of what happened to the essence of David's personhood and the losses that he experienced in his early relationships. He has spent his life feeling unseen and unsupported, not allowed to feel what he felt and or to be who he was. He coped by splitting off his unmet needs for connection and validation, denying his pain and anger, and experiencing his life as a shell of a person. Susan helps David reconnect with his spark of life, that desire for love and connection, which has been banished throughout much of his life. Trauma processing for him, then, involves both grieving his losses and reclaiming disowned parts of himself to build a more cohesive sense of himself and his life. As the therapy moves into this deeper work, all of the CBP components come into play: the therapeutic relationship is providing the holding environment David needs in order to explore some of his more vulnerable parts of self and the different regulatory patterns and narratives held by these parts.

Stuck Places in Therapy: Unconscious Collusion in Avoidance

Long-term therapy with adults who have been emotionally abused or neglected does not tend to progress at a steady rate. Instead, there are often periods of rapid progress and emerging insights, interspersed with periods of repetition or apparent stagnation. Let's move ahead a year into David's therapy. After a long period of apparent progress, the therapy begins to focus increasingly on David's relationship with his wife, whom he describes as increasingly critical and sometimes even hostile toward him. Susan notices that she is feeling less engaged in therapy and sometimes feels bored. David begins to miss sessions—something that has never happened before. She feels a sense of relief when David calls to cancel a session, followed by shame about her lack of engagement. Susan's supervisor reflects that it is unusual that they have not talked about David for some time. Susan initially dismisses this reflection, saying that other clients have had more pressing issues, but then, with a slight sense of guilt, she reluctantly acknowledges that she has been feeling bored and unengaged in the therapy with David. With the support of her supervisor, Susan recognizes that David's apparent hopelessness is activating a part of her that feels helpless and frustrated. Because this part of herself is at odds with her strong self-identification as a caring and effective professional, she has disconnected from her internal experience and from the therapy process in general. As they explore this process in supervision, Susan realizes the potential that David's interactions with his wife have been triggering an early and almost automatic dissociative coping process in him. When he is triggered, this part of him feels inadequate and collapses inward, in an attempt to disappear. In this enactment, both Susan and David are experiencing hopelessness and are unconsciously colluding to avoid these difficult feelings. Once Susan recognizes this pattern, she is able to step out of the enactment and to raise the issue of this shift in therapy with David, allowing them to acknowledge their feelings. This opens the door for them to reconnect and to access other, more hopeful parts of self.

Parts Work and Trauma Processing

Well into his therapy, David is able to explore the feeling of "deadness" in his body without feeling swallowed by it. He feels a deep sadness begin to well up and has an image of the neglected, frightened boy inside who was waiting for his father to come home while his mother was passed out on the couch. Very gradually, with much support from Susan, he comes to have sympathy for the young boy he had been. David begins to notice when this younger part of him becomes activated, as well as to recognize when a protective, defensive part of himself berates this younger self for his vulnerability. When Susan introduces an experiential parts work exercise, David is able to use imagery to bring Susan and his adult self together with this young part, in order to comfort him. This young part of him is sitting alone and expresses loneliness and sadness. He wonders if his adoptive parents would have loved him if he had been nicer or better behaved—or maybe if he had just been white. In a later session, after some time of engaging with this young part, the boy shifts away from this self-blame and begins to question why his biological mother had him when she was so young and obviously ill equipped to care for him, and why his adoptive parents took him in if they couldn't accept him. David's adult self tells the boy that he deserves to be loved and cared for. The boy is able to accept reassurance and support from David's adult self and begins to seem more playful. Through direct engagement with his younger parts of self, David begins to increasingly acknowledge and tolerate many feelings that he previously tried to ignore or control.

During the period when he is actively engaged in parts work, David impulsively stops by a basketball court for a pick-up game, something he used to do as a boy. As he plays, he feels a sense of freedom and joy and is mindful of the boy inside of him. He shares with Susan that this felt like a healing experience for him and for this young part of him; he decides that he wants to start playing basketball again and wonders if his daughter might enjoy it too.

Saying Goodbye

Therapy can end for many reasons. The ending may be abrupt or planned, for external reasons or because a piece of work has been completed. Imagine that David and Susan have worked together for almost 2 years; David has made a great deal of progress in therapy and feels like he needs a "break" from this type of self-exploration. They explore David's different parts of self and all of his different reactions to the thought of ending the therapy. In parallel, Susan explores her own responses to his declaration. Along with her pride and confidence in him, she notices some sadness about his decision and an anxious desire to protect him. By acknowledging and working through these reactions in supervision, Susan is able to come back into the therapy in a more regulated and open state and to support David in exploring his own reactions to the ending of treatment.

Susan provides the frame for David that the process of ending is a major aspect of therapy, and they spend their last 2 months of therapy reviewing their work together and saying goodbye. They talk about how their relationship has developed over time and about how David has changed through the therapy, including regulatory skills he has internalized, his different relationship with parts of himself, and his overall sense of himself and his life. David raises his fear that he will shut down emotionally and revert to his old ways of coping, and they consider ways that he can be aware of this and encourage himself to continue to be present, self-reflective, and expressive. David says that he often hears Susan's voice outside of session, when he is confronting difficult situations and that this will help him. They write cards to each other that they share at their last session. Susan invites David to call her in the future, should he decide that he could benefit from another piece of work, and he says, "You know, I just might do that," and they part with a warm handshake, eye contact, and a smile.

NICOLE

As in the case of David, Nicole's therapist Katherine begins by trying to understand Nicole. As a newer therapist, Katherine tends to put more effort into trying to cognitively understand Nicole, versus Susan, who seems to operate by developing a "felt sense" of David. As in David's case, we can consider Nicole along the various continuums of CBP as a basis for discussing Katherine's thoughts around the therapeutic process (see Figure 12.2). Because Nicole has quite dissociated parts of self, she seems to present differently at different times and has rather ambivalent internal experiences.

Case Conceptualization and Initial Approach

As opposed to David's early engagement in therapy, Nicole and Katherine connect rather quickly and easily. Katherine is struck by Nicole's "capacity to connect interpersonally and evoke empathy from their first meeting" and her "engaging, disarming, and highly protective facility with humor." Nicole

Relationship

Overly Open/Vulnerable ----X---------------- (Open) --X--- Guarded

Uncontained ----------X-------------------- (Expressive) --------------------------------- Unexpressive

Enmeshed -----------------------X-------- (Connected) ----------------------X--- Alienated/Isolated

Aggressive/Self-focused -----X------------ (Assertive) ------------------X- Compliant/Other-focused

Regulation

Hypoaroused ------------------------------- (Alert/Calm) -----------------X------------- Hyperaroused

Volatile ---------------X------------------------ (Flexible) --------------------------------------- Fixed

Internalizing ------------------ (Adaptable Expressions of Distress) --------------X---- Externalizing

Controlled ------------------------------ (Active Acceptance) ---------------------X------ Uncontrolled

Parts

Fragmented ------------X--- Cohesive

Disengaged ----------------------X--X------- Engaged

Disembodied ----------X---X-------------- Embodied

Underresourced --------------------X--- Resourced

Narrative

Intrusions ----X-------------------- (Acceptance of Memories) -------------X-- Avoidance/Numbing

Secretive about Trauma --------X------ (Mindful Sharing) ---------X-- Spilling Trauma Narrative

Identity Disavows Trauma ----------X (Defined by Trauma) ------------ Identity Beyond Trauma

Compartmentalized Trauma Narrative ----X----------------------------- Integrated Life Narrative

FIGURE 12.2. Nicole's early presentation on component continuums.

is comforted by Katherine's attentiveness and careful attention to pacing: she reflects on her pleasure that Katherine didn't miss much, as well as her relief that Katherine "did not push [her] too hard about things she wasn't ready to talk about." Although Nicole engages quickly, there are also early signs that the therapy is likely to be rife with enactments. Her instability in her perception of others suggests an ambivalent attachment style. Even before meeting Katherine, Nicole experiences both admiration and envy, based on Katherine's name, biographical sketch, and website photo. She vacillates between seeing Katherine as "someone who will finally understand me" to anticipating rejection from her.

Because the therapeutic relationship is immediately intense and fraught with meaning for Nicole, the relationship component is likely to be central in their work together. Nicole highlights a difficult relational pattern in which her attempts to be a "good person" result in her being "taken for granted or taken advantage of in her relationships: with family, friends, and work colleagues." Throughout their therapy together, Katherine will need to be alert for repetitions of this relational dynamic within the therapy. Nicole may have a tendency to ignore her own feelings and desires as she attempts to please Katherine but then to feel invisible or unimportant as a result. Katherine's own need to be a "good person" creates a parallel process that complicates the therapeutic relationship. She will need to be aware of her vulnerability to accepting agreement and praise from Nicole as a reflection of her own skill as a therapist, rather than as a relational strategy that Nicole uses to manage uncertainty and anxiety. Early use of the therapeutic relationship is likely to be implicit, as Katherine creates a therapeutic environment by being highly engaged and attuned, noticing verbal and nonverbal communications, and encouraging and inviting disclosures. As the therapy progresses, the relationship will likely be used in a more explicit way, in which Katherine and Nicole actively explore their interactional patterns and enactments that occur.

On the continuum of regulatory capacity, Nicole seems to have a great deal of dissociated emotion bubbling just under the surface that is not well controlled. Her anxiety is apparent, and she struggles with a sense of hopelessness and emptiness. Shame is also central in Nicole's presentation. She holds her trauma in her body, and it shows up through behavioral dysregulation and enactments. Consider, for example, Nicole's somatically rigid, defensive posture. She is generally not consciously aware of pushing people away and does not link this rigid somatic state to her need to defend herself from emotional assaults as a child. In order to shift this engrained somatic state and relational response, she will need to develop a conscious awareness of her internal experiences. Katherine helps Nicole become more conscious of her somatic tension, while holding the larger perspective of the link between Nicole's current-day somatic tension and the likely early chronic activation of her survival response system in the face of her mother's repeated attacks. Over time, Katherine and Nicole will make more explicit links between the early chronic activation of Nicole's threat response and her current somatic, emotional, and cognitive states. Because the therapeutic relationship is important in co-regulation as Nicole acknowledges and increasingly tolerates distress, Katherine may choose to reflect that Nicole is not facing these emotions alone—that Katherine is there with her. In conjunction with this exploration, she teaches Nicole a number of regulatory tools that she quickly learns and readily practices in session, although she has difficulty accessing these tools when Katherine is not there to prompt her.

Nicole's regulatory capacity is intricately intertwined with her "many layers," and a parts perspective proves to be very helpful in conceptualizing Nicole's struggles. She talks about the "good girl" part of her that attempts to please people and puts others first. This part seems to be highly controlled and self-punitive. The somatic state of this part of self is frozen and constricted. Nicole describes an overcontrolled behavior of restricting food that began early in her childhood. She refers to her inability to feel anger, which may prompt Katherine to wonder whether there is a dissociated part of Nicole that is holding anger or rage. She describes feeling "empty and alone" in her marriage and "trapped and controlled" by her life. This part of Nicole emerges in therapy before she even makes it to her first appointment. When she considers canceling her appointment, she is filled with shame and self-loathing, realizing that "if she doesn't show, she will have wasted Ms. Silvester's time."

It seems that Nicole has a dissociative response to her trauma history, leaving her without a coherent narrative or sense of self. Nicole tells stories easily and shares aspects of her history very quickly; however, she has a tendency to disclose details without being connected to her internal experience and without attention to her regulation. Katherine recognizes very early the need to attend to the pacing of the sessions and at times to slow the process down. For instance, when Nicole broadly describes her early childhood as troubled, Katherine suggests, and she agrees, that they will come back to this topic at length in a later session. This approach maintains the early focus on current-day issues and allows Nicole to "settle in" with Katherine before sharing more emotionally difficult memories. She also uses humor at times to create a break in the intensity of the emotional disclosures that Nicole makes at the beginning of therapy. This regulatory tool increases Nicole's comfort in the moment, helping her to stay within her window of tolerance, and strengthens the therapeutic relationship. Thus, in her work with Katherine, the early focus is not narrative in nature. Instead, the work is led by the regulation and parts components, with elements of relationship weaving strongly throughout.

Relational Development and Relationally Based Somatic Resourcing

Katherine's early focus is on learning more about Nicole's many layers, including the relational and regulatory capacity of each of these parts of self. She constantly brings her attention to the emotional and somatic states behind the stories that Nicole is sharing.

Katherine pays close attention to subtle nonverbal communications from Nicole, such as the "imploring" eye contact she makes when talking about trying to please everyone and the "earnest expression of pain on Nicole's face" when she talks about how exhausting this constant effort is for her.

As Katherine repeatedly invites Nicole to share feelings of disappointment, anger, alienation, and hurt about the therapeutic relationship, she begins to become more comfortable openly expressing her feelings rather than acting out her feelings through shutting down and withdrawing from the relationship. She realizes cognitively that she is hypersensitive to any sign of rejection from Katherine, but she continues to experience these fears on a very regular basis. They often lead her to feel a sense of shame, berating herself for being so sensitive and ruminating that there is something fundamentally and irreversibly wrong with her. Katherine works to invite and accept Nicole's feelings, to manage her own reactions to Nicole's anger or self-blame, and to acknowledge her own role in the interactions they have. As they process these enactments, Katherine uses the language of parts to help Nicole explore the ambivalence in her reactions. Over time, Nicole is more able to acknowledge feelings of disappointment and sometimes even anger, building regulatory capacity within this relational frame.

Because of the extent of Nicole's dysregulation, dissociation, and shame, Katherine recognizes the importance of identifying and building up Nicole's resources before engaging in a great deal of exploratory work. The therapeutic relationship is a major resource that is being developed early in therapy. In fact, Nicole and Katherine explicitly use the therapeutic relationship itself as a resource when Nicole identifies memories of feeling accepted by Katherine. She guides Nicole in noticing the emotional, cognitive, and somatic states associated with these memories. As she is thinking of an instance of feeling accepted by Katherine, Nicole feels her chin lifting and notices a warm feeling in her chest. She feels calm and settled and thinks, "I am okay." She describes feeling a "glow" inside of her. Katherine helps Nicole strengthen this resource by further noticing her somatic and emotional reactions to this memory. The more time that is spent on noticing this memory and the greater the repetition, the more easily Nicole is able to access these sensations. Later in therapy, she is able to call up these sensations of feeling accepted by eliciting this memory.

Emergence of Parts Work

Nicole and Katherine have a very informative discussion about Nicole's phobic response to feelings of anger. When Katherine asks if she has found any other outlets for the pain, Nicole offhandedly mentions her "bad side." This reference hints at what becomes a central issue in the therapy—Nicole's need to split off her "bad side," which holds anger, desire, and vitality, so that she could go unnoticed and avoid the emotional and verbal abuse in her home.

Nicole's sense of shame over her "bad side" is apparent. In the moment, Katherine creates space for this part of Nicole to enter into the therapy.

With a curious and empathetic approach, all of Katherine's energy is directed toward being receptive to Nicole's emotional state and her internal conflict over sharing this rejected part of herself. This disclosure opens the door to two potential benefits: relief from the shame, alienation, and secrecy elicited by her "bad side," and an increase in felt safety from the "good girl" part of her who is afraid of losing control.

Nicole's "bad side" provides a counterpoint to her more typical presentation, which is a more passive, constricted part of self. This "bad side" holds a lot of Nicole's energy and her desire to feel "a thrill, a rush, a bit of a spark." As they explore her parts of self, Nicole recognizes that she lives in two extremes: the anxious part of her keeps her emotionally shut down and in a loveless marriage, while her more impulsive side is dysregulated in her thoughts, feelings, somatic experiences, and behavior. With support, she begins to understand the adaptive value of each of these sides of her. Her "good girl" side helped her to avoid abuse and mistreatment and has maintained some stability in her life, while her "bad side" holds self-protective anger and her passion and vitality. Nicole has other parts that emerge over time, as her relationship with Katherine deepens, including a young part of her that is seeking love and affection. This is the part of her that sometimes smiles warmly at Katherine when she feels supported or connected. It is also likely the part of her that was motivated to seek therapy in the first place. This part of her looks at Katherine with "an imploring, searching, almost desperate" look and discloses, "I don't know the limits of how far I will go to feel something, and I'm starting to scare myself. That's why I forced myself to come here."

Changes Outside of Therapy: A Marker for Progress

Often, changes in a client's life will reflect progress made in therapy. Because these changes may be subtle, Katherine tries to help Nicole acknowledge the importance of small moments that have a larger meaning for her. Imagine that, after many months of increasing awareness of her emotional states and her underlying desire for connection, Nicole begins to notice her pattern of disengagement from her husband. She recognizes that she easily interprets ambiguous behaviors of his as cold or discounting, and she preemptively withdraws in order to avoid feeling rejected by him. She comes in one week and tells Katherine about a new experience that she had with her husband. Nicole describes how she came home after a stressful encounter with an acquaintance and said offhandedly, "Phew! That was a long day!" Her husband was on the computer and did not respond to her. In fact, he didn't even look up. Nicole noticed a strong urge to turn around and walk upstairs. Instead, she used a skill that she had worked on with Katherine and took three deep breaths before reacting. She decided to try an experiment—something she had also been working on in sessions with Katherine. She forced herself to walk over to her husband and say, "I'm really upset because of something that happened today, and I'd like to talk about it with you when you have time." Nicole's husband turned around and asked her what had happened and seemed concerned about her feelings when she explained. She reflected that this was the first time she can remember feeling connected with him in months. Katherine reflected what a wonderful interaction that was and praised Nicole for being aware of her initial impulse and having the strength to take a risk by being vulnerable with her husband.

Enactments, Parts Work, and Trauma Processing

For almost a year, Nicole has not had any affairs or one-night stands. Periodically, she points out how long it has been since she has engaged in this behavior, looking forward to the reinforcement she gets from Katherine. In each instance, Katherine notices that Nicole looks at her eagerly, waiting for her response. As Katherine reflects back on her apparent feeling of pride, Nicole smiles, pleased at the praise. Their developing relationship often elicits a young part of Nicole that is anxious for reinforcement.

However, as Nicole's daughter begins applying for colleges, her behavior becomes more erratic, and she is more emotionally dysregulated. She comes in one week, bitterly and angrily announcing, "Well, I did it again. Maybe we should just call this done. It's obviously not working." When Katherine clarifies that she had a one-night stand that week, Nicole says, "I don't know what you expect of me. This is just what I do. I've always done this. Everyone is always trying to judge me, tell me what I shouldn't do, how bad I am. Well, I don't get any love or affection from anyone else, so what do you expect? I'm starving to death. I'm dying, and no one cares."

Katherine holds her breath for a beat, with a momentary fear that Nicole is going to walk out and do something dangerous. As she realizes that Nicole is not moving, she notices a sense of frustration and slight defensiveness that she is being lumped in with "everyone." As she checks herself, she tries to look beyond Nicole's apparent anger. Katherine wonders whether Nicole views her as judgmental or does not experience her as warm or affectionate. She also begins to wonder about possible triggers for Nicole. As she notices these reactions in herself, she tries to sit back and invite a curious, open, and accepting part of herself.

As Katherine wonders about Nicole's somatic and affective states, Nicole is able to acknowledge feelings of rage toward Katherine. Katherine notices both of her feet on the floor and then invites Nicole to be curious about this part of her. Nicole's anger intensifies but then subsides, allowing her to explore different parts of herself that are activated. She acknowledges a sad and hopeless part of her that anticipates being "abandoned and alone" after her daughter leaves home. She reflects that these feelings are intolerable because they remind her of her mother's depression and helplessness. Nicole expresses an overwhelming sense of shame over recent bitter, biting comments that she'd made to her daughter, as she recalls hearing her mother's voice come out of her own mouth.

Nicole notes that when her "bad side" comes out and she has an affair, the physiological and emotional "rush" helps her not to feel the panic and despair. Katherine and Nicole spend some time identifying the connection between Nicole's current dysregulated emotions and behaviors and her early traumatic experiences. At this point, the narrative component is primary, with relationship, regulation, and parts components supporting this early trauma-processing work. Trauma processing here is not a separate phase of the work but rather is intricately interwoven with other elements of the therapy. Dipping into and out of references to earlier traumatic experiences builds tolerance for the exposure and increases the likelihood that these exposures are experienced as "successful" or healing.

Although a great deal of important information is emerging here, Katherine is not so easily led away from the brief reference that Nicole made to the rage that she was feeling toward her. The intensity of Nicole's feelings, and Katherine's response, lead her to wonder whether an enactment of Nicole's trauma is occurring. She invites Nicole to share more about this feeling. Nicole reflects that, as she sat in the waiting room that morning, her fear and hopelessness were reactivated, and she began imagining that Katherine would be angry and disgusted and would kick her out of therapy when she learned about Nicole's recent one-night stand. Nicole wonders whether she might have even had the one-night stand to test Katherine. She expresses resentment that she needs to be "perfect" or to act in a certain way in order to receive love or affection. She says that sometimes it just feels easier to be alone than to try so desperately to avoid being rejected. These fears reflect Nicole's early experiences of neglect, rejection, and condemnation from her parents.

Katherine is struck by the similarity between Nicole's fears and her early misinterpretation of her "bad side." She shares this reaction, which runs parallel to Nicole's own rejection of this part of her. Katherine shares the work that she did in supervision to help her recognize her own role in that perspective and reflects on her recognition of the essential strength and energy of this part of Nicole. She assures Nicole that it is okay to have all of these feelings and that all parts of her are important and are welcome in the therapy.

After some time engaging in parts work, Nicole and Katherine begin to explore the use of imagery to communicate with and support Nicole's younger parts of self. They use imagery to bring Nicole's adult self into connection with a young and frequently silenced part of her, with Katherine's presence and support. This vulnerable, fearful part is able to express her sense of connection to Katherine and her worry that she will be abandoned or rejected. Katherine supports Nicole's adult self in being able to witness, accept, and support this vulnerable part of her. Together, they also spend time getting to know the resentful, angry part of Nicole, building empathy for this part and coming to understand that this part tries to protect Nicole from feeling hurt by preemptively rejecting people to avoid intimacy. Nicole begins to not only have empathy for this part, but to appreciate the essential energy and vitality that she holds. They start to consider other ways that this part of her might be able to feel alive, without the negative consequences of the affairs.

Throughout this parts work, the therapeutic relationship provides safety and containment, allowing Nicole to acknowledge how much of her dysregulation is reflective of her younger parts of self. As she gets to know these parts of herself better, she is able to understand the dynamics underlying her behavioral patterns. As she develops her ability to notice and tolerate uncomfortable sensations, Nicole is increasingly able to acknowledge her emotions without acting them out. Instead of ignoring or rejecting the young part of her that feels abandoned, Nicole can begin to identify these feelings as a sign that she needs to take care of herself and reach out to others for support. As she honors the self-protective impulse of the part of her that acts out in rage, this part may learn different ways of protecting herself, including through assertion and setting clear boundaries in relationships. Over time, Nicole may also begin to tap into the part of her that is a caretaker for others, using this as a source of self-nurturance. The process of getting to know, accept, and support all of the parts of her supports the development of Nicole's regulatory and relational capacities, as she accepts her difficult past and begins to build greater hope for the future.

CONCLUSION

As is reflected in David and Nicole's therapies, work with survivors of early emotional abuse and neglect is complex and nuanced. The CBP framework provides a general approach to progressive stages of treatment with survivors of complex trauma, including emotional abuse and neglect; recommendations on adapting the work to unique factors of both the client and therapist; and guidance on timing and pacing in this work. David and Nicole follow different paths toward similar goals: increasing self-knowledge, becoming more interpersonally connected, accepting and caring for themselves, and developing efficacy about themselves and their future. In CBP, the client and therapist are challenged to reach across the abyss, taking risks to connect more fully with themselves and each other and creating opportunities for healing, growth, and vitality.

APPENDIX

Component-Based Psychotherapy

Clinician Self-Assessment

with Jana Pressley

For each item, please rate how you would currently describe your level of proficiency to engage in each of the following clinical skills or therapeutic stances.

Intervention Strategies for Relationship Component of CBP				
Clinical skill				
	Minimal proficiency			High proficiency
1. Establishing a relational stance; maintaining empathic attunement with clients.	1　　2	3	4	5
2. Offering a consistent, predictable, safe relationship in therapy.	1　　2	3	4	5
3. Assisting the client in building awareness of attachment style and implications for relational patterns.	1　　2	3	4	5
4. Supporting the client in developing relational skills, such as communication, attunement, assertiveness, problem solving, and boundary setting; practicing in the context of the therapeutic relationship to generalize to other relationships.	1　　2	3	4	5
5. Learning through therapeutic ruptures and repairs.	1　　2	3	4	5

Jana Pressley, PsyD, is Director of Training and Education at the Trauma Center at Justice Resource Institute and Adjunct Associate Professor at Richmont Graduate University. She is a national ARC trainer and consultant and also trains on the impact of trauma on adult spirituality.

Therapist self-reflective capacity

	Minimal proficiency			High proficiency	
1. Maintaining present-moment relational attunement and engagement while concurrently developing meta-awareness of the client's and therapist's individual processes and interaction patterns.	1	2	3	4	5
2. Developing balance in regard to boundaries, self-disclosure, level of action, "holding" experiences, and meeting clients' needs.	1	2	3	4	5
3. Understanding personal attachment style(s) and relational patterns and how these impact the therapeutic process.	1	2	3	4	5
4. Exploring the ways in which cultural and other contextual factors influence worldviews of the client and therapist and impact the therapeutic process.	1	2	3	4	5

Supervision *(only fill out if you serve as a supervisor; leave blank if you do not)*

	Minimal proficiency			High proficiency	
1. Providing a holding environment for the supervisee and the therapy itself.	1	2	3	4	5
2. Reflecting on parallel processes (between client's relationships, the therapeutic relationship, and the supervisory relationship).	1	2	3	4	5

Intervention Strategies for Regulation Component of CBP

Clinical skill

Regulation	Minimal proficiency			High proficiency	
1. Supporting the client in building/expanding self-regulatory capacity, including awareness of, tolerance for, linkages among, skills to regulate, and ability to express aspects of experience: affect, cognition, somatic, and behavioral.	1	2	3	4	5
2. Teaching the client affective, cognitive, somatic, or behavioral tools for regulation:	1	2	3	4	5
a. Applying standard regulation tools/utilizing existing tools (grounding, imagery, breathing, mind–body tools, yoga).	1	2	3	4	5
b. Working with client to tailor tools (modifying standard tools or creating new tools collaboratively).	1	2	3	4	5
3. Matching regulatory tool to type of current client dysregulation (affective, cognitive, somatic, behavioral).	1	2	3	4	5
4. Supporting the client in expanding client window of tolerance.	1	2	3	4	5
Regulation × Relationship					
1. Using the therapeutic relationship to facilitate containment, reflection/self-awareness, and co-regulation.					

2. Progressing in the regulatory role of the therapeutic relationship—from providing containment, to supporting exploration, to encouraging client's internalization of skills.	1	2	3	4	5
3. Assisting the client in developing regulatory tools that emerge organically from the therapeutic relationship.	1	2	3	4	5
4. Working through ways in which the therapeutic relationship acts as a dysregulating force with the client (e.g., intimacy as dysregulating).	1	2	3	4	5

Therapist self-reflective capacity

Regulation	**Minimal proficiency**			**High proficiency**	
1. Managing personal reactivity, including affective, somatic, cognitive, and behavioral reactivity.	1	2	3	4	5
2. Expanding therapist window of tolerance.	1	2	3	4	5
Regulation × Relationship					
1. Maintaining an optimal window of engagement with the client (therapeutic relationship feels safe at a given time for both client need and therapist capacity).	1	2	3	4	5
2. Recognizing personal reactivity to clients.	1	2	3	4	5
3. Understanding the impact of personal tendencies regarding pacing (colluding with avoidance or pressure to "do" more in treatment).	1	2	3	4	5

Supervision (*only fill out if you serve as a supervisor; leave blank if you do not*)

	Minimal proficiency			**High proficiency**	
1. Use of reflection to increase awareness of regulatory processes of client, clinician, supervisor, and their interactions.	1	2	3	4	5
2. Supporting supervisee's regulatory processes and proactive self-care; addressing vicarious trauma responses.	1	2	3	4	5

Intervention Strategies for Parts Component of CBP

Clinical skill

Parts work	**Minimal proficiency**			**High proficiency**	
1. Maintaining awareness that the current client presentation might be reflecting only one part of self; understanding that parts hold, embody, and/or express unresolved traumatic material.	1	2	3	4	5
2. Developing a curious, compassionate stance toward all parts of client; building empathic engagement toward fragmented self-states.	1	2	3	4	5
3. Acknowledging and supporting strengths of client parts.	1	2	3	4	5
4. Working with the client to reduce fragmentation; building cohesion, linkages, and communication among parts of self.	1	2	3	4	5

	Minimal proficiency				High proficiency
5. Engaging in indirect work with client parts.	1	2	3	4	5
6. Working directly with client parts.	1	2	3	4	5

Parts × Relationship

	Minimal proficiency				High proficiency
1. Engaging relational parts of the client as resources.	1	2	3	4	5
2. Identifying and learning to meet client parts' relational needs.	1	2	3	4	5
	1	2	3	4	5
3. Using the therapeutic relationship to co-regulate parts of client self and to facilitate direct engagement with dissociated parts.					
4. Exploring enactments with the client in therapy.	1	2	3	4	5

Parts × Regulation

1. Recognizing client patterns in affective, cognitive, somatic, and/or behavioral responses that may reflect parts of client's self.	1	2	3	4	5
2. Assisting the client in expanding each part's repertoire of coping skills.	1	2	3	4	5
3. Reflecting and soothing client dysregulated parts; regulating the whole by regulating specific parts.	1	2	3	4	5
4. Tailoring regulatory tools and strategies to developmental stage of parts.	1	2	3	4	5

Therapist self-reflective capacity

Parts	Minimal proficiency				High proficiency
1. Developing a curious, compassionate stance toward all parts of self and toward all parts of the client, honoring the role they have served.	1	2	3	4	5

Parts × Relationship

1. Maintaining compassion for all parts of client.	1	2	3	4	5
2. Building awareness of the ways in which therapist parts are activated through interactions with client parts.	1	2	3	4	5
3. Acknowledging and communicating with clients about therapist role in enactment.	1	2	3	4	5

Parts × Regulation

1. Noticing activation of parts of self and engaging in self-regulation in the moment.	1	2	3	4	5
2. Identifying and drawing on parts as therapeutic resources.	1	2	3	4	5

Supervision *(only fill out if you serve as a supervisor; leave blank if you do not)*				
	Minimal proficiency			**High proficiency**
1. Offering a mindful, reflective environment to build awareness of all parts of the client and supervisee.	1	2	3	4 5
2. Exploring interactions between supervisee and supervisor parts of self.	1	2	3	4 5

Intervention Strategies for Narrative Component of CBP

Clinical skill

Narrative	**Minimal proficiency**			**High proficiency**
1. Assisting the client in linking triggers to past traumas.	1	2	3	4 5
2. Assisting the client in reframing behaviors as survival adaptations.	1	2	3	4 5
3. Supporting the client in the development of a trauma narrative; integrating aspects of trauma-related experience and decreasing related distress (verbal, affective, sensory/somatic, cognitive, behavioral).	1	2	3	4 5
4. Supporting the client in the process of integrating traumatic experience and evolving the trauma narrative into a life narrative.	1	2	3	4 5
5. Redefining narrative work: moving beyond memory processing to meaning-making and identity development.	1	2	3	4 5
Narrative × Relationship				
1. Assisting the client in developing a narrative about relational patterns, using a trauma-informed lens.	1	2	3	4 5
2. Supporting the client in building new relational patterns and a new story about self-in-relationship.	1	2	3	4 5
3. Bearing witness and "holding" the developing client narrative.	1	2	3	4 5
4. Building the story of the therapy and the therapeutic relationship over time.	1	2	3	4 5
Narrative × Regulation				
1. Providing the client with psychoeducation about trauma reactions and regulatory processes.	1	2	3	4 5
2. Paying careful attention to the client window of tolerance and window of engagement during trauma processing.	1	2	3	4 5
3. Supporting the client in the process of achieving regulation through narrative work or memory processing, including relief of alienation and shame that can emerge from being seen or witnessed.	1	2	3	4 5

Narrative × Parts					
1. Listening for one-sentence stories that may hold the defensive stance and defining narrative of a part of self.	1	2	3	4	5
2. Providing psychoeducation about dissociation and parts work.	1	2	3	4	5
3. Helping the client recognize implicit trauma narratives that are organizing identity and driving behavior.	1	2	3	4	5

Therapist self-reflective capacity

Narrative	**Minimal proficiency**				**High proficiency**
1. Recognizing personal stance or orientation to trauma work.	1	2	3	4	5
2. Acknowledging that therapist self-narrative is always present, even when it is implicit or unspeakable; understanding that there is no singular narrative.	1	2	3	4	5
3. Actively working on personal trauma or life narrative (building self-awareness), with growing recognition of professional narrative integrated into a larger self-narrative.	1	2	3	4	5
4. Recognizing the presence, operations, advantages, and limitations of the professional identities and organizing narratives that influence and at times drive work as a trauma therapist; working to shift and temper these as needed to increase therapeutic effectiveness in general and with particular clients.	1	2	3	4	5
Narrative × Relationship					
1. Using self-disclosure appropriately with the client.	1	2	3	4	5
2. Codeveloping the therapeutic narrative with the client.	1	2	3	4	5
3. Acknowledging the intersections of traumatic experiencing and broader cultures and context of oppression and integrating recognition of these into the treatment process.	1	2	3	4	5
Narrative × Regulation					
1. Understanding self-regulatory patterns and challenges as therapist.	1	2	3	4	5
2. Maintaining effective pacing regarding trauma processing; not colluding in avoidance or overfocusing on traumatic experiences.	1	2	3	4	5
Narrative × Parts					
1. Recognizing implicit narratives in identity as a trauma therapist.	1	2	3	4	5
2. Cultivating the ability to be flexible around self-narrative as a therapist; drawing on different identities/roles in response to the unique needs of different clients.					

Supervision *(only fill out if you serve as a supervisor; leave blank if you do not)*

	Minimal proficiency			High proficiency	
1. Bringing attention to pacing of narrative work in supervisee cases.	1	2	3	4	5
2. Fostering increased supervisee awareness of latent identities and implicit narratives driving their general approach to trauma treatment, or held by less integrated parts of self.	1	2	3	4	5
3. Assisting supervisee in obtaining and cultivating the personal supports and resources to manage internal experiences in order to increase attunement to and effective response with clients.	1	2	3	4	5
4. Maintaining a grounded stance in the meaning of supervisory work; building mindful awareness of the impact personal and professional experiences and worldview has on supervisory style.	1	2	3	4	5

Interactions among CBP Components

Clinical skill

	Minimal proficiency			High proficiency	
1. Incorporating assessment of the four components into conceptualization and treatment planning.	1	2	3	4	5
2. Individually tailoring treatment by prioritizing among components for different client presentations.	1	2	3	4	5
3. Developing an in-depth understanding of client's parts of self, regulatory processes, relational patterns, and life narrative.	1	2	3	4	5
4. Attending to timing and pacing; shifting between CBP components and between macro focus and present-moment experience to contribute to effective pacing.	1	2	3	4	5
5. Supporting the client in developing greater sense of connection to self and others, improving general functioning, and increasing sense of meaning and engagement with life.	1	2	3	4	5
6. Reflecting on the therapeutic process and progress.	1	2	3	4	5

Therapist self-reflective capacity

	Minimal proficiency			High proficiency	
1. Cultivating personal ability to be actively engaged in moment-to-moment therapeutic interactions, while simultaneously maintaining meta-awareness of all parts of the client, self, and contextual factors that influence the therapeutic process over time.	1	2	3	4	5
2. Parallel to client experience, developing therapist capacity to "show up" in professional and personal life, continually developing self-awareness, regulatory and relational capacity, and cohesive identity that includes all parts of self.	1	2	3	4	5

Supervision *(only fill out if you serve as a supervisor; leave blank if you do not)*				
	Minimal proficiency			**High proficiency**
1. Raising awareness about relational enactments, regulatory challenges, dissociative processes, and narrative development, involving the client and/or supervisee.	1	2	3	4 5
2. Supporting the supervisee's present-moment attunement (to client and to self) and meta-awareness of the larger therapeutic process and the ability to effectively toggle between the two.	1	2	3	4 5
3. Attending to parallel processes in the supervisory relationship that informs CBP work.	1	2	3	4 5

References

Adults Surviving Child Abuse. (2012). *Practice guidelines for treatment of complex trauma and trauma-informed care and service delivery.* Kirribilli, Australia: Author.

Agorastos, A., Pittman, J. O., Angkaw, A. C., Nievergelt, C. M., Hansen, C. J., Aversa, L. H., et al. (2014). The cumulative effect of different childhood trauma types on self-reported symptoms of adult male depression and PTSD, substance abuse and health-related quality of life in a large active-duty military cohort. *Journal of Psychiatric Research, 58,* 46–54.

Allen, P. B. (2007). Wielding the shield: The art therapist as conscious witness in the realm of social action. In F. F. Kaplan (Ed.), *Art therapy and social action* (pp. 72–85). Philadelphia: Jessica Kingsley.

Alpert, J. (1995). *Sexual abuse recalled.* Northvale, NJ: Jason Aronson.

American Professional Society on the Abuse of Children (APSAC). (1995). *Guidelines for the psychosocial evaluation of suspected psychological maltreatment in children and adolescents.* Chicago: Author.

American Psychiatric Association. (1980). *Diagnostic and statistical manual of mental disorders* (3rd ed.). Washington, DC: Author.

American Psychiatric Association. (1994). *Diagnostic and statistical manual of mental disorders* (4th ed.). Washington, DC: Author.

American Psychiatric Association. (2013). *Diagnostic and statistical manual of mental disorders* (5th ed.). Arlington, VA: Author.

Barnett, D., Manly, J. T., & Cicchetti, D. (1993). Defining child maltreatment: The interface between policy and research. In D. Cicchetti & S. L. Toth (Eds.), *Child abuse, child development, and social policy: Advances in developmental psychology* (Vol. 8, pp. 7–73). Norwood, NJ: Ablex.

Barth, P., Lee, B., Lindsey, M., Collins, K., Strieder, F., Chorpita, B., et al. (2012). Evidence-based practice at a crossroads: The timely emergence of common elements and common factors. *Research on Social Work Practice, 22*(1), 108–119.

Bartlett, F. (1932). *Remembering.* Oxford, UK: Oxford University Press.

Benish, S. G., Imel, Z. E., & Wampold, B. E. (2008). The relative efficacy of bona fide psychotherapies for treating post-traumatic stress disorder: A meta-analysis of direct comparisons. *Clinical Psychology Review, 28,* 746–758.

Blaustein, M., & Kinniburgh, K. (2010). *Treating traumatic stress in children and adolescents: How to foster resilience through attachment, self-regulation, and competence.* New York: Guilford Press.

Boll, P. (2008). *Who does she think she is?* [Film]. Mystic Artists Film Productions.

Bowen, M. S. (2013). Through the looking-glass: Exploring identity development for a beginning therapist and her late adolescent patient. *Journal of Infant, Child, and Adolescent Psychotherapy, 12*(4), 286–300.

Bowlby, J. (1973). *Attachment and loss: Vol. 2. Separation: Anxiety and anger.* New York: Basic Books.

Bowlby, J. (1980). *Attachment and loss: Vol. 3. Loss, sadness and depression.* New York: Basic Books.

Bowlby, J. (1982). *Attachment and loss: Vol. 1. Attachment* (2nd ed.). New York: Basic Books. (Original work published 1969)

Briere, J., Kaltman, S., & Green, B. (2008). Accumulated childhood trauma and symptom complexity. *Journal of Traumatic Stress, 21*, 223–226.

Briere, J., & Scott, C. (2012). *Principles of trauma therapy: A guide to symptoms, evaluation, and treatment* (2nd ed.). Thousand Oaks, CA: Sage.

Briere, J., & Scott, C. (2015). Complex trauma in adolescents and adults: Effects and treatment. *Psychiatric Clinics of North America, 38*, 515–527.

Briere, J., & Spinazzola, J. (2005). Phenomenology and psychological assessment of complex posttraumatic states. *Journal of Traumatic Stress, 18*, 401–412.

Briggs, E. C., Fairbank, J. A., Greeson, J. K. P., Layne, C. M., Steinberg, A. M., Amaya-Jackson, L. M., et al. (2012). Links between child and adolescent trauma exposure and service use histories in a national clinic-referred sample. *Psychological Trauma: Theory, Research, Practice, and Policy, 5*(2), 101–109.

Brom, D., Kleber, R. J., & Defares, P. B. (1989). Brief psychotherapy for posttraumatic stress disorders. *Journal of Consulting and Clinical Psychology, 57*, 607–612.

Bromberg, P. (1994). "Speak! That I may see you": Some reflections on dissociation, reality, and psychoanalytic listening. *Psychoanalytic Dialogues, 4*, 517–547.

Bromberg, P. M. (2001). *Standing in the spaces: Essays on clinical process, trauma, and dissociation.* New York: Routledge.

Bromberg, P. (2009). Multiple self-states, the relational mind, and dissociation: A psychoanalytic perspective. In P. Dell & J. O'Neill (Eds.), *Dissociation and the dissociative disorders* (pp. 637–652). Florence, KY: Routledge.

Bronfenbrenner, U. (1989). Ecological systems theory. *Annals of Child Development, 6*, 124–187.

Brown, D., & Fromm, E. (1986). *Hypnotherapy and hypnoanalysis.* Hillsdale, NJ: Erlbaum.

Bruner, J. (1990) *Acts of meaning.* Cambridge, MA: Harvard University Press.

Buber, M. (1965). *The knowledge of man: Selected essays* (R. Smith & M. Friedman, Trans.). New York: Harper & Row.

Cahill, S. P., Rothbaum, B. O., Resick, P., & Follette, V. M. (2009). Cognitive-behavioral therapy for adults. In E. B. Foa, T. M. Keane, M. J. Friedman, & J. A. Cohen (Eds.), *Effective treatments for PTSD: Practice guidelines from the International Society for Traumatic Stress Studies* (2nd ed., pp. 139–222). New York: Guilford Press.

Cardemil, E. V., & Battle, C. I. (2003). Guess who's coming to therapy?: Getting comfortable with conversations about race and ethnicity in psychotherapy. *Professional Psychology: Research and Practice, 34*(3), 278–286.

Caruth, C. (1996). *Unclaimed experience: Trauma, narrative and history.* Baltimore: Johns Hopkins University Press.

Cerney, M. S. (1995). Treating the "heroic treaters." In C. R. Figley, *Compassion fatigue: Coping with secondary traumatic stress disorder in those who treat the traumatized* (131–149). New York: Brunner/Mazel.

Chamberland, C., Laporte, L., Lavergne, C., Tourigny, M., Wright, J., Helie, S., et al. (2005). Psychological maltreatment of children reported to youth protection services: A situation of grave concern. *Journal of Emotional Abuse, 5*(1), 65–94.

Chefetz, R. A. (2015). *Intensive psychotherapy for persistent dissociative processes.* New York: Norton.

Chefetz, R. A., & Bromberg, P. M. (2004). Talking with "me" and "not me": A dialogue. *Contemporary Psychoanalysis, 40*(3), 409–464.

Chu, J. (2011). *Rebuilding shattered lives: Treating complex PTSD and dissociative disorders* (2nd ed.). Hoboken, NJ: Wiley.

Cloitre, M. (2015). The "one size fits all" approach to trauma treatment: Should we be satisfied? *European Journal of Psychotraumatology, 6*(1). Retrieved from *www.tandfonline.com/doi/full/10.3402/ejpt.v6.27344.*

Cloitre, M., Cohen, L., & Koenen, K. (2006). *Treating survivors of childhood abuse: Psychotherapy for the interrupted life.* New York: Guilford Press.

Cloitre, M., Courtois, C. A., Charuvastra, A., Carapezza, R., Stolbach, B. C., & Green, B. L. (2011). Treatment of complex PTSD: Results of the ISTSS expert clinician survey on best practices. *Journal of Traumatic Stress, 24*(6), 615–627.

Cloitre, M., Courtois, C., Ford, J., Green, B., Alexander, P., Briere, J., et al. (2012). The ISTSS expert consensus treatment guidelines for complex PTSD in adults. Retrieved from *www.istss.org/ISTSS_Main/media/Documents/ISTSS-Expert-Concesnsus-Guidelines-for-Complex-PTSD-Updated-060315.pdf.*

Cloitre, M., Garvert, D. W., Brewin, C. R., Bryant, R. A., & Maercker, A. (2013). Evidence for proposed ICD-11 PTSD and complex PTSD: A latent profile analysis. *European Journal of Psychotraumatology, 4*(1). Retrieved from *www.tandfonline.com/doi/full/10.3402/ejpt.v4i0.20706.*

Cloitre, M., Koenen, K. C., Cohen, L. R., & Han, H. (2002). Skills training in affective and interpersonal regulation followed by exposure: A phase-based treatment for PTSD related to childhood abuse. *Journal of Consulting and Clinical Psychology, 70*(5), 1067–1074.

Cloitre, M., Stolbach, B., Herman, J., van der Kolk, B., Pynoos, R., Wang, J., et al. (2009). A developmental approach to complex PTSD: Childhood and adult cumulative trauma as predictors of symptom complexity. *Journal of Traumatic Stress, 22*(5), 399–408.

Cloitre, M., Stovall-McClough, K., Miranda, R., & Chemtob, C. (2004). Therapeutic alliance, negative mood regulation, and treatment outcome in child abuse-related posttraumatic stress disorder. *Journal of Consulting and Clinical Psychology, 72*(3), 411–416.

Cloitre, M., Stovall-McClough, K. C., Nooner, K., Zorbas, P., Cherry, S., Jackson, C. L., et al. (2010). Treatment for PTSD related to childhood abuse: A randomized controlled trial. *American Journal of Psychiatry, 167*(8), 915–924.

Cohler, B. J. (1991). The life story and the study of resilience and response to adversity. *Journal of Narrative and Life History, 1,* 169–200.

Cook, A., Spinazzola, J., Ford, J., Lanktree, C., Balustein, M., Sprague, C., et al. (2007). Complex trauma in children and adolescents. *Focal Point, 21*(1), 4–8.

Courtois, C. (2004). Complex trauma, complex reactions: Assessment and treatment. *Psychotherapy: Theory, Research, Practice, Training, 41*(4), 412–425.

Courtois, C. (2010). *Healing the incest wound: Adult survivors in therapy* (2nd ed.). New York: Norton.

Courtois, C. A., & Ford, J. D. (Eds.). (2009). *Treating complex traumatic stress disorders: Scientific foundations and therapeutic models.* New York: Guilford Press.

Courtois, C. A., & Ford, J. D. (2013). *Treatment of complex trauma: A sequenced, relationship-based approach.* New York: Guilford Press.

Crenshaw, K. (1989). Demarginalizing the intersection of race and sex: A black feminist critique of antidiscrimination doctrine, feminist theory and antiracist politics. *University of Chicago Legal Forum, 1989*(1), 139–167.

Crittenden, P. (1985). Attachment and psychopathology. In, S. Goldberg, R. Muir, & J. Kerr (Eds.), *Attachment theory: Social, developmental and clinical perspectives.* Hillsdale, NJ: Analytic Press.

Dalenberg, C. (2000). *Countertransference and the treatment of trauma.* Washington, DC: American Psychological Association Press.

D'Andrea, W., Ford, J., Stolbach, B., Spinazzola, J., & van der Kolk, B. A. (2012). Understanding interpersonal trauma in children: Why we need a developmentally appropriate trauma diagnosis. *American Journal of Orthopsychiatry, 82*(2), 187–200.

Davies, J. M., & Frawley, M. G. (1994). *Treating the adult survivor of childhood sexual abuse: A psychoanalytic perspective.* New York: Basic Books.

de Jong, J. T. V. M., Komproe, I., Spinazzola, J., van der Kolk, B., & van Ommeren, M. H. (2005). DESNOS in three post conflict settings: Assessing cross-cultural construct equivalence. *Journal of Traumatic Stress, 18*(1), 13–21.

DeJongh, A., Resick, P. A., Zoellner, L. A., van Minnen, A., Lee, C. W., Monson, C. M., et al. (2016). Critical analysis of the current treatment guidelines for complex PTSD in adults. *Depression and Anxiety, 33*(5), 359–369.

Dell, P. F., & O'Neil, J. A. (Eds.). (2009). *Dissociation and the dissociative disorders: DMS-V and beyond.* New York: Routledge.

Duncan, B. L., Miller, S. D., Wampold, B. E., & Hubble, M. A. (Eds.). (2010). *The heart and soul of change: Delivering what works in therapy* (2nd ed.). Washington, DC: American Psychological Association.

Dunmore, E., Clark, D. M., & Ehlers, A. (2001). A prospective investigation of the role of cognitive factors in persistent posttraumatic stress disorder (PTSD) after physical or sexual assault. *Behaviour Research and Therapy, 39,* 1063–1084.

Emerson, D., & Hopper, E. (2011). *Overcoming trauma through yoga: Reclaiming your body.* Berkeley, CA: North Atlantic Books.

Erickson, M. F., Egeland, B., & Pianta, R. (1989). The effects of maltreatment on the development of young children. In V. Carlson (Ed.), *Child maltreatment: Theory and research on the causes and consequences of child abuse and neglect* (pp. 647–684). New York: Cambridge University Press.

Espín, O. M. (1993). Giving voice to silence—the psychologist as witness. *American Psychologist, 48*(4), 408.

Feinauer, L. L., & Stuart, D. A., (1996). Blame and resilience in women sexually abused as children. *American Journal of Family Therapy, 24,* 31–40.

Felitti, V. J., Anda, R. F., Nordenberg, D., Williamson, D. F., Spitz, A. M., Edwards, V., et al. (1998). Relationship of childhood abuse and household dysfunction to many of the leading causes of death in adults: The Adverse Childhood Experiences (ACE) Study. *American Journal of Preventive Medicine, 14*(4), 245–258.

Ferenczi, S. (1980). Confusion of tongues between adults and the child: The language of tenderness and passion. In M. Balint (Ed.), *Final contributions to the problems and methods of psychoanalysis* (pp. 156–167). New York: Brunner/Mazel. (Original work published 1933)

Finkelhor, D., Ormrod, R. K., & Turner, H. A. (2007). Poly-victimization: A neglected component in child victimization. *Child Abuse and Neglect, 31*(1), 7–26.

Finn, H., Warner, E., Price, M., & Spinazzola, J. (2017). The boy who was hit in the face: The role of somatic regulation and trauma processing in treatment of preverbal complex trauma. *Journal of Child and Adolescent Trauma.* [Epub ahead of print]

Foa, E. B., Chrestman, K. R., & Gilboa-Schectman, E. (2009). *Prolonged exposure therapy for adolescents with PTSD: Emotional processing of traumatic experiences* (Therapist guide). New York: Oxford University Press.

Foa, E. B., Hembree, E. A., & Rothbaum, B. (2007). *Prolonged exposure therapy for PTSD: Emotional processing of traumatic experiences therapist guide.* New York: Oxford University Press.

Foa, E. B., Keane, T. M., Friedman, M. J., & Cohen, J. A. (Eds.). (2008). *Effective treatments for PTSD: Practice guidelines from the International Society for Traumatic Stress Studies* (2nd ed.). New York: Guilford Press.

Foa, E. B., Rothbaum, B. O., Riggs, D. S., & Murdock, T. (1991). Treatment of posttraumatic stress disorder in rape victims: A comparison between cognitive-behavioral procedures and counseling. *Journal of Consulting and Clinical Psychology, 59*(5), 715–723.

Fogel, A. (1993). *Developing through relationships: Origins of communication, self and culture.* Chicago: University of Chicago Press.

Ford, J. (2015). An affective cognitive neuroscience-based approach to PTSD psychotherapy: The TARGET model. *Journal of Cognitive Psychotherapy, 29*(1), 69–91.

Ford, J., & Courtois, C. (2009). Defining and understanding complex trauma and complex traumatic stress disorders. In C. A. Courtois & J. D. Ford (Eds.), *Treatment of complex traumatic stress disorders: Scientific foundations and therapeutic models* (pp. 13–30). New York: Guilford Press.

Ford, J., & Gómez, J. (2015). Self-injury and suicidality: The impact of trauma and dissociation. *Journal of Trauma and Dissociation, 16*(3), 225–231.

Ford, J., Grasso, D., Green, C., Levine, J., Spinazzola, J., & van der Kolk, B. (2013). Clinical significance of a proposed developmental trauma diagnosis: Results of an international survey of clinicians. *Journal of Clinical Psychiatry, 74*(8), 841–849.

Ford, J., & Kidd, P. (1998). Early childhood trauma and disorders of extreme stress as predictors of treatment outcome with chronic posttraumatic stress disorder. *Journal of Traumatic Stress, 11*(4), 743–761.

Ford, J., & Smith, S. (2008). Complex posttraumatic stress disorder in trauma-exposed adults receiving public sector outpatient substance abuse disorder treatment. *Addiction Research and Theory, 16*(2), 193–203.

Ford, J. D., Steinberg, K. L., & Zhang, W. (2011). A randomized clinical trial comparing affect regulation and social-problem solving psychotherapies for mothers with victimization-related PTSD. *Behavior Therapy, 42,* 560–578.

Ford, J., Stockton, P., Kaltman, S., & Green, B. (2006). Disorders of extreme stress (DESNOS) symptoms are associated with interpersonal trauma exposure in a sample of healthy young women. *Journal of Interpersonal Violence, 21,* 1399–1416.

Fosha, D. (2000). *The transforming power of affect: A model for accelerated change.* New York: Basic Books.

Fosha, D., Paivio, S. C., Gleiser, K., & Ford, J. D. (2009). Experiential and emotion-focused therapy. In C. A. Courtois & J. D. Ford (Eds.), *Treating complex traumatic stress disorders: An evidence-based guide* (pp. 286–311). New York: Guilford Press.

Fosha, D., & Slowiaczek, M. L. (1997). Techniques to accelerate dynamic psychotherapy. *American Journal of Psychotherapy, 51*(2), 229–249.

Fraser, G. A. (1991). The dissociative table technique: A strategy for working with ego states in dissociative disorders and ego state therapy. *Dissociation, 4,* 205–213.

Freud, S. (1896). The etiology of hysteria. In J. Strachey (Ed. & Trans.), *The standard edition of the complete psychological works of Sigmund Freud* (Vol. 3, pp. 191–221). London: Hogarth Press.

Friedman, M. J. (2013). Finalizing PTSD in *DSM-5*: Getting here from there and where to go next. *Journal of Traumatic Stress, 26,* 548–556.

Gapen, M., van der Kolk, B., Hamlin, E., Hirshberg, L., Suvak, M., & Spinazzola, J. (2016). A pilot study of neurofeedback for chronic PTSD. *Applied Psychophysiology and Biofeedback, 40*(4), 1–11.

Garbarino, J., & Bedard, C. (1996). Spiritual challenges to children facing violent trauma. *Childhood, 3*(4), 467–478.

Garner, A. S., Shonkoff, J. P., Siegel, B. S., Dobbins, M. I., Earls, M. F., McGuinn, L., et al. (2012). Early childhood adversity, toxic stress, and the role of the pediatrician: Translating developmental science into lifelong health. *Pediatrics, 129*(1), e224–e231.

Gartner, R. B. (2005). *Beyond Betrayal: Taking charge of your life after boyhood sexual abuse.* Hoboken, NJ: Wiley.

Gelinas, D. (1983). The persistent negative effects of incest. *Psychiatry, 46,* 312–322.

Grand, S. (2000). *The reproduction of evil.* Hillsdale, NJ: Analyic Press.

Greenspan, M. (1983). *A new approach to women and therapy.* New York: McGraw-Hill.

Grossman, F. K., Cook, A. B., Kepkep, S. S., & Koenen, K. C. (1999). *With the Phoenix rising: Lessons from ten resilient women who overcame the trauma of childhood sexual abuse.* San Francisco: Jossey-Bass.

Grossman, F. K., Sorsoli, L., & Kia-Keating, M. (2006). A gale force wind: Meaning making by male survivors of childhood sexual abuse. *American Journal of Orthopsychiatry, 76*(4), 434–443.

Grossman, F., Spinazzola, J., Zucker, M., & Hopper, E. (2017). Treating adult survivors of childhood emotional abuse and neglect: A new framework. *American Journal of Orthopsychiatry, 87*(1), 86–93.

Grossman, F., & Zucker, M. (2010, May). *Relational parts work: A model of working with dissociative parts.* Workshop presented at the annual International Trauma Conference on Psychological Trauma, Boston, MA.

Guina, J., Rossetter, S. R., Derhodes, B. J., Nahhas, R. W., & Welton, R. S. (2015). Benzodiaz-epines for PTSD: A systematic review and meta-analysis. *Journal of Psychiatric Practice*, *21*(4), 281–303.

Harlow, H. (1958). The nature of love. *American Psychologist*, *13*, 673–685.

Harney, P. A. (2007). Resilience processes in context. *Journal of Aggression, Maltreatment and Trauma*, *14*(3), 73–87.

Harvey, J. D., Orbuch, T. L., & Weber, A. L. (1990). A social psychological model of account making: In response to severe stress. *Journal of Language and Social Psychology*, *9*(3), 191–207.

Hays, P. A. (2001). *Addressing cultural complexities in practice: A framework for clinicians and counselors*. Washington, DC: American Psychological Association.

Herman, J. L. (1992a). Complex PTSD: A syndrome in survivors of prolonged and repeated trauma. *Journal of Traumatic Stress*, *3*, 377–391.

Herman, J. L. (1992b). *Trauma and recovery: The aftermath of violence from domestic abuse to political terror*. New York: Basic Books.

Herman, J. L. (2009). Foreword. In C. A. Courtois & J. D. Ford (Eds.), *Treating complex trau-matic stress disorders: An evidence-based guide* (p. xiii). New York: Guilford Press.

Hersoug, A. G., Høglend, P., Havik, O., von der Lippe, A., & Monsen, J. (2009). Therapist characteristics influencing the quality of alliance in long-term psychotherapy. *Clinical Psychology and Psychotherapy*, *16*(2), 100–110.

Hibbard, R., Barlow, J., MacMillan, H., & the Committee on Child Abuse and Neglect, Ameri-can Academy of Pediatrics. (2012). Psychological maltreatment. *Pediatrics*, *130*, 372–378.

Hodgdon, H., Suvak, M., Zinoviev, D., Liebman, R., Briggs, E., & Spinazzola, J. (in press). Net-work analysis of cumulative exposure to trauma and adverse events in a clinical sample of children and adolescents. *Psychological Assessment*.

Hodges, M., Godbout ,N., Briere ,J., Lanktree, C., Gilbert, A., & Kletzka, N. (2013). Cumu-lative trauma and symptom complexity in children: A path analysis. *Child Abuse and Neglect*, *37*, 891–898.

Holmes, D. (2012). Multicultural competence: A practitioner-scholar's reflections on its reality and its stubborn and longstanding elusiveness. *The Register Report*, *8*(1). Retrieved from *www.nationalregister.org/trr_spring12_Holmes.html*.

Hopper, J. W., Spinazzola, J., Simpson, W., & van der Kolk, B. (2006). Preliminary evidence of parasympathetic influence on basal heart rate in posttraumatic stress disorder. *Journal of Psychosomatic Research*, *60*, 83–90.

Howell, E. F. (2005). *The dissociative mind*. New York: Routledge.

Janet, P. (1889). *L'automatisme psychologique*. Paris: Felix Alcan. [Reprint: Paris: Societe Pierre Janet, 1973.]

Janoff-Bulman, R. (1992). *Shattered assumptions: Towards a new psychology of trauma*. New York: Free Press.

Jordan, J. (1987). Clarity in connection: Empathic knowing, desire and sexuality. *Works in Progress*, No. 29. Wellesley, MA: Stone Center, Wellesley College.

Kairys, S. W., Johnson, C. F., & Committee on Child Abuse and Neglect. (2002). The psycho-logical maltreatment of children—technical report. *Pediatrics*, *109*(4), e68.

Kaiser, E., Gillette, C., & Spinazzola, J. (2010). A controlled pilot-outcome study of sensory integration (SI) in the treatment of complex adaptation to traumatic stress. *Journal of Aggression, Maltreatment, and Trauma*, *19*, 699–720.

Karam, E. G., Friedman, M. J., Hill, E. D., Kessler, R. C., McLaughlin, K. A., Petukhova, M., et al. (2013). Cumulative traumas and risk thresholds: 12-month PTSD in the World Mental Health (WMH) Surveys. *Depression and Anxiety*, *31*, 130–142.

Karatzias, T., Shevlin, M., Fyvie, C., Hyland, P., Efthymiadou, E., Wilson, D., et al. (2017). Evidence of distinct profiles of posttraumatic stress disorder (PTSD) and complex post-traumatic stress disorder (CPTSD) based on the new ICD-11 Trauma Questionnaire (ICD-TQ). *Journal of Affective Disorders*, *207*, 181–187.

Kendall, P. C., & Beidas, R. S. (2007). Smoothing the trail for dissemination of evidence-based practices for youth: Flexibility within fidelity. *Professional Psychology: Research and Prac-tice*, *38*(1), 13–20.

Kia-Keating, M., Grossman, F. K., Sorsoli, L., & Epstein, M. (2005). Containing and resist-
ing masculinity: Narratives of renegotiation among resilient male survivors of childhood
sexual abuse. *Psychology of Men and Masculinity, 6*(3), 169–185.

Kingsbury, S. J. (1988). Hypnosis in the treatment of posttraumatic stress disorder: An isomor-
phic intervention. *American Journal of Clinical Hypnosis, 31*(2), 81–90.

Kinniburgh, K. J., Blaustein, M., Spinazzola, J., & van der Kolk, B. A. (2005). Attachment, self
regulation and competency (ARC): A comprehensive framework for intervention with
complexly traumatized youth. *Psychiatric Annals, 35*(5), 424–430.

Kluft, R. P. (2006). Dealing with alters: A pragmatic clinical perspective. *Psychiatric Clinics of
North America, 29,* 281–304.

Korn, D., & Leeds, A. (2002). Preliminary evidence of efficacy for EMDR resource development and installation in the stabilization phase of treatment of complex posttraumatic
stress disorder. *Journal of Clinical Psychology, 58*(12), 1465–1487.

La Roche, M., Davis, T., & D'Angelo, E. (2015). Challenges in developing a cultural evidence
based psychotherapy in the USA: Suggestions for international studies. *Australian Psychologist, 50*(2), 95–101.

Lanius, R., Hopper, J., & Menon, R. (2003). Individual differences in a husband and wife who
developed PTSD after a motor vehicle accident: A functional MRI case study. *American
Journal of Psychiatry 160*(4), 667–669.

Laub, D., & Auerhahn, N. (1993). Knowing and not knowing massive psychic trauma: Forms
of traumatic memory. *International Journal of Psychoanalysis, 74,* 287–302.

Layne, C. M., Ippen, C. G., Strand, V., Stuber, M., Abramovitz, R., Reyes, G., et al. (2011). The
core curriculum on childhood trauma: A tool for training a trauma-informed workforce.
Psychological Trauma: Theory, Research, Practice, and Policy, 3(3), 243–252.

LeDoux, J. (2000). Emotion circuits in the brain. *Annual Review of Neuroscience, 23*(1), 155–
184.

Levine, P. A. (1997). *Waking the tiger: Healing trauma: The innate capacity to transform overwhelming experiences.* Berkeley, CA: North Atlantic Books.

Lew, M. (2004). *Victims no longer: The classic guide for men recovering from childhood sexual
abuse* (2nd ed.). New York: Quill.

Linehan, M. M. (1993). *Skills training manual for treatment of borderline personality disorder.* New
York: Guilford Press.

Loewenstein, R. J. (1993). Posttraumatic and dissociative aspects of transference and counter-
transference in the treatment of multiple personality disorder. In R. P. Kluft & S. C. Fine
(Eds.), *Clinical perspectives on multiple personality disorder* (pp. 51–86). Washington, DC:
American Psychiatric Association.

Lonergan, B. A., O'Halloran, M. S., & Crane, S. (2004). The development of the trauma
therapist: A qualitative study of the child therapist's perspectives and experiences. *Brief
Treatment and Crisis Intervention, 4*(4), 353–366.

Lyons-Ruth, K. (1999). Two-person unconscious: Intersubjective dialogue, enactive relational
representation, and the emergence of new forms of relational organization. *Psychoanalytic
Inquiry, 19,* 576–617.

Lyons-Ruth, K. (2003). The two-person construction of defenses: Disorganized attachment
strategies, unintegrated mental states, and hostile/helpless relational processes. *Journal of
Infant, Child, and Adolescent Psychotherapy, 2,* 105–114.

Lyons-Ruth, K., & Jacobvitz, D. (1999). Attachment disorganization: Unresolved loss, relational violence, and lapses in behavioral and attentional strategies. In J. Cassidy & P. R.
Shaver (Eds.), *Handbook of attachment: Theory, research and clinical application* (pp. 520–
554). New York: Guilford Press.

Main, M. (1995). Recent studies in attachment: Overview, with selected implications for clinical work. In S. Goldberg, R. Muir, & J. Kerr (Eds.), *Attachment theory: Social, developmental and clinical perspectives.* Hillsdale, NJ: Analytic Press.

Main, M., & Cassidy, J. (1988). Categories of response to reunion with the parent at age six:
Predictable from infant attachment classifications and stable over a 1-month period.
Developmental Psychology, 24, 415–426.

Main, M., & Solomon, J. (1986). Discovery of a new insecure-disoriented/disorganized attachment pattern. In T. B. Brazelton & M. Yogman (Eds.), *Affective development in infants* (pp. 95–124). Norwood, NJ: Ablex.

Malcolm, J. (1981). *Psychoanalysis: The impossible profession*. New York: Knopf.

McAdams, D. (2008). Personal narratives and the life story. In O. Johns, R. Robins, & L. Pervin (Eds.), *Handbook of personality: Theory and research* (3rd ed.). New York: Guilford Press.

McCann, L., & Pearlman, L. (1990a). *Psychology trauma and the adult survivor: Theory, therapy and transformation*. New York: Brunner/Mazel.

McCann, L., & Pearlman, L. (1990b). Vicarious traumatization: A framework for understanding the psychological effects of working with victims. *Journal of Traumatic Stress, 3*(1), 131–149.

McDonagh, A., Friedman, M., McHugo, G., Ford, J., Sengupta, A., Mueser, K., et al. (2005). Randomized trial of cognitive-behavioral therapy for chronic posttraumatic stress disorder in adult female survivors of childhood sexual abuse. *Journal of Consulting and Clinical Psychology, 73*, 515–524.

Miller, J. B. (1976). *Toward a new psychology of women*. Boston: Beacon Press.

Morton, N. (1985). *The journey is home*. Boston: Beacon Press.

Myers, J. E., Berliner, L., Briere, J., Hendrix, C. T., Jenny, C., & Reid, T. (2002). *The APSAC handbook on child maltreatment* (2nd ed.). Thousand Oaks, CA: Sage.

Nezu, A. M. (2010). Cultural influences on the process of conducting psychotherapy: Personal reflections of an ethnic minority psychologist. *Psychotherapy: Theory, Research, Practice, Training, 47*(2), 169–176.

Nissen-Lie, H. A., Havik, O. E., Høglend, P. A., Monsen, J. T., & Ronnestad, M. H. (2013). The contribution of the quality of therapists' personal lives to the development of the working alliance. *Journal of Counseling Psychology, 60*(4), 483–495.

Norcross, J., Krebs, P., & Prochaska, J. O. (2011). Stages of change. *Journal of Clinical Psychology 67*(2), 143–154.

Ogden, P., & Fisher, J. (2015). *Sensorimotor psychotherapy: Interventions for trauma and attachment*. New York: Norton.

Ogden, P., Minton, K., & Pain, C. (2006). *Trauma and the body: A sensorimotor approach to psychotherapy*. New York: Norton.

Ogden, T. H. (1979). On projective identification. *International Journal of Psycho-Analysis, 60*, 357–373.

Omaha, J. (2004). *Psychotherapeutic interventions for emotion regulation*. New York: Norton.

Paivio, S. C., & Angus, L. E. (2017). *Narrative processes in emotion-focused therapy for trauma*. Washington, DC: American Psychological Association.

Paivio, S. C., & Pascual-Leone, A. (2010). *Emotion-focused therapy for complex trauma: An integrative approach*. Washington, DC: American Psychological Association.

Pearlman, L. A., & Caringi, J. (2009). Living and working self-reflectively to address vicarious trauma. In C. A. Courtois & J. D. Ford (Eds.), *Treating complex traumatic stress disorders: An evidence-based guide* (pp. 202–224). New York: Guilford Press.

Pearlman, L. A., & Mac Ian, P. S. (1995). Vicarious traumatization: An empirical study of the effects of trauma work on trauma therapists. *Professional Psychology: Research and Practice, 26*(6), 558.

Pearlman, L., & Saakvitne, K. W. (1995a). *Trauma and the therapist: Countertransference and vicarious traumatization in psychotherapy with incest survivors*. New York: Norton.

Pearlman, L. A., & Saakvitne, K. W. (1995b). Treating therapists with vicarious traumatization and secondary traumatic stress disorders. In C. R. Figley, *Compassion fatigue: Coping with secondary traumatic stress disorder in those who treat the traumatized* (pp. 150–177). New York: Brunner/Mazel.

Pechtel, P., & Pizzagalli, D. A. (2011). Effects of early life stress on cognitive and affective function: an integrated review of human literature. *Psychopharmacology, 214*(1), 55–70.

Pedersen, P., Crethar, H., & Carlson, J. (2008). *Inclusive cultural empathy: Making relationships central in counseling and psychotherapy*, Washington, DC: American Psychological Association.

Pelcovitz, D., van der Kolk, B. A., Roth, S., Mandel, F., Kaplan, S., & Resick, P. (1997).

Development of a criteria set and structured interview for disorders of extreme stress. *Journal of Traumatic Stress, 10,* 3–16.

Pennebaker, J., & Evans, J. (2014). *Expressive writing: Words that heal.* Enumclaw, WA: Idyll Arbor.

Perlman, S. (1998). *The therapist's emotional survival: Dealing with the pain of exploring trauma.* Lanham, MD: Jason Aronson.

Perry, B. D., & Hambrick, E. P. (2008). The neurosequential model of therapeutics. *Reclaiming Children and Youth, 17*(3), 38–43.

Pesso, A., Boyden-Pesso, D., & Cooper, D. E. (2013). *Sharing the practical wisdom: A compendium of PBSP concepts and insights.* Amazon Digital Services.

Pipher, M. (2002, January/February). Healing wisdom: The universals of human resilience. *Psychotherapy Networker,* pp. 59–61.

Polkinghorne, D. (1988) *Narrative knowing and the human sciences.* Albany: State University of New York Press.

Porges, S. W. (2011). *The polyvagal theory: Neurophysiological foundations of emotions, attachment, communication, and self-regulation.* New York: Norton.

Pressley, J., & Spinazzola, J. (2015). Beyond survival: Application of a complex trauma treatment model in the Christian context. *Journal of Psychology and Theology, 43*(1), 8–22.

Pressley, J., & Spinazzola, J. (2017). Treating complex trauma among adult survivors of Christian faith. In J. Aten & D. Walker (Eds.), *Treating trauma in Christian counseling and psychotherapy* (pp. 211–231). Downers Grove, IL: InterVarsity Press.

Price, M., Spinazzola, J., Musicaro, R., Turner, J., Suvak, M., Emerson, D., et al. (2017). Effectiveness of an extended yoga treatment for women with chronic posttraumatic stress disorder. *Journal of Alternative and Complementary Medicine, 23*(4), 300–309.

Putnam, F. W. (1989). *Diagnosis and treatment of multiple personality disorder.* New York: Guilford Press.

Putnam, F. W. (1994). The switch process in multiple personality disorder and other state change disorders. In R. M. Klein & B. K. Doane (Eds.), *Psychological concepts and dissociative disorders* (pp. 283–304). New York: Erlbaum.

Raio, C., Orederu, T., Palazzolo, L., Shurick, A., & Phelps, E. (2013). Cognitive emotion regulation fails the stress test. *Proceedings of the National Academy of Sciences of the USA, 110*(37), 15139–15144.

Reed, G. M. (2010). Toward *ICD-11:* Improving the clinical utility of WHO's International Classification of Mental Disorders. *Professional Psychology: Research and Practice, 41,* 457–464.

Reis, B. (2009). Performative and enactive features of psychoanalytic witnessing: The transference as the scene of address. *International Journal of Psychoanalysis, 90*(6), 1359–1372.

Resick, P. A., Bovin, M. J., Calloway, A. L., Dick, A. M., King, M. W., Mitchell, K. S., et al. (2012). A critical evaluation of the complex PTSD literature: Implications for the *DSM-5. Journal of Traumatic Stress, 25*(3), 241–251.

Resick, P., & Schnicke, M. (1993). *Cognitive processing therapy for rape victims: A treatment manual.* Thousand Oaks, CA: Sage.

Rhodes, A., Spinazzola, J., & van der Kolk, B. (2016). Yoga for adult women with chronic PTSD: A long-term follow-up study. *Journal of Alternative and Complementary Medicine, 22*(3), 189–196.

Rizzolatti, G., & Sinigaglia, C. (2008). *Mirrors in the brain. How we share our actions and emotions.* Oxford, UK: Oxford University Press.

Rogers, A. (2007). *The unsayable: The hidden language of trauma.* New York: Ballantine Books.

Rosenberg, M. S. (1987). New directions for research on the psychological maltreatment of children. *American Psychologist, 42*(2), 166–171.

Rosenzweig, S. (1936). Some implicit common factors in diverse methods of psychotherapy. *American Journal of Orthopsychiatry, 6*(3), 412–415.

Roth, S., & Batson, R. (1997). *Naming the shadows: A new approach to individual and group psychotherapy for adult survivors of childhood incest.* New York: Free Press.

Sands, S. (1997). Self psychology and projective identification—Wither shall they meet?: A reply to the editors. *Psychoanalytic Dialogues, 7,* 651–666.

Sapolsky, R. (2009). Any kind of mother in a storm. *Nature Neuroscience, 12,* 1355–1356.

Schauer, M., Neuner, F., & Elbert T. (2011). *Narrative exposure therapy: A short term treatment for traumatic stress disorders* (2nd ed.). Cambridge, MA: Hogrefe.

Schore, A. (1996). The experience-dependent maturation of a regulatory system in the orbital prefrontal cortex and the origin of developmental psychopathology. *Development and Psychopathology, 8,* 59–87.

Schore, A. (2003a). *Affect dysregulation and disorders of the self.* New York: Norton.

Schore, A. (2003b). *Affect regulation and the repair of the self.* New York: Norton.

Schore, A. (2010). The right brain implicit self: A central mechanism of the psychotherapy change process. In J. Petrucelli (Ed.), *Knowing, not-knowing and sort of knowing: Psychoanalysis and the experience of uncertainty* (pp. 177–202). London: Karnac.

Schwartz, R. C. (1995). *Internal family systems therapy.* New York: Guilford Press.

Sedlak, A. J., Mettenburg, J., Basena, M., Petta, I., McPherson, K., Greene, A., et al. (2010). *Fourth National Incidence Study of Child Abuse and Neglect (NIS-4).* Washington, DC: U.S. Department of Health and Human Services (DHHS), Administration for Children and Families.

Shapiro, F. (2001). *Eye movement desensitization and reprocessing (EMDR): Basic principles, protocols, and procedures* (2nd ed.). New York: Guilford Press.

Shin, L., Rauch, S., & Pitman, R. (2006). Amygdala, medial prefrontal cortex, and hippocampal function in PTSD. *Annuals of the New York Academy of Sciences, 1071,* 67–79.

Shusta-Hochberg, S. R. (2004). Therapeutic hazards of treating child alters as real children in dissociative identity disorder. *Journal of Trauma and Dissociation, 5*(1), 13–27.

Siegel, D. J. (1999). *The developing mind: Toward a neurobiology of interpersonal experience.* New York: Guilford Press.

Siegel, D. J. (2007). *The mindful brain: Reflection and attunement in the cultivation of well being.* New York: Norton.

Silver, R. L., Boon, C., & Stone, M. H. (1983). Search for meaning in misfortune: Making sense of incest. *Journal of Social Issues, 39,* 81–101.

Singh, A., & Dickey, L. (2016). *Affirmative counseling and psychological practice with transgender and gender nonconforming clients.* Washington, DC: American Psychological Association.

Slochower, J. (2013) Analytic enclaves and analytic outcome: A clinical mystery. *Psychoanalytic Dialogues, 23,* 243–258.

Smith, L. (2009). Enhancing training and practice in the context of poverty. *Training and Education in Professional Psychology, 3*(2), 84–93.

Solomon, E., & Heide, K. (1999). Type III trauma: Toward a more effective conceptualization of psychological trauma. *International Journal of Offender Therapy and Comparative Criminology, 43*(2), 202–210.

Sorsoli, L. (2010). "I remember," "I thought," "I know I didn't say": Silence and memory in trauma narratives. *Memory, 18,* 129–141.

Sorsoli, L., Kia-Keating, M., & Grossman, F. K. (2008). "I keep that hush hush": Male survivors of sexual abuse and the challenges of disclosure. *Journal of Counseling Psychology, 55*(3), 333–345.

Spinazzola, J., Blaustein, M., & van der Kolk, B. (2005). PTSD treatment outcome research: The study of unrepresentative samples? *Journal of Traumatic Stress, 18*(5), 425–436.

Spinazzola, J., Ford, J., Zucker, M., van der Kolk, B., Silva, S., Smith, S., et al. (2005). National survey of complex trauma exposure, outcome and intervention for children and adolescents. *Psychiatric Annals, 35*(5), 433–439.

Spinazzola, J., Habib, M., Knoverek, A., Arvidson, J., Nisenbaum, J., Wentworth, R., et al. (2013, Winter). The heart of the matter: Complex trauma in child welfare. *Child Welfare 360°* [Special Issue: Trauma-Informed Child Welfare Practice], pp. 8–9, 37.

Spinazzola, J., Hodgdon, H., Liang, L., Ford, J., Layne, C., Pynoos, R., et al. (2014). Unseen wounds: The contribution of psychological maltreatment to child and adolescent mental health and risk outcomes in a national sample. *Psychological Trauma: Theory, Research, Practice and Policy, 6*(S1), S18–S28.

Stark, M. (2000). *Modes of therapeutic action.* Lanham, MD: Rowman & Littlefield.

Steele, C. S., & van der Hart, O. (2009). Treating dissociation. In C. A. Courtois & J. D. Ford

(Eds.), *Treating complex traumatic stress disorders: An evidence-based guide* (pp. 145–165). New York: Guilford Press.

Steele, C. S., van der Hart, O., & Nijenhuis, E. R. S. (2001). Dependency in the treatment of complex posttraumatic stress disorder and dissociative disorders. *Journal of Trauma and Dissociation, 2*(4), 79–116.

Stein, J., Wilmot, D., & Solomon, Z. (2016). Does one size fit all?: Nosological, clinical, and scientific implications of variations in PTSD Criterion A. *Journal of Anxiety Disorders, 43,* 106–117.

Stern, D. (2004). *The present moment in psychotherapy and everyday life.* New York: Norton.

Stern, D. B. (1997). *Unformulated experience: From dissociation to imagination in psychoanalysis.* Hillsdale, NJ: Analytic Press.

Stiles, W., Honos-Webb, L., & Lani, J. (1999). Some functions of narrative in the assimilation of problematic experiences. *Journal of Clinical Psychology, 55,* 1213–1226.

Stoltenberg, C. D., & Delworth, U. (1987). *Supervising counselors and therapists: A developmental approach:* Hoboken, NJ: Jossey-Bass.

Sue, S. (1998). In search of cultural competence in psychotherapy and counseling. *American Psychologist, 53*(4), 440–448.

Sullivan, H. S. (1953). *Interpersonal theory of psychiatry.* New York: Norton.

Summit, R. C. (1983). The child sexual abuse accommodation syndrome. *Child Abuse and Neglect, 7,* 177–193.

Sykes, W. (2004). The limits of talk: Bessel van der Kolk wants to transform the treatment of trauma. *Psychotherapy Networker, 28*(1), 30–41.

Teicher, M., & Sampson, J. (2016). Annual research review: Enduring neurobiological effects of childhood abuse and neglect. *Journal of Child Psychology and Psychiatry, 57,* 241–266.

Teicher, M., Sampson, J., Polcari, A., & McGreenery, C. (2006). Sticks, stones and hurtful words: Relative effects of various forms of childhood maltreatment. *American Journal of Psychiatry, 163,* 993–1000.

Terr, L. (1991). Childhood traumas: An outline and overview. *American Journal of Psychiatry, 148*(1), 10–20.

Trickett, P. K., Mennen, F. E., Kim, K., & Sang, J. (2009). Emotional abuse in a sample of multiply maltreated urban adolescents: Issues of definition and identification. *Child Abuse and Neglect, 33*(1), 27–35.

Tronick, E. Z., & Weinberg, M. K. (1997). Depressed mothers and infants: Failure to form dyadic states of consciousness. In L. Murray & P. J. Cooper (Eds.), Postpartum depression and child development (pp. 54–81). New York: Guilford Press.

Ursano, R. J., Bell, C., Eth, S., Friedman, M., Norwood, A., Pfefferbaum, B., et al. (2004). Practice guideline for the treatment of patients with acute stress disorder and posttraumatic stress disorder. *American Journal of Psychiatry, 161*(11, Suppl.), 3–31.

van der Hart, O., Brown, P., & van der Kolk, B. (1989). Pierre Janet's treatment of post traumatic stress. *Journal of Traumatic Stress, 2*(4), 379–395.

van der Hart, O., Nijenhuis, E., & Steele, K. (2006). *The haunted self: Structural dissociation and the treatment of chronic traumatization.* New York: Norton.

van der Kolk, B. (1989). The compulsion to repeat the trauma: Re-enactment, revictimization and masochism. *Psychiatric Clinics of North America, 12*(2), 389–411.

van der Kolk, B. A. (2005). Developmental trauma disorder: Toward a rational diagnosis for children with complex trauma histories. *Psychiatric Annals, 35*(5), 401–408.

van der Kolk, B. (2014). *The body keeps the score: Mind, brain and body in the healing of trauma.* New York: Viking Press.

van der Kolk, B. A., & Fisler, R. (1995). Dissociation and the fragmentary nature of traumatic memories: Overview and exploratory study. *Journal of Traumatic Stress, 8*(4), 505–525.

van der Kolk, B. A., Hodgdon, H., Gapen, M., Musicaro, R., Suvak, M. K., Hamlin, E., et al. (2016). A randomized controlled study of neurofeedback for chronic PTSD. *PLOS ONE, 11*(12), e0166752.

van der Kolk, B. A., & McFarlane, A. C. (1996). The black hole of trauma. In B. A. van der Kolk, A. C. McFarlane, & L. Weisaeth (Eds.), *Traumatic stress: The effects of overwhelming experience on mind, body, and society* (pp. 3–23). New York: Guilford Press.

van der Kolk, B., McFarlane, A., & van der Hart, O. (1996a). A general approach to treatment of posttraumatic stress disorder. In B. van der Kolk, A. McFarlane, & L Weisaeth (Eds.), *Traumatic stress: The effects of overwhelming experience on mind, body and society* (pp. 417–440). New York: Guilford Press.

van der Kolk, B., McFarlane, A., & Weisaeth, L. (Eds.). (1996b). *Traumatic stress: The effects of overwhelming experience on mind, body and society*. New York: Guilford Press.

van der Kolk, B., Roth, S., Pelcovitz, D., Sunday, S., & Spinazzola, J. (2005). Disorders of extreme stress: The empirical foundation of a complex adaptation to trauma. *Journal of Traumatic Stress, 18*(5), 389–399.

van der Kolk, B., Spinazzola, J., Hopper, J., Blaustein, M., Hopper, E., Korn, D., et al. (2007). A randomized clinical trial of eye movement desensitization and reprocessing (EMDR), fluoxetine, and pill placebo in the treatment of posttraumatic stress disorder: Treatment effects and long-term maintenance. *Journal of Clinical Psychiatry, 68*(1), 37–46.

van der Kolk, B., Stone, L., West, J., Rhodes, A., Emerson, D., Suvak, M., et al. (2014). Yoga as an adjunctive treatment for posttraumatic stress disorder: A randomized controlled trial. *Journal of Clinical Psychiatry, 75*(6), e559–e565.

Vissing, Y., Strauss, M., Gelles, R., & Harrop, J. (1991). Verbal aggression by parents and psychosocial problems of children. *Child Abuse and Neglect, 15*, 223–238.

Vocisano, C., Klein, D. N., Arnow, B., Rivera, C., Blalock, J. A., Rothbaum, R., et al. (2004). Therapist variables that predict symptom change in psychotherapy with chronically depressed outpatients. *Psychotherapy: Theory, Research, Practice, Training, 41*, 255–265.

Walker, D., Reid, H. W., O'Neill, T., & Brown, L. (2009). Changes in personal religion/spirituality during and after childhood abuse: A review and synthesis. *Psychological Trauma: Theory, Research, Practice, and Policy. 1*(2), 130–145.

Warner, E., Spinazzola, J., Westcott, A., Gunn, C., & Hodgdon, H. (2014). The body can change the score: Empirical support for somatic regulation in the treatment of traumatized adolescents. *Journal of Child and Adolescent Trauma, 7*(4), 237–246.

Waters, E., Hamilton, C. E., & Weinfield, N. S. (2000). The stability of attachment security from infancy to adolescence and early adulthood: General introduction. *Child Development, 71*(3), 678–683.

Waters, E., Merrick, S., Treboux, D., Crowell, J., & Albersheim, L. (2000). Attachment security in infancy and early adulthood: A twenty-year longitudinal study. *Child Development, 71*(3), 684–689.

Watkins, J. G. (1971). The affect bridge: A hypnoanalytic technique. *International Journal of Clinical and Experimental Hypnosis, 19*, 21–27.

West, J., Liang, B., & Spinazzola, J. (2016). Trauma sensitive yoga as a complementary treatment for posttraumatic stress disorder: A qualitative descriptive analysis. *International Journal of Stress Management*. [Epub ahead of print]

Wigren, J. (1994). Narrative completion in the treatment of trauma. *Psychotherapy, 31*, 415–423.

Winnicott, D. W. (1965). *The maturational process and the facilitating environment: Studies in the theory of emotional development*. New York: International Universities Press.

Wolf, E., Miller, M., Kilpatrick, D., Resnick, H., Badour, C., Marx, B., et al. (2015). ICD-11 complex PTSD in U.S. national and veteran samples prevalence and structural associations with PTSD. *Clinical Psychological Science, 3*(2), 215–229.

Wolfe, D. A., & McIsaac, C. (2011). Distinguishing between poor/dysfunctional parenting and child emotional maltreatment. *Child Abuse and Neglect, 35*, 802–813.

Wolff, P. H. (1987). *The development of behavioral states and the expression of emotions in early infancy*. Chicago: University of Chicago Press.

Wrye, H., & Welles, J. (1994) *The narration of desire*. Hillsdale, NJ: Analytic Press.

Wylie, M. (2004). The limits of talk: Bessel van der Kolk wants to transform the treatment of trauma. *Psychotherapy Networker, 28*(1), 30–41.

Zlotnick, C., Shea, T. M., Rosen, K., Simpson, E., Mulrenin, K., Begin, A., et al. (1997). An affect-management group for women with posttraumatic stress disorder and histories of childhood sexual abuse. *Journal of Traumatic Stress, 10*, 425–436.

Zucker, M., Spinazzola, J., Blaustein, M., & van der Kolk, B. (2006). Dissociative symptomatology in posttraumatic stress disorder and disorders of extreme stress. *Journal of Trauma and Dissociation, 7*(1), 19–31.

Index

Note. Page numbers that appear in *italic* indicate a figure or a table